Photographic Manual of
Regional Orthopaedic
and Neurological Tests

Fourth Edition

PHOTOGRAPHIC MANUAL OF
REGIONAL ORTHOPAEDIC AND NEUROLOGICAL TESTS

FOURTH EDITION

JOSEPH J. CIPRIANO, D.C.
Atlanta, Georgia

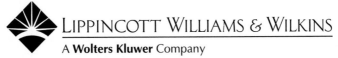

LIPPINCOTT WILLIAMS & WILKINS
A **Wolters Kluwer** Company
Philadelphia • Baltimore • New York • London
Buenos Aires • Hong Kong • Sydney • Tokyo

Editor: Peter J. Darcy
Managing Editor: Linda S. Napora
Marketing Manager: Paul Jarecha
Production Editor: Jennifer Ajello
Designer: Armen Kojoyian
Compositor: Graphic World
Printer: Maple Vail Book Manufacturing Group

351 West Camden Street
Baltimore, MD 21201
530 Walnut Street
Philadelphia, PA 19106

Printed in the United States of America

First Edition, 1985
Second Edition, 1991
Third Edition, 1997

Library of Congress Cataloging-in-Publication Data

Cipriano, Joseph J.
    Photographic manual of regional orthopaedic and neurological tests / Joseph J.
    Cipriano.—4th ed.
        p. cm.
    Includes index.
    ISBN 0-7817-3552-1
    1. Physical orthopedic tests—Atlases. 2. Neurologic examination—Atlases. I. Title.
    RD734.5.P58 C57 2003
    617.3—dc21   2002072497

To purchase additional copies of this book, call our customer service department at
(800) 638-3030 or fax orders to **(301) 824-7390**. International customers should call
(301) 714-2324.

Visit Lippincott Williams & Wilkins on the Internet: http://www.LWW.com. Lippincott Williams & Wilkins customer service representatives are available from 8:30 am to 6:00 pm, EST.

To
Jenny, my loving wife,
Maria, my encouraging mother, and
in memory of Vincent, my Father,
who gave me the courage to follow my dreams.

Without their love, encouragement, compassion,
and courage this manual would not exist.

PREFACE

After four editions and nearly 20 years from the beginning of *Photographic Manual of Regional Orthopaedic and Neurological Tests,* I have come to realize that when information is presented in a logical and concise way, readers will master it quickly. For this reason, the format of this manual has remained the same over four editions, successfully providing instruction for the clinician or student of orthopaedics and neurology in the proper performance and evaluation of physical orthopaedic and neurological tests. The tests are categorized in terms of anatomical applications and subcategorized in terms of diagnostic entities. This arrangement assists the clinician and student in evaluating various orthopaedic and neurological conditions.

The 4th edition continues to be user-friendly. Each test is accompanied by appropriate photographs that illustrate the performance of the test. Where applicable, anatomic illustrations provide enhanced clarity of concept. All of the information for each test is on one page or two facing pages so the user can view all of the information without turning the page.

This new edition includes approximately 30 new tests with 90 new photographs and 20 new anatomical illustrations. Two new features are: Clinical Description, a brief clinical description for each diagnostic entity, and Suggested Imaging Procedures, suggested diagnostic imaging for each condition; these feature are presented in a convenient, easy-to-see format. In addition, there is a Sensitivity/Reliability Scale. The tests are rated based on the biomechanics of the movement that produces the desired outcome of each test, and the Sensitivity/Reliability scale rating provides a logical order for selecting tests more efficiently by indicating the more sensitive/reliable tests first.

This 4th edition will keep readers abreast of new physical orthopaedic and neurological testing while learning and using the classic and standard tests more efficiently. I believe this material will enhance your clinical skills. Ultimately, the benefit will be the enhanced well-being of the patients who have sought our help.

Joseph J. Cipriano, D.C.

ACKNOWLEDGMENTS

I thank the following people for their contributions to this book:

J. Randazzo, D.C., Mark E. White, D.C. and Warren T. Jahn, Sr., D.C., F.A.C.O—their technical review of the manuscript and suggestions have been greatly appreciated.

Mark DelSantro , Steve Hite, Dr. L.F. Jernigan and Michelle Larson—their expertise is evident in the photographs that enhance the accuracy of this text.

Anthony Conticelli, John Michie, Barry Silverstein, Joseph Castellana, Mark E. White and Lucas Wells—their time and professionalism as models have my gratitude.

Lydia V. Kibiuk—her fine artwork and 20 additional illustrations continue to enhance the readers' comprehension of anatomy throughout the book.

Steven P. Weiniger, D.C.—his experience and professionalism are evident in his significant chapter on postural assessment

Pete Darcy, Linda Napora, and Jenn Ajello at Lippincott Williams & Wilkins—their patience and support have been constant during the publication process.

CONTENTS

CLINICAL ASSESSMENT PROTOCOL

A thorough understanding of anatomic and biomechanical principles provides the foundation for accurate evaluation of orthopaedic and related neurologic conditions. Knowledge of these principles is required to understand the relationship between structure and function and the role it plays in assessing orthopaedic and neurologic dysfunction. The examiner must also be familiar with anatomic and biomechanical variants that may be normal to a particular patient.

This text deals primarily with physical examination procedures, which are an integral part of any orthopaedic or related neurologic examination. Complete assessment is not limited to physical examination; it includes other standard procedures, such as plain film radiography, computed tomography (CT), and magnetic resonance imaging (MRI). The clinician must perform the appropriate protocol to evaluate the patient's condition.

This chapter discusses the appropriate protocol for evaluating orthopaedic and related neurologic problems. These procedures, when followed properly, allow the clinician to assemble parts of a puzzle so that he or she can visualize the picture, in this case, the patient's condition. Each piece of the puzzle is analogous to the information gathered by each particular procedure in the clinical assessment protocol. The clinical assessment protocol is shown in Box 1-1.

Box 1-1   Clinical Assessment Protocol

- Patient history
- Inspection/observation
- Palpation
- Range of motion
- Orthopaedic and neurologic testing
- Diagnostic imaging
- Functional testing

During the clinical assessment, it is necessary to document findings. The most common method to record the outcome of the assessment is through a problem-oriented records method that uses a SOAP (subjective, objective, assessment, plan) note format (Box 1-2).

Box 1-2   SOAP Notes

Subjective   The subjective portion is evaluated by taking the patient's history.

Objective   The objective portion is evaluated by observation and special tests that measure an objective component.

Assessment   The assessment is based on the compilation of the subjective and objective findings and the examination.

Plan   The plan may include further testing and/or treatment options.

The clinical assessment protocol is a comprehensive, organized, and reproducible system. This protocol is an essential tool for evaluating musculoskeletal and neurologic disorders.

PATIENT HISTORY

A complete history is one of the most important aspects of the clinical assessment protocol. A complete and thorough history is invaluable in assessing the patient's condition. At times, a history alone may lead to a proper diagnosis. The examiner should place emphasis on the aspect of the patient's history with the greatest clinical significance. Although concentrating on the area of greatest clinical significance, the examiner must not forget to acquire **all** of the patient's history, whether or not it seems relevant at the time. There may come a time during the clinical assessment that the information that seemed irrelevant is quite useful.

History may also help to determine the personality type of the patient and his or her ability or willingness to follow directions. Patients who have a history of using an inordinate number of clinicians for the same disorder and receiving little or no help from them may be unwilling or unable to perform certain functions to better their condition.

It is important that the examiner keep the patient focused on the problem and discourage wandering from the presenting condition. To achieve a good history it is essential to listen carefully to the patient's concerns about his or her problem and the expectations for diagnosis and treatment. When acquiring information from the patient the examiner must not lead the patient into answering questions, such as, "Is this movement painful?" Instead the examiner should say something like, "What do you feel with this movement?"

This history should concentrate on, but not be limited to, the patient's chief complaint, past history, family history, occupational history, and social history. History taking should be accomplished in two steps:

Closed-Ended History

The first step is a closed-ended question and answer format in which the patient answers direct, pointed questions. This step can be accomplished in a written form that the patient fills out.

Open-Ended History

After the closed-ended history is complete, the patient and examiner should engage in an open dialog to discuss the patient's condition. A closed-ended history may lead the examiner to the patient's problem but may not address the patient's fears or concerns regarding this condition. The patient may also have other problems either directly or indirectly related to the presenting complaint that may not be addressed by a closed-ended history.

An open-ended history may take on a discussion format in which the examiner and patient ask questions of each other. In this way, the examiner acquires extra needed information about the patient and the patient's complaint. All aspects of the patient's complaint should be explored and evaluated to its fullest. The examiner should develop a good rapport with the patient, keeping the patient focused on the presenting problem and discouraging irrelevant topics. The pneumonic OPQRST (onset, provoking or palliative concerns, quality of pain, radiating, site and severity, time) may be incorporated into this evaluation (Box 1-3).

Box 1-3 **OPQRST Mnemonic**
• **O**nset of complaint
• **P**rovoking or palliative concerns
• **Q**uality of pain
• **R**adiating to a particular area
• **S**ite and severity of complaint
• **T**ime frame of complaint

Once the examiner has determined all aspects of the presenting complaint, it is time to focus on the history. Has the patient had prior problems with this or any other complaint? This information may assist with both assessment of the problem and insight on how to treat the problem.

Family history can give a clue about the patient's propensity of inheriting familial diseases. A significant number of neurologic problems and many orthopaedic problems can be traced to family members.

Occupational and social histories are also important because they may lead to a factor causing the patient's problem, such as an overuse syndrome. They can also help to determine whether the patient's condition will respond more favorably if the patient refrains from performing certain work or social functions. For example, lifting, bending, and playing tennis or golf may be contraindicated. The patient may also need to be retrained for other types of work.

OBSERVATION/INSPECTION

Observe the patient for general appearance and functional status. Note the body type, such as slim, obese, short, or tall, and postural deviations for general appearance, gait, muscle guarding, compensatory or substitute movements, and assistive devices for functional status.

Inspection should be divided into three layers: skin, subcutaneous soft tissue, and bony structure. Each layer has its own special characteristics for determining underlying pathology or dysfunction.

Skin

Skin assessment should begin with common and obvious findings, such as bruising, scarring, and evidence of trauma or surgery. Then look for changes in color, either from vascular changes accompanying inflammation or from vascular deficiency, such as pallor or cyanosis. Large, brownish, pigmented areas and/or hairy regions, especially on or near the spine, may indicate a bony defect such as spina bifida. Changes in texture may accompany reflex sympathetic dystrophies. Open wounds should be evaluated for either traumatic or insidious origin, which may accompany diabetes.

Subcutaneous Soft Tissue

Subcutaneous soft tissue abnormalities usually involve either inflammation and swelling or atrophy. When evaluating for an increase in size, attempt to identify edema, articular effusion, muscle hypertrophy, or other hypertrophic changes. Also note any nodules, lymph nodes, or cysts. Establish any inflammation by comparing bilateral symmetry for the torso and circumferential measurements for the extremities.

Bony Structure

Bony structure should be evaluated, especially when the patient presents with a functional abnormality, such as a gait deviance or an altered range of motion. Bony inspection in the spine should focus on items such as scoliosis, pelvic tilt, and shoulder height. Note and possibly measure malformations in the extremities that may be congenital or traumatic. Two examples of congenital malformations are genu varus and genu valgus. Traumatic malformations include a healed Colles' fracture with residual angulation. All bony structures should be visually assessed for abnormalities and documented.

PALPATION

Palpate the patient in conjunction with inspection; the structures being inspected are the same ones that should be palpated. The layers are the same for palpation as for inspection, skin, subcutaneous soft tissue, and bony structures.

When palpating the skin, begin with a light touch, especially if nerve pressure is suspected. Pressure on a nerve may result in dysesthesia, which may feel like an exaggerated burning sensation to the patient.

Skin

Evaluate skin temperature first. High skin temperature may indicate an underlying inflammatory process. Low skin temperature may indicate a vascular deficiency. Also, evaluate skin mobility for adhesions, especially after surgery or trauma.

Subcutaneous Soft Tissue

The subcutaneous soft tissue consists of fat, fascia, tendons, muscles, ligaments, joint capsules, nerves, and blood vessels. Palpate these structures with more pressure than for skin. Tenderness is a subjective complaint that should be noted. It may be caused by (a) injury; (b) pathology that correlates directly to the tenderness, such as tenderness at the supraspinatus ligament for supraspinatus tendinitis; or (*c*) a referred component, such as tenderness in the buttock area from a lumbar injury or pathology. Determine tenderness by applying pressure to the area and grade it according to the patient's response (Box 1-4).

Evaluate swelling or edema according to its origin. Determine if the inflammation is intra-articular or extra-articular. In intra-articular effusion, the fluid is confined to the joint capsule. In extra-articular effusion, the fluid is in the surrounding tissues. Various palpation techniques are discussed in detail in the chapters on specific areas of the body.

Box 1-4	Tenderness Grading Scale
Grade I	Patient complains of pain.
Grade II	Patient complains of pain and winces.
Grade III	Patient winces and withdraws the joint.
Grade IV	Patient will not allow palpation of the joint.

There are different types of swelling or edema, according to onset and palpation feel. If swelling occurs immediately after an injury and feels hard and warm, the swelling contains blood. If the swelling occurs 8 to 24 hours after an injury and feels boggy or spongy, the swelling contains synovial fluid. If the swelling feels tough and dry, it is most likely a callus. If the feeling is thickened or leathery, it is most likely chronic swelling. If the swelling or edema is soft and fluctuating, it is most likely acute. If the feeling is hard, it is most likely bone. If the feeling is thick and slow moving, it is most likely pitting edema.

Pulse

Pulse amplitude in certain arteries is important. It is used to assess the vascular integrity of an area and plays an integral part in certain tests for thoracic outlet syndrome, arterial insufficiency, and vertebrobasilar compromise.

Bony Structures

Bony structure palpation is critical for the detection of alignment problems, such as dislocations, luxations, subluxations, and fractures. When you palpate bony structures, you must also identify the ligaments and tendons that attach to those structures. Tenderness is a major finding in bony palpation. It may indicate periosteoligamentous sprain. It also may indicate fracture. Bony enlargements usually are associated with healing of fractures and degenerative joint disease.

RANGE OF MOTION EVALUATION

Range of motion evaluation is not only a measurement of function but also an important part of biomechanical analysis. Range of motion is evaluated for three separate types of functions: passive motion, active motion, and resisted motion.

Passive Range of Motion

In passive motion, the examiner moves the body part for the patient without the patient's help. It can yield a significant amount of information about the underlying pathology. The goal obviously depends on which joint is being tested and what pathology or injury is suspected. In evaluating such motion, first note whether the movement is normal, increased, or decreased and in which planes. Second, note any pain. Classically, pain on passive range of motion indicates a capsular or ligamentous lesion on the side of movement and/or a muscle lesion on the opposite side of movement. Various other problems may be detected, depending on the degree of mobility and pain. Six possible variations of range of motion pain are shown in Box 1-5.

Box 1-5	Six Range of Motion and Pain Variations

1. **Normal mobility with no pain** indicates a normal joint with no lesion.
2. **Normal mobility with pain elicited** may indicate a minor sprain of a ligament or capsular lesion.
3. **Hypomobility with no pain** may indicate an adhesion of a particular tested structure.
4. **Hypomobility with pain elicited** may indicate an acute sprain of a ligament or capsular lesion. When an injury is severe, hypomobility and pain may also be a sign of muscle spasm caused by guarding or by muscle strain opposite the side of movement.
5. **Hypermobility with no pain** suggests a complete tear of a structure with no fibers intact where pain can be elicited. It may also be normal if other joints in the absence of trauma are also hypermobile.
6. **Hypermobility with pain elicited** indicates a partial tear with some fibers still intact. Normal pressure by the weight of structure that is attached to the ligament or capsule is being exerted. This pressure on the intact fibers can elicit pain.

After you determine the degree of passive range of motion and evaluate for pain, evaluate for an end feel. To determine end feel, passively move the joint to the end of its range of motion and then apply slight overpressure to the joint. The quality of the feeling that this elicits is the end feel, assessed as either normal (physiologic) or abnormal (pathologic) (Table 1-1).

TABLE 1-1   END FEEL EVALUATION

Category	Normal Physiologic End Feels	Abnormal Pathologic End Feels
Hard	Abrupt hard to stop movement when bone contacts bone. Example: passive elbow extension. Olecranon process contracts the olecranon fossa	Abrupt stopping movement before normal expected passive movement. Example: Cervical flexion hard end feel due to severe degenerative joint disease.
Soft	When two body surfaces come together, a soft compression of tissue is felt. Example: Passive elbow flexion. Anterior aspect of the forearm approximates the biceps muscle.	A soft boggy sensation resulting from synovitis or soft tissue edema. Example: Ligamentous sprain.
Firm	A firm or spongy sensation that has some give when a muscle, ligament, or tendon is stretched. Example: Passive wrist flexion, passive external shoulder rotation.	A firm springy sensation to movement with a slight amount of give in capsular joints. Example: Frozen shoulder.
Springy, block		Rebound effect with limited motion; usually in joints with a meniscus. Example: Torn meniscus.
Empty		An empty feel in a joint with severe pain when passively moved. The movement cannot be performed because of the pain. Example: Fracture, subacromial bursitis, neoplasm, joint inflammation.

Active Range of Motion

Active range of motion evaluates the physical function of a body part. This type of range will yield general information regarding the patient's general ability and willingness to use the part. If a patient is asked to move a joint through a full arc of movement and cannot, it is impossible to distinguish whether the loss of function is caused by pain, weakness caused by a neurologic motor dysfunction, stiffness, or the conscious unwillingness of the patient to perform the full function. Therefore, the assessment value of active range of motion in and of itself is vague and limited. Active motion is a basic test for the integrity of the muscle or muscles used in the action and the nerve supply attached to the muscle. Obviously, the integrity of the joint being tested must be intact to evaluate muscular or neurologic dysfunction. This integrity is best evaluated by passive range of motion.

When evaluating active motion, note the degree of motion in the tested plane as well as any pain associated with the movement. The pain should be correlated with the movement, such as pain in the full arc or only in the extreme range of motion. Crepitus should also be noted when performing active range of motion. Crepitus is a crackling sound that usually indicates a roughening of joint surfaces or increased friction between a tendon and its sheath (caused by swelling or roughening).

Joint range of motion should be measured and recorded by commonly accepted reproducible means. To measure the range of motion of the spine, the most accurate instrument is the inclinometer (Fig. 1-1). This instrument measures angular displacement relative to gravity as opposed to arcs. The reason for inclinometer measurement of the spine is that the spine is composed of multiple joints that function in unison to produce movement. A device that measures arcs, such as a goniometer (Fig. 1-2), cannot distinguish the difference between sacral flexion and lumbar flexion in the lower back when the patient is bending forward. In this particular instance, the inclinometer can distinguish between true lumbar flexion and sacral or hip flexion (see inclinometer range of motion in Chapters 3, 9, and 10). Goniometers are best suited to measure extremity range of motion.

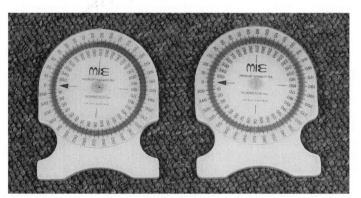

Figure 1-1

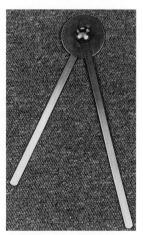

Figure 1-2

Resisted Range of Motion

Resisted range of motion is useful in assessing musculotendinous and neurologic structures. It is primarily used to test neurologic function (see nerve root lesions). The tests are graded 5 to 0, a scale that has been adopted by the American Academy of Orthopaedic Surgeons (Box 1-6).

Musculotendinous injuries are generally more painful than they are weak. Neurologic lesions are generally more weak than they are painful. The four general pain-related reactions to resisted range of motion testing are listed in Box 1-7.

Box 1-6	Muscle Grading Scale
5	Complete range of motion against gravity with full resistance
4	Complete range of motion against gravity with some resistance
3	Complete range of motion against gravity
2	Complete range of motion with gravity eliminated (movement in the horizontal plane)
1	Evidence of slight contractility
0	No evidence of contractility

Box 1-7   Resistant Range of Motion Reactions

1. Strong with no pain elicited is normal and not indicative of any lesions.
2. Strong with pain elicited may indicate a minor lesion of the muscle or tendon.
3. Weak and painless may indicate a neurologic lesion, which must be evaluated with the previous chart. It may also indicate a complete rupture of a tendon or muscle because there are no fibers intact from which pain can be elicited.
4. Weak and painful may indicate a partial rupture of a muscle or tendon because intact fibers may be stressed to produce pain. Fracture, neoplasm, and acute inflammation are also possibilities.

SPECIAL PHYSICAL, ORTHOPAEDIC, AND NEUROLOGIC TESTING

Special physical, orthopaedic, and neurologic testing is designed to place functional stress on isolated tissue structures in terms of the underlying pathology. Positive physical testing is not diagnostic in itself but rather a biomechanical assessment to be used as part of a complete clinical evaluation.

Before performing certain special tests, you must ascertain that they will not be detrimental to the patient's condition. Box 1-8 lists the conditions for which care must be taken when performing either range of motion testing or special physical orthopaedic and neurologic testing.

Box 1-8   Physical Examination Precautions

- Dislocation
- Unhealed fracture
- Myositis ossificans/ ectopic ossification
- Joint infection
- Marked osteoporosis
- Bony ankylosis
- Newly united fracture
- After surgery

If it is determined that special physical testing may indeed harm the patient, structural and/or functional testing, such as radiography, CT, MRI, or electromyography (EMG), should be employed before any physical testing.

The subsequent chapters contain a collection of special physical orthopaedic and neurologic tests organized anatomically and subcategorized by diagnostic entity. This system is best suited for expedient evaluation of musculoskeletal and orthopaedic neurologic conditions. Each test illustrates and discusses the procedures for correct performance of the test. Each test is accompanied by an explanation that indicates the positive indicators for that test and what they may mean in terms of an underlying pathology or injury. Biomechanical considerations that may not be evident in the classical interpretation of a particular test are also explored.

Sensitivity/Reliability Scale

I have chosen to add a sensitivity/reliability scale to each of the tests described in this text. For each diagnosis presented, there are multiple tests. Some of those tests are more sensitive/reliable than others. I have attempted to rate each test based on the biomechanics of the movement to isolate the affected structures. The scale is numbered from 0 to 4, with 1 to 2 being poorly sensitive/reliable, 2 to 3 being moderately sensitive/reliable and 3 to 4 being very sensitive/reliable. Those tests that are very sensitive/reliable should be performed first. This will help in evaluating the patient's condition more expeditiously.

DIAGNOSTIC IMAGING AND OTHER SPECIALIZED STRUCTURAL TESTING

Diagnostic imaging or structural testing entails the use of specialized equipment to visualize certain anatomic structures. The most common diagnostic imaging procedures include plain film radiology (x-ray), CT), MRI), and skeletal scintigraphy (bone scan). Each type of structural test may be best suited to visualize various structures in specific ways.

Plain Film Radiology

Plain film radiology dates to 1895, and its fundamentals are still used in practice today. X-rays are a form of radiant energy that have a short wavelength and can penetrate many substances (Fig. 1-3). The x-ray is produced by bombarding a tungsten target with an electron beam in an x-ray tube. Plain film radiography demonstrates five basic densities: air, fat, subcutaneous tissue, bone, and metal. Anatomic structures are seen on radiographs as outlines in whole or as part of different tissue densities. These differences in densities are the key to determining the normal or pathologic state of tissues shown on radiographic film. Bone is the best-seen tissue on plain film radiography.

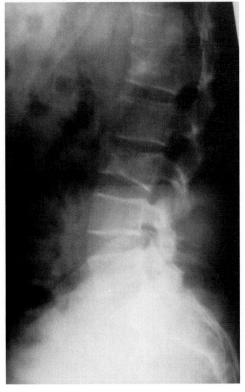

Figure 1-3

Computed Tomography

Computed tomography is a cross-sectional imaging technique that uses x-ray as its energy (Fig. 1-4). A computer is used to reconstruct a cross-sectional image from measurements of x-ray transmission. Most CT units allow for a slice thickness between 1 and 10 mm and are generally limited to the axial plane. CT is best used for bone detail and demonstration of calcifications. Intervertebral disc defects may also be visualized on CT, but not as well as with MRI.

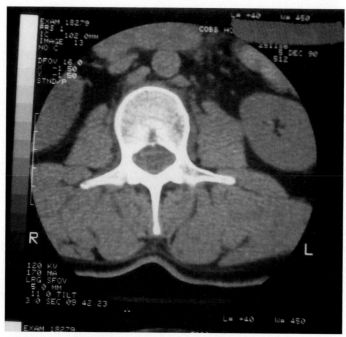

Figure 1-4

Magnetic Resonance Imaging

MRI is also a cross-sectional imaging technique (Fig. 1-5). It uses magnetic fields and radio waves instead of x-rays to produce its images. MRI is based on the ability of the body to absorb and emit radio waves when the body is in a strong magnetic field. The absorption and release of this energy is different and detectable in each individual type of tissue. Hence, MRI is invaluable in contrasting soft tissue structures in many planes without the use of ionizing radiation. It poorly demonstrates bone density detail or calcifications; this is the advantage of CT. MRI is superior in visualizing an intervertebral disc or other soft tissue structure for pathology.

Patients with any metallic implants or metal fragments (e.g., cardiac pacemakers, insulin pumps, vascular clips, skin staples, bullets, or shrapnel) are advised not to undergo MRI because of the strong magnetic field emitted by the scanner. This field may move or dislodge metallic implants or objects in an individual whose body is being scanned.

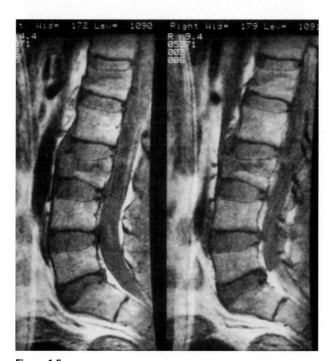

Figure 1-5

Myelography

Myelography introduces a small amount of water-soluble contrast medium into the subarachnoid space (Fig. 1-6). Standard x-ray films of the spine are then taken to evaluate and defects of the spinal canal, such as spinal stenosis, spinal cord lesions, and dural tears.

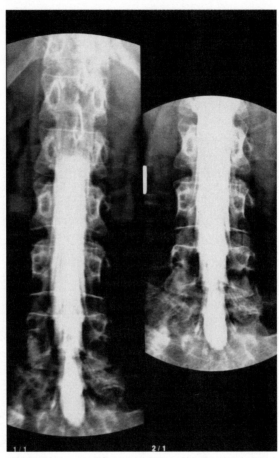

Figure 1-6

1

Skeletal Scintigraphy

Skeletal scintigraphy, or bone scan, uses an intravenous radiopharmaceutical, technetium-99m, which is attracted to osteoblastic activity in bone tissue and is detected by a gamma camera (Fig. 1-7). Vigorous osteoblastic activity, such as healing fractures and pathologic conditions, stimulate skeletal blood flow and bone repair. In turn, more of the radiopharmaceutical attaches to the area, marking the increased activity for evaluation. Bone scans are best suited for undetectable fractures on x-ray and arthropathies, such as early degenerative changes in joints, osteomyelitis, bony dysplasias, primary bone tumors, and metastatic malignancy.

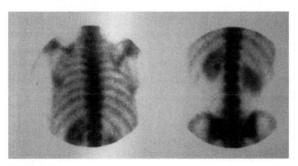

Figure 1-7

FUNCTIONAL TESTING

Functional testing for musculoskeletal and neurologic pathology entails testing neurologic function by assessing electrical activity of specific neurologic structures, such as electroencephalography (EEG), EMG, and somatosensory evoked potential studies (SSEP).

Electroencephalography

EEG records the electrical activity of the brain through the skull by surface electrodes. Abnormal electrical activity may indicate cerebral pathology, such as epilepsy, inflammatory encephalopathies, infarction, trauma, or tumor, that may not be detectable by structural testing.

Electromyography

EMG measures the electrical activity of contracting muscles and is recorded either via surface electrodes or through needles inserted directly into the muscle itself. The surface electrodes record and average the activity from many motor units, whereas needle EMG can detect the activity from a single motor unit. The recordings are used to detect the cause of muscle weakness. They are also useful in detecting neuropathies, denervation, and entrapment syndromes.

Somatosensory Evoked Potential

SSEP studies measure electrical activity from a distal nerve to a more proximal point on the nerve, spinal cord, or brain stem. A stimulus is given peripherally, and responses are recorded and averaged proximal to the stimulated area. The purpose of the test is to determine and quantify nerve, cord, or brain stem lesions. It is used most commonly to detect trauma, tumors, and demyelinating diseases of the nervous system.

Suggested Diagnostic Imaging

Each chapter contains a suggested diagnostic imaging section for each diagnostic entity. These suggestions start from the most basic diagnostic imaging and move on to more advanced testing procedures. If diagnostic imaging is needed, the clinician should start with the most basic tests and move forward based on the outcome of those first tests. Secondly, the clinician should not advance to other diagnostic tests if the results of the basic diagnostic imaging reveal that injury may result from further testing, such as flexion/extension plain film radiography to the cervical spine if instability is noted on static scout films. Remember that there is no substitution for a complete history and physical examination and that the suggested diagnostic imaging sections are just that— "suggested," based on the history and examination of the presenting patient.

SUMMARY

The examining clinician should employ the techniques discussed in this chapter to assess the patient's condition. Not all segments of the clinical assessment protocol need be employed for each patient and complaint. History, inspection, palpation, range of motion, and physical testing are core requirements. Whether to use diagnostic imaging and functional testing is based on the outcomes of the core requirements and the clinical judgment and experience of the examiner.

General References

1. Adams JC, Hamblen DL. Outline of Orthopaedics. 11th ed. Edinburgh: Churchill Livingstone, 1990.
2. American Academy of Orthopaedic Surgeons. The Clinical Measurement of Joint Motion. Chicago: American Academy of Orthopaedic Surgeons, 1994.
3. Bates B. Bates' Guide to Physical Examination and History Taking. 7th ed. Philadelphia: Lippincott Williams & Wilkins, 1999.
4. Clarkson HM. Musculoskeletal Assessment: Joint Range of Motion and Manual Muscle Strength. 2nd ed. Baltimore: Lippincott Williams & Wilkins, 2000.
5. Corrigan B, Maitland GD. Practical Orthopaedic Medicine. London: Butterworth, 1983.
6. Cyriax J. Textbook of Orthopaedic Medicine. Vol 1. Diagnosis of Soft Tissue Lesions. 8th ed. London: Bailliere Tindall, 1982.
7. Dambro MR, Griffith JA. Griffith's 5 Minute Clinical Consult. Baltimore: Williams & Wilkins, 1997.
8. Endow AJ, Swisher SN. Interviewing and Patient Care. New York: Oxford University, 1992.
9. French S. History Taking in Physiotherapy Assessment. Physiotherapy 1988;74:158–160.
10. Greenstein GM. Clinical Assessment of Musculoskeletal Disorders. St. Louis: Mosby, 1997.
11. Hawkins RJ. An Organized Approach to Musculoskeletal Examination and History Taking. St. Louis: Mosby, 1995.
12. Hertling D, Kessler RM. Management of Common Musculoskeletal Disorders: Physical Therapy Principles and Methods. 3rd ed. Philadelphia: Lippincott Williams & Wilkins, 1996.
13. Hoppenfeld S. Physical Examination of the Spine and Extremities. New York: Appleton-Century-Crofts, 1976.
14. Kendall FP, McCreary EK, Provance PG. Muscles: Testing and Function. 4th ed. Baltimore: Williams & Wilkins, 1993.
15. Krejci VP. Koch muscle and tendon injuries. Chicago: Year Book, 1979.
16. Magee DJ. Orthopaedic physical assessment. 3rd ed. Philadelphia: WB Saunders, 1997.
17. Minor MAD, Minor SD. Patient Evaluation Methods for the Health Professional. Reston, VA: Reston, 1985.
18. Mooney V. Where is the Pain Coming From? Spine 1989;12:8:754–759.
19. Nordin M, Frankel VH. Basic biomechanics of the musculoskeletal system. 3rd ed. Philadelphia: Lippincott Williams & Wilkins, 2001.
20. Post M. Physical Examination of the Musculoskeletal System. Chicago: Year Book, 1987.
21. Salter RB. Textbook of disorders and injuries of the musculoskeletal system. 3rd ed. Baltimore: Williams & Wilkins, 1999.
22. Starkey C, Ryan J. Evaluation of Orthopedic and Athletic Injuries. Philadelphia. FA Davis, 1996.

POSTURAL ASSESSMENT

*Steven P. Weiniger, DC**

*Private practice in Conyers, Georgia; founder, BodyZone.com.

WHY POSTURE IS IMPORTANT

Posture is how a body balances. If a body doesn't balance, it falls down. To analyze posture it is necessary to observe how the body is balancing. Posture is more than muscles and bones. The spine, with its ligaments intact but devoid of muscles, is an extremely unstable structure. Muscles and their complex neuromuscular control are required (*a*) to provide stability of the trunk in a given posture and (*b*) to produce movement during physiologic activity (1). The motor system and the nervous system function as one entity (2). Therefore, postural analysis is an assessment of the function of the motor system (bones, muscles, and ligaments) and the nervous system's control of the motor system.

Postural observations are organic; that is, they deal with the whole organism. Unlike most orthopaedic or neurologic tests, which focus on identifying the specific nature of an injury, illness, or other clinical problem, a postural evaluation looks at the whole person and attempts to assess the relative contributions of myriad postural observations. Posture comprises an accumulation of adaptations and compensations from injuries and habits to allow the body to balance and function effectively.

An individual's neutral posture occurs when the brain and nervous system use information from three sources to balance the body in space when standing, sitting, or moving:

Eyes: We see what is level.

Ears: The vestibular apparatus gives the brain information about the relative position and motion of each inner ear.

Muscles and joints: Proprioceptors in the muscles, ligaments, and tendons tell the brain how hard each is being stressed.

The brain integrates the information it receives to balance the body.

ARCHITECTURAL VERSUS ADAPTIVE POSTURAL CHANGES: BODY TYPES, INJURY, AND HABIT

Postural compensations and adaptations can be both a cause and an effect of a clinical problem. Orthopedic problems frequently cause a postural change, which in turn worsens the orthopaedic problem. Asymptomatic postural problems can cause undue mechanical stress, predisposing an individual to either injury or chronic mechanical stress syndrome.

There is no one "normal" posture. An ideal posture is used as a reference point, but rarely does a patient have "perfect posture." Since the posture is how the body balances, the ideal posture for an individual distributes the forces of gravity for balanced muscle function. Joints should move in their mid range so as to minimize undue stress and strain on ligaments at the joint's end range of motion and fully distribute stress on the joint surfaces. A biomechanically efficient posture is maximally effective in that individual's activities of daily living and avoids injury.

People come in various shapes and sizes and live unique lives, and their postures differ accordingly (Fig. 2-1). An individual learns during childhood to balance the body's unique architecture. The child's habits affect his or her posture. Good habits can create a strong and stable posture. Bad habits can train the body for poor posture and instability. Excessive sitting, carrying a heavy backpack, slumping, or poor sleeping position trains the body to a folded-forward posture. Habitual one-sided activities, such as carrying a heavy purse, sitting on a wallet, or facing sidewise to view a poorly placed computer monitor train the body to be asymmetrical from left to right.

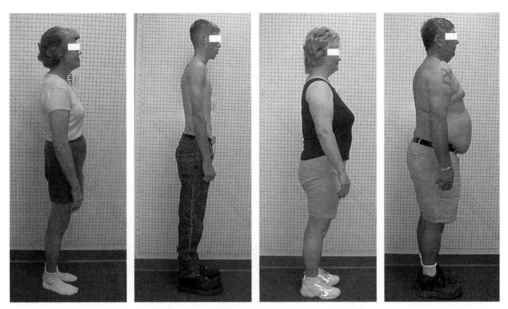

Figure 2-1. Posture varies by individual body type, history of injury, and habits.

Poor posture creates adaptive patterns of body motion. Poor posture and body motion stress the musculoskeletal system, resulting in premature joint wear and susceptibility to injury. Studies show that sports injuries correlate with deviations of body mechanics (3). The incidence of injury in athletes has been linked to postural distortions associated with the site of injury, and those with more than two types of injury have significantly worse postural symmetry.

The human bipedal posture is extremely effective and "the most economical of antigravity mechanisms once the upright posture is attained" (4). However, when there is an illness or injury, the body adapts and moves differently. The body must balance, so the posture adapts to changes in muscle and joint motion and resting positions. Overstressed muscles strengthen and favored muscles weaken.

Posture and body motion are like a fold in a piece of paper. Once folded, the paper will bend along the fold when it is stressed. Similarly, once posture and body motion change to compensate for poor habits or injury, the body continues to assume the same uneven resting posture and follows the same adaptive pattern of motion. Biomechanically speaking, this adaptive posture is almost always inefficient. Mother was right about molding good posture in a child by standing straight with head and shoulders back.

Clinically, a postural change begins a cascade of compensating causes and effects. Subjectively, the patient usually believes he or she is standing straight and balanced, even if a visual inspection shows otherwise. If the brain believes the body is balanced when it is not, posture adaptations cause uneven stress and predisposition to future injury. Over a lifetime, people's history of injury, daily activities, and habits shape their unique posture.

Spinal distortions occur in all directions of three-dimensional space and are more than a sum of the front, back, and side views of the spine. When viewed from above, the helical nature of spinal adaptations becomes apparent (Fig. 2-2) (1). However, according to White and Panjabi (1), present knowledge and technology do not allow effective evaluation of helical adaptations. Nonetheless, posture analysis can provide valuable clinical information that must be correlated with a patient's history and reported symptoms.

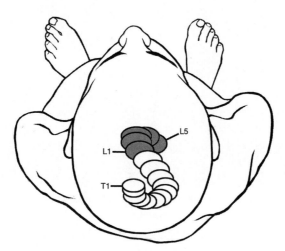

Figure 2-2. Helical spine adaptation.

POSTURE EVALUATION: METHODS AND OBSERVATIONS

A suggested posture evaluation mindset is to think of the body as a stack of children's blocks (Fig. 2-3). When the blocks are all balanced, the stack is stable. But when one is out of place, the stack wobbles. To balance a stack of blocks, you put the second block on top of the first. When you place the third block on the second, it can be only as stable as the second. Placing a forth block requires stability of the blocks below, and so on. This bottom-to-top arrangement is how human beings balance. That is why shoulder corrections tend to follow correction of lateral pelvic tilt, but the reverse does not necessarily occur.

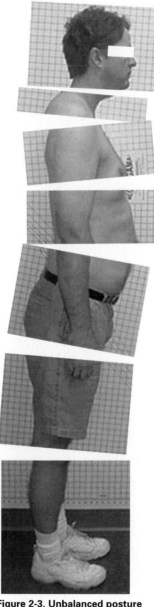

Figure 2-3. Unbalanced posture creates instability.

Additionally, in posture analysis and clinical treatment, it is important to determine whether a muscle is weak or inhibited. A weak muscle is unused because it is unstressed and should therefore be strengthened with exercise. An inhibited muscle is not used because its antagonist is being adaptively overused. The neurologic reciprocal inhibition of a muscle by its antagonist results in overdevelopment of the muscles most used in posture and underdevelopment of their antagonists (2).

Clinically, the goal is to identify the most important fault in the kinetic chain. Since postural analysis can be diagnostic and possibly suggest therapeutic actions, it is imperative to differentiate between actions and reactions. Unbalanced postures have compensating reactions. When observing the posture, the examiner should note any inconsistencies or imbalances, both from left to right and from front to back. Mentally integrate the patient's complaint and history with the mechanics of the body's balance. Palpation can help differentiate longstanding adaptive muscle hypertrophy (unilaterally tight muscles without significant reactive pain on palpation) from acute muscle spasm (with reactive pain on palpation).

Prior to postural evaluation, the examiner should obtain all pertinent history, including a description of symptoms, fractures, injuries, congenital abnormalities, and the patient's dominant hand. It is important to note any gross structural asymmetries, scoliosis, or other condition that creates imbalance.

The patient should be as minimally clothed as possible so that the examiner may clearly visualize the contours, bony prominences, and other anatomical landmarks from the front (anteroposterior [AP] view), back (posteroanterior [PA] view) and sides (left and right lateral views) (Fig. 2-4).

The patient should be told to stand straight and look straight ahead. The patient who adopts a rigid standing straight posture (i.e. bilateral shoulder or abdominal tightening on assuming a straight posture) should be told to relax and assume a comfortable position. Patients will try to assume a "good" posture, so to observe a true resting posture it is important not to coach patients by asking them to straighten up what is misaligned.

If there is poor alignment of the feet and the torso or if both feet are not facing at the same angle, instruct the patient to march in place for five steps. A postural distortion is indicated if the feet and torso are still misaligned.

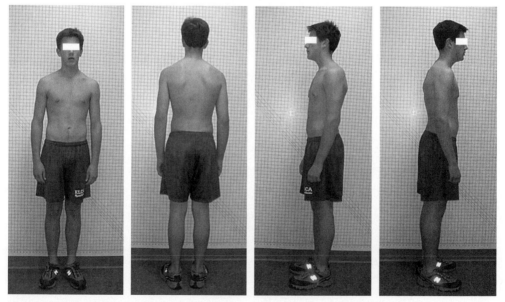

Figure 2-4. Posture should be viewed from the front, back, left side, and right side.

Posterior View Evaluation

In a balanced posture, the body appears equal from left to right. A vertical plumb line over the center of the body (Fig. 2-5) should show alignment of the occipital protuberance; cervical, thoracic, and lumbar spinous processes; coccyx; and gluteal folds. The arms should hang equally from the torso, with an equal and small amount of the palms visible. The space between the arms and the body should be the same on both sides. The legs should appear equally abducted from the centerline, and the backs of the knees should appear the same. The ankles and feet should display bilaterally symmetric alignment (e.g., no pronation or supination) and toe out. In balanced posture, the following structures should be level and equal: tips of the mastoid processes, acromia, scapula, lower margins of the 12th ribs, iliac crests, posterior superior iliac spines, and ischial tuberosities.

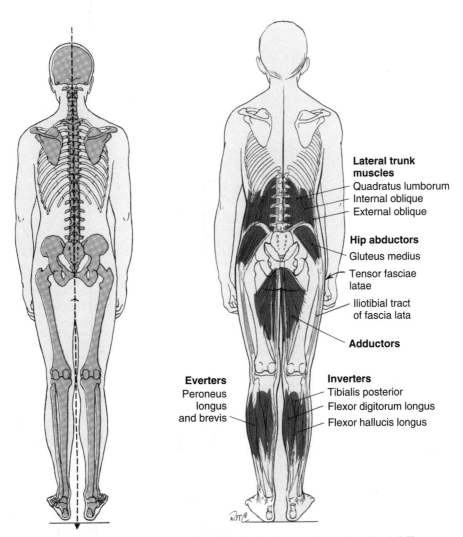

Lateral trunk muscles
Quadratus lumborum
Internal oblique
External oblique

Hip abductors
Gluteus medius

Tensor fasciae latae

Iliotibial tract of fascia lata

Adductors

Everters
Peroneus longus and brevis

Inverters
Tibialis posterior
Flexor digitorum longus
Flexor hallucis longus

Figure 2-5. Ideal alignment, posterior view. (Modified with permission from Kendall FP, McCreary EK, Provance PG. Muscles: Testing and Function. 4th ed. Baltimore: Williams & Wilkins, 1993:88.)

Most people have a slight postural distortion because of left- or right-hand dominance. Right-handed people tend to have a high right hip and a low right shoulder (Fig. 2-6). Left-handed ones tend to have a high left hip and a low left shoulder. In addition, the normal AP spine has a slight right convex thoracic curve, most likely due to an individual's left or right-handedness (1).

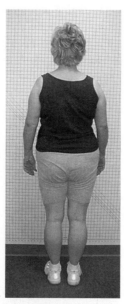

Figure 2-6. Right-handed postural pattern.

Lateral View

The examiner should evaluate the patient from both sides. From the side view, a plumb line should show alignment between the external auditory canal, acromion process of the shoulder, axillary line, midpoint of the iliac crest, greater trochanter of the hip, lateral condyles of the femur, and tibia slightly anterior to the lateral malleolus.

The head, chest, pelvis, and lower extremities should be in alignment and balanced. There should be a normal cervical lordosis, thoracic kyphosis, and lumbar lordosis (Fig. 2-7). The head is balanced when a horizontal line can be drawn from the occipital protuberance to the lower margin of the zygomatic arch. In neutral posture the head should be above the shoulders, not forward. The eyes have a strong tendency to seek level, so if there is postural distortion, the head position may tilt forward or backward to compensate (Fig. 2-8).

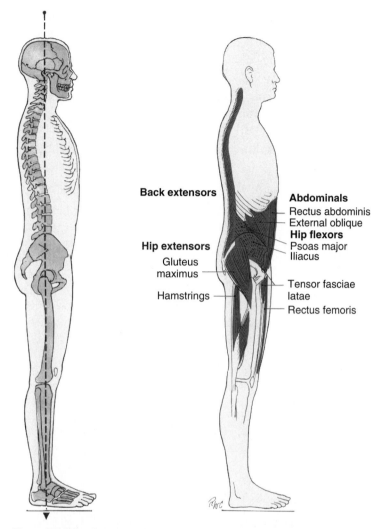

Back extensors

Abdominals
Rectus abdominis
External oblique
Hip flexors
Psoas major
Iliacus

Hip extensors
Gluteus
maximus

Hamstrings

Tensor fasciae
latae

Rectus femoris

Figure 2-7. Lateral posture alignment. (Modified with permission from Kendall FP, McCreary EK, Provance PG. Muscles: Testing and Function. 4th ed. Baltimore: Williams & Wilkins, 1993:83.)

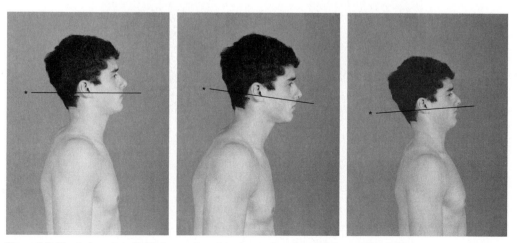

Figure 2-8. Neutral posture (left), forward posture (center), and cervical retraction (right).

On a lateral view, the shoulder girdle and torso are balanced when a horizontal line can be drawn from the medial end of the spine of the scapula to the head of the humerus and then to the medial end of the clavicle. The scapulae should appear equal and lie symmetrically against the torso (Fig. 2-9).

The pelvis is level and balanced when a horizontal line can be drawn from just below the anterior superior iliac spine to the posterior superior iliac spine. Ideally, the anterior superior iliac spine should be vertically aligned with the symphysis pubes (Fig. 2-9).

The lower extremities should be vertically aligned with the knee joints neutral (e.g., not locked in hyperextension). The legs should be equally vertical and at a right angle to the sole of the foot (Fig. 2-9).

Anteroposterior/Front View

Balanced posture should appear equal from left to right. A vertical plumb line over the center of the body will show alignment of the bridge of the nose, center of the chin, episternal notch, xiphoid process, umbilicus, and pubes. The arms should be hanging similarly, both palms at the side of the thighs. Shoulder girdle symmetry is indicated if the hands show similar rotation and placement on the body. The legs should appear equally abducted from the centerline, with the feet displaying bilaterally symmetric alignment (e.g., no pronation or supination) and toe out. The knees should be forward and bilaterally symmetric in their alignment and orientation on the lower extremity (Fig. 2-10).

In balanced posture, anterior examination will show the following structures to be equal bilaterally and level: eyes, clavicles, lower margins of the ribcage, anterior superior iliac spines, femoral trochanters, knees, and ankles.

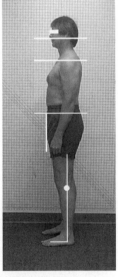

Figure 2-9. Balanced shoulder girdle and torso.

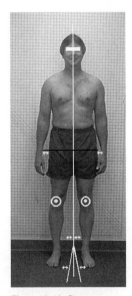

Figure 2-10. Posture balanced left to right.

POSTURE TYPES

A postural distortion is an adaptation, or change, in the way the body is balancing. This is accompanied by characteristic patterns of dysfunctional muscle tightness and weakness. Significant clinical information can be deduced from observing and correlating different posture types and distortions.

Kendall and Kendall's posture typing system categorizes posture types by lateral view into four types: military, kypholordotic, swayback, and flat back (Fig. 2-11). Each posture type's characteristic patterns of muscle overactivity and underactivity are shown, with tight muscles dark and weak muscles lightly drawn. Observing head position (neutral or forward) and pelvic posture (neutral or posterior) allows posture to be categorized into the four types. Table 2-1 correlates with the posture types in Fig. 2-11 and summarizes the posture types and their associated patterns of muscle weakness (Table 2-1).

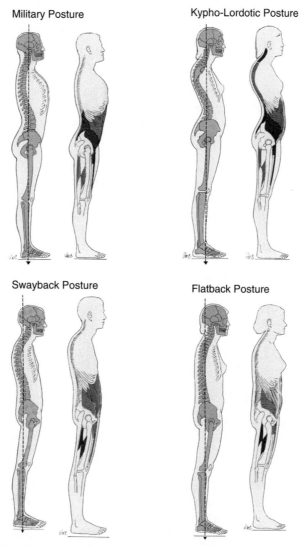

Military Posture

Kypho-Lordotic Posture

Swayback Posture

Flatback Posture

Figure 2-11. Four posture types. (Modified with permission from Kendall FP, McCreary EK, Provance PG. Muscles: Testing and Function. 4th ed. Baltimore: Williams & Wilkins, 1993:84–87.)

TABLE 2-1	POSTURE TYPE CLASSIFICATION BY PELVIC TILT AND HEAD POSTURE	
	Neutral Head Postures	**Forward Head Postures**

Posterior Pelvic Tilt	**Military Posture**
	Anterior body structure
	  Chest; pelvis if lordosis is
	    marked
	Tight muscles
	  Low back
	  Hip flexors
	Weak muscles
	  Anterior abdominals initially,
	    hamstrings lengthen, then
	    adaptively shorten
		Kypholordotic Posture
		Anterior body structure
		  Head (forward head posture)
		  Abdomen
		Tight muscles
		  Suboccipital neck extensors
		  Hip flexors
		  Serratus anterior
		  Pectorals
		  Upper trapezius (if scapulae are
		    abducted)
		Weak muscles
		  Neck flexors
		  Upper thoracic spinae
		  External abdominal oblique
		  Mid and lower trap (if scapulae are
		    abducted)

Forward Pelvic Tilt	**Swayback Posture**
	Anterior body structure
	  Pelvis or femur heads with
	    compensating long kyphosis
	Tight muscles
	Hamstrings
	  Internal abdominal obliques
	  Low back erector spinae
	  Same side TFL (if lateral pelvic
	    distortion)
	Weak muscles
	  1 hip joint flexors
	  External abdominal obliques
	  Lower and mid trapezius
	  Deep neck flexors
	  Same side gluteus medius (if
	    lateral pelvic distortion)
		Flat Back Posture
		Anterior body structure
		  Head
		Tight muscles
		  Hamstrings
		  Abdominals
		Weak muscles
		  1 joint hip flexors

POSTURAL SYNDROMES

The body moves in patterns of motion. Unbalanced overuse of the postural muscles (e.g., the muscles used to maintain posture) is accompanied by weakening of the opposing antagonist muscles. This weakening is due to lack of use and a neurologic reciprocal inhibition. This pattern of overuse and weakening results in distinct postural syndromes. The upper crossed syndrome affects the head, neck, and shoulders, while the lower crossed syndrome affects the lumbar spine and pelvis. They frequently exist simultaneously and combine to create chronic musculoskeletal stress.

This upper crossed posture syndrome is the source of computer user's (and others in long-term seated postures) complaint of chronic neck and shoulder tightness and pain. The upper crossed posture is characterized by rolled-in and forward shoulders with increased thoracic kyphosis, a forward head posture, and loss of the cervical lordosis (Fig. 2-12). The tightness in anterior shoulder muscles results in weak and inhibited infraspinatus, teres minor, rhomboids, and thoracic erector spinae muscles. Neck, upper and middle back, and shoulder girdle muscles are shortened and tight from overuse, while their antagonists are weak and stretched. Trigger points are frequently found in the

2

overused neck extensor muscles, the upper trapezius, and the levator scapulae muscles. The opposing longus colli, capitis, and lower trapezius muscles are weak (Table 2-2).

The lower crossed syndrome is the other modern postural pattern. The lower crossed posture is characterized by an anterior pelvis and increased lumbar lordosis with tightness in the psoas and lumbar erector spinae (Fig. 2-13). Sitting shortens the psoas and other hip flexor muscles when the thigh is flexed. Long-term sitting at work and play, along with driving between the two, creates muscle imbalance between these overused hip flexors and the underused hip extensors. The gluteus maximus, the primary hip extensor, opposes the hip flexors and therefore becomes adaptively weak. To maintain erect posture and balance, the lumbar erector spinae muscles compensate and extend the spine, resulting in hypertonicity of the lumbar erector spinae and adaptive weakening of the opposing abdominal muscles. Also, the hip adductor muscles are frequently tight, with compensating weakness of the gluteus medius and minimus muscles (Table 2-2).

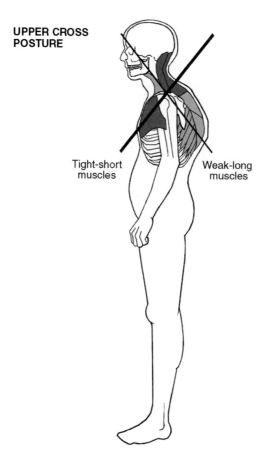

UPPER CROSS POSTURE

Tight-short muscles

Weak-long muscles

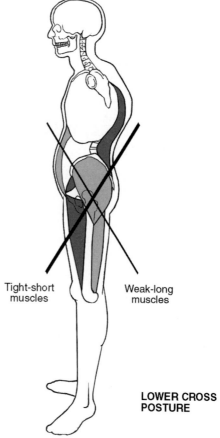

Tight-short muscles

Weak-long muscles

LOWER CROSS POSTURE

Figure 2-12.
  Upper cross posture
  Forward head
  Loss of cervical lordosis
  Shoulders rolled in and forward
  Increased thoracic kyphosis
  Tight-short muscles
    Suboccipitals
    Pectorals, anterior shoulder
    Upper trapezius
  Weak-long muscles
    Mid, lower trapezius
    Serratus anterior

Figure 2-13.
  Lower cross posture
  Anterior pelvis
  Protruding abdomen
  Increased lumbar lordosis
  Feet turned out
  Tight-short muscles
    Psoas
    Lumbar erector spinae
    Hip adductor
  Weak-long muscles
    Hip extensors, gluteus maximus
    Abdominal
    Gluteus medius, minimus

TABLE 2-2	POSTURAL SIGNS OF UPPER AND LOWER CROSSED SYNDROME
Postural Finding	**Dysfunction**
Upper crossed syndrome	
Round shoulders	Shortened pectorals
Forward-drawn head	Kyphotic upper thoracic spine
C0-C1 hyperextension	Shortened suboccipitals
Elevation of shoulders	Shortened upper trapezius, levator scapulae, weak lower, middle trapezius
Winging of scapulae	Weak serratus anterior
Lower crossed syndrome	
Lumbar hyperlordosis	Shortened erector spinae
Anterior pelvic tilt	Weak gluteus maximus
Protruding abdomen	Weak abdominals
Foot turned out	Shortened piriformis
Hypertrophy of thoracolumbar junction	Hypermobile lumbosacral junction
Groove in iliotibial band	Shortened tensor fascia latae

Adapted with permission from Liebenson C, ed. Rehabilitation of the Spine. Baltimore: Williams & Wilkins, 1996:363–364.

OTHER POSTURAL DISTORTIONS, ADAPTATIONS, AND PATHOLOGIES

Because postural evaluation is a global evaluation of how the body balances, faults and postures from one part of the kinetic chain can cause a compensating postural distortion in a different region. The overall posture is the sum of all distortions and resulting compensations necessary to allow the individual to balance and avoid painful positions and motions. In the interest of providing a comprehensive summary, primarily local muscular involvements are detailed below. Also, a normal skeletal system without vertebral compression fractures or congenital abnormalities such as hemivertebra is assumed.

Forward Head Posture

Forward head posture is probably the most common posture distortion (Fig. 2-14). For every inch that the head moves forward of neutral posture, the weight carried by the lower neck increases by the additional weight of the entire head (Fig. 2-15). Many patients' symptoms of neck, shoulder, and arm pain; headaches; and stress are associated with the faulty biomechanics of carrying the skull too far forward of the torso. Observations associated with forward head posture include (*a*) external auditory meatus anterior of the acromion and (*b*) sternocleidomastoideus usually hypertrophied.

Possible tight, overactive muscles: SCM and/or suboccipitals, anterior cervical flexors; upper trapezius, levator scapulae, pectorals.

Possible weak, underactive muscles: Cervical extensors, lower and mid trapezius, serratus anterior. Also possible deep neck flexors (longus colli) inhibition.

Clinical correlate: Palpate the suboccipitals when sitting and standing (Figs. 2-16 and 2-17). If there is less tension when sitting, pelvic postural stress is contributing to the forward head posture.

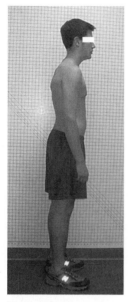

Figure 2-14. Forward head posture.

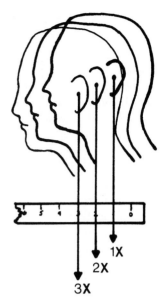

Figure 2-15. For every inch the head moves forward of neutral posture, the weight carried by the lower neck increases by the additional weight of the entire head. (Adapted from Liebenson C, ed. Rehabilitation of the Spine. Baltimore: Williams & Wilkins, 1996:177.)

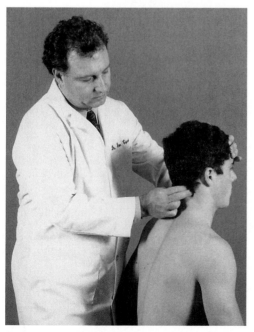

Figure 2-16. Palpation of the suboccipitals with the subject seated.

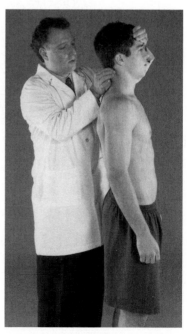

Figure 2-17. Palpation of the suboccipitals with the subject standing.

Head Tilt and/or Rotation

PA view: The line between tips of the mastoid processes is unlevel (Fig. 2-18). The occipital protuberance is to one side of a center line bisecting the pelvis and spine. The skull is not evenly bisected by a centerline.

Possible tight, overactive muscles: Lateral neck flexors on the flexed side, scalene or intrinsic rotator muscles on the opposite side of head rotation. Sternocleidomastoideus, upper trapezius.

Possible weak, underactive muscles: Lateral neck flexors on the opposite side of head flexion. Intrinsic rotator muscles on the side of head rotation.

Unlevel Shoulders

Observations: The horizontal line between the acromia is not level. Shoulder imbalance is also observed with thoracic scoliosis and hand dominance (Fig. 2-19).

Possible tight overactive muscles: On the side of the high shoulder, upper trapezius and/or levator scapulae muscles; on the side of the low shoulder, lower trapezius and pectoralis minor muscles, tight rhomboid and/or latissimus dorsi muscles.

Possible weak, underactive muscles: On the side of the high shoulder, lower and mid trapezius; on the side of the low shoulder, upper trapezius.

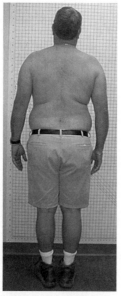

Figure 2-18. Right head tilt and rotation.

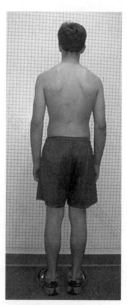

Figure 2-19. High left shoulder.

Observation: The neck–shoulder line is not contoured normally (Fig. 2-20). A straightening of the neck–shoulder line indicates a tight trapezius muscle. This is known as a gothic shoulders appearance because it looks like a Gothic church tower.

Observation: A double wave appearance at the lateral scapula at the insertion of the levator scapula indicates tightness of the levator scapula (Fig. 2-21).

2

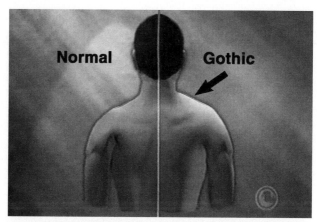

Figure 2-20. Elevated, or Gothic, shoulders. (Reprinted with permission from Liebenson C, Chapman S. Cervico-Thoracic Spine: Making a Rehabilitation Prescription, Tape 2. Baltimore: Williams & Wilkins, 1998, Fig 3.)

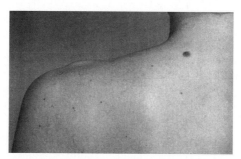

Figure 2-21. Tightness of the levator scapula. (Reprinted with permission from Liebenson C, ed. Rehabilitation of the Spine. Baltimore: Williams & Wilkins, 1996:108.)

Scapula Winging

The medial borders of the scapulae are lifted posteriorly from the ribs.

Possible tight, overactive muscles: Rhomboid.

Possible weak, underactive muscles: serratus anterior.

Clinical correlate: Push-up test. Observe whether scapula winging increases when the person does a pushup (Fig. 2-22).

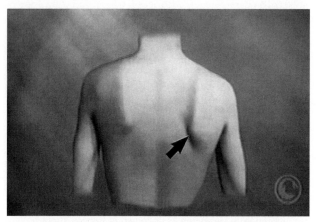

Figure 2-22. Winged scapula. (Reprinted with permission from Liebenson C, Chapman S. Cervico-Thoracic Spine: Making a Rehabilitation Prescription, Tape 2. Baltimore: Williams & Wilkins, 1998, Fig 2.)

Scapula Rotation

The scapula are unevenly centered on the torso. Usually one is abducted (more lateral from thoracic spine midline) and one is adducted (more medial to the thoracic spine midline) (Fig. 2-23). Scapular rotation is also observed with thoracic scoliosis and hand dominance.

Possible tight, overactive muscles: Side of the abducted scapula: serratus anterior. Side of the adducted scapula: rhomboid.

Possible weak, underactive muscles: Side of the abducted scapula: rhomboid and middle trapezius; side of the adducted scapula: pectoralis major or minor.

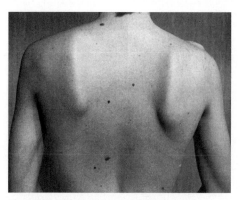

Figure 2-23. Right scapula abduction and winging. (Reprinted with permission from Liebenson C, ed. Rehabilitation of the Spine. Baltimore: Williams & Wilkins, 1996:108.)

2

Round Shoulders/Internal Rotation of the Upper Extremity

In addition to having a rounded appearance of the shoulders, the back of the hands may be visible on an anterior view as the thumbs point across the body instead of to the anterior. The palm of the hands may be visible from the posterior (Fig. 2-24).

Possible tight, overactive muscles: Latissimus dorsi and/or pectorals.
Possible weak, underactive muscles: Mid trapezius.
Clinical correlate: Usually observed with forward head posture.

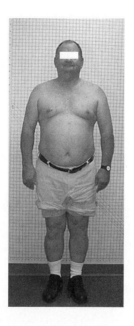

Figure 2-24. Round shoulders with internal rotation of the arms.

Lateral Spinal Deviation/Scoliosis

Scoliosis is a lateral curvature of the spine that may be acquired or congenital. Congenital scoliosis is due to some architectural asymmetry, such as a wedge vertebra or other anatomic variant. Most acquired scoliosis is idiopathic, or of unknown origin. Scoliosis evaluation, management, and treatment continually progress but are still controversial. On visual evaluation, the spinous processes are lateral to the midline of the trunk (Fig. 2-25).

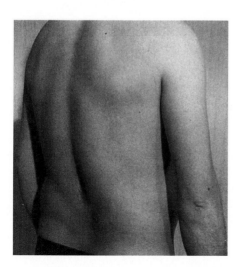

Figure 2-25. Right thoracolumbar erector spinae hypertrophy. (Reprinted with permission from Liebenson C, ed. Rehabilitation of the Spine. Baltimore: Williams & Wilkins, 1996:107.)

Possible tight, overactive muscles: Shortened intrinsic paraspinal muscles on the side of concavity.

Possible weak, underactive muscles: Lengthened intrinsic paraspinal muscles on the side of convexity.

Clinical correlate: Thoracolumbar erector spinae hypertrophy indicates a longstanding adaptive change. Most AP spines have a slight right convex thoracic curve due to the individual's right-handedness. It is important to rule out congenital abnormalities and factor in leg length discrepancies and other distortions.

Lateral Pelvic Tilt/Abdominal Asymmetry

The horizontal line connecting the left and right iliac crests are unlevel (Fig. 2-26)

Possible tight, over-active muscles:

High side: PA—quadratus lumborum muscle; AP—abdominal obliques

Low side: hip adductor.

Possible weak/underactive muscles:

High side: gluteus maximus, abductor muscles

Low side: opposite side abdominal obliques.

Clinical correlates: Leg length discrepancies and other distortions are usually present. Trendelenburg test may be positive on the side of laterality. Scoliosis may be present.

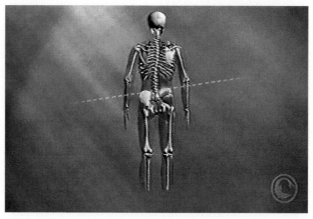

Figure 2-26. Pelvic unleveling. (Reprinted with permission from Liebenson C, Chapman S. Lumbar Spine: Making a Rehabilitation Prescription, Tape 1. Baltimore: Williams & Wilkins, 1998, Fig 5.)

Anterior or Posterior Pelvic Tilt

Neutral and stable pelvic position is the range of possible stable positions, which are the base upon which spinal posture rests. The anterior superior spines of the innominates should be vertically aligned with the symphysis pubes. On a lateral view, the waist line (or belt line) should be level to tilting slightly forward with a normal anterior lumbar lordosis providing stable posture.

2

Anterior pelvis: The pelvis tilts forward, with an associated increased lumbar lordosis (Figs. 2-27 and 2-28).

Possible tight, overactive muscles: Psoas, lumbar erector spinae.

Possible weak, underactive muscles: Gluteus maximus; abdominals.

Posterior Pelvis: (Fig. 2-29) There is a flattened lumbar curve with the pelvis tilting posteriorly or slightly forward of level.

Possible tight, overactive muscles: Hamstrings, abdominals, low back erector spinae.

Possible weak, underactive muscles: Hip flexors, quadriceps.

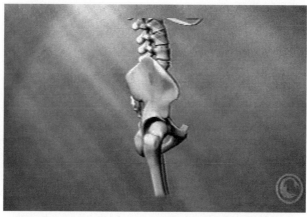

Figure 2-27. Anterior pelvic tilt. (Reprinted with permission from Liebenson C, Chapman S. Lumbar Spine: Making a Rehabilitation Prescription, Tape 1. Baltimore: Williams & Wilkins, 1998, Fig 4.)

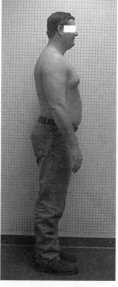

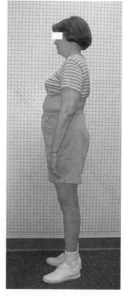

Figure 2-28. Anterior pelvic tilt.

Figure 2-29. Posterior pelvic tilt.

Abdomen Protrusion (Figs. 2-30 and 2-31)

Possible associated findings: Lateral buttock flattening in the lateral or superior quadrant.

Possible tight, overactive muscles: Erector spinae, iliopsoas.

Possible weak, underactive muscles: Gluteus maximus, abdominals.

Clinical correlate: Because of the marked anterior pelvic tilt usually associated with abdominal protrusion, weakness and limited range of motion on hip extension and hip abduction are common.

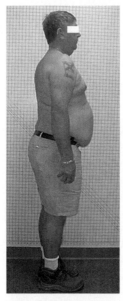

Figure 2-30. Abdominal protrusion.

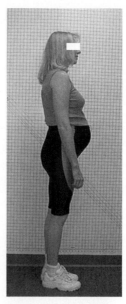

Figure 2-31. Abdominal protrusion in pregnancy.

Knock Knees: Genu Valga (Fig. 2-32)

Associated observations:

Pronation

Prominence of iliotibial tract

Observation: Lateral deviation of the patellae.

Possible tight, overactive muscles: TFL

Possible weak underactive muscles: Adductors, sartorius

Clinical correlate: Correlate with wear patterns of shoes

2

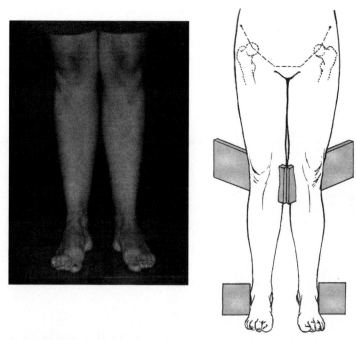

Figure 2-32. Knock-knees (genu valga). (Reprinted with permission from Kendall FP, McCreary EK, Provance PG. Muscles: Testing and Function. 4th ed. Baltimore: Williams & Wilkins, 1993:97.)

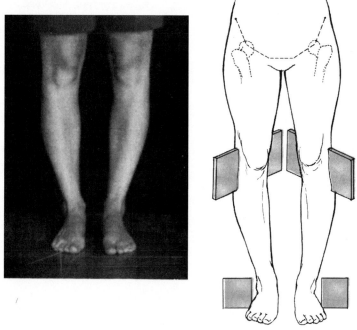

Figure 2-33. Bowlegs (genu vara). (Reprinted with permission from Kendall FP, McCreary EK, Provance PG. Muscles: Testing and Function. 4th ed. Baltimore: Williams & Wilkins, 1993:97.)

Observation: Bowleg (genu vara) (Fig. 2-33).
Possible weak underactive muscles: Weak hip rotators.
Observation: Pronation of the feet (Figs. 2-34 and 2-35)
Possible tight, overactive muscles: Soleus (on the right).
Possible weak underactive muscles: Anterior tibialis, Gluteus medius and maximus.
Clinical correlate: Flat feet.

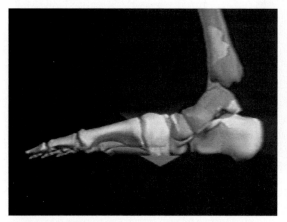

Figure 2-34. Pronation of the foot. (Reprinted with permission from Liebenson C, Chapman S. Lumbar Spine: Making a Rehabilitation Prescription, Tape 1. Baltimore: Williams & Wilkins, 1998, Fig 1.)

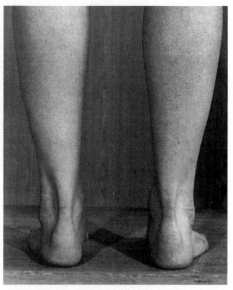

Figure 2-35. Pronation with soleus tightness on the right. (Reprinted with permission from Liebenson C, ed. Rehabilitation of the Spine. Baltimore: Williams & Wilkins, 1996:107.)

References

1. White AA, Panjabi MM. Clinical Biomechanics of the Spine. 2nd ed. Philadelphia: JB Lippincott, 1990:58, 86–91, 116, 162.
2. Janda V. Functional Pathology of the Motor System Seminars. Atlanta: 1999; Greenville, SC: 2000; Prague: 2000.
3. Watson J. Relationship between injuries & body mechanics in soccer and rugby players. Sports Med Physical Fitn 1995;35:289–294.
4. Basmajian JV, De Luca DJ. Muscles Alive. 5th ed. Baltimore: Williams & Wilkins, 1985:255, 414, P71, 328.

General References

Kendall FP, McCreary EK, Provance PG. Muscles: Testing and Function. 4th ed. Baltimore: Williams & Wilkins, 1993:20, 70–119, 354–356.

Janda V. Functional Pathology of the Motor System Seminars. Atlanta: 1999; Greenville, SC: 2000; Prague: 2000.

Jull G, Janda V, Muscles and motor control in low back pain. In: Twomey LT, Taylor JR, eds. Physical Therapy for the Low Back. Clinics in Physical Therapy. New York: Churchill Livingstone, 1987.

Liebenson C, ed. Rehabilitation of the Spine. Baltimore: Williams & Wilkins, 1996

CERVICAL ORTHOPAEDIC TESTS

Cervical Orthopaedic Examination

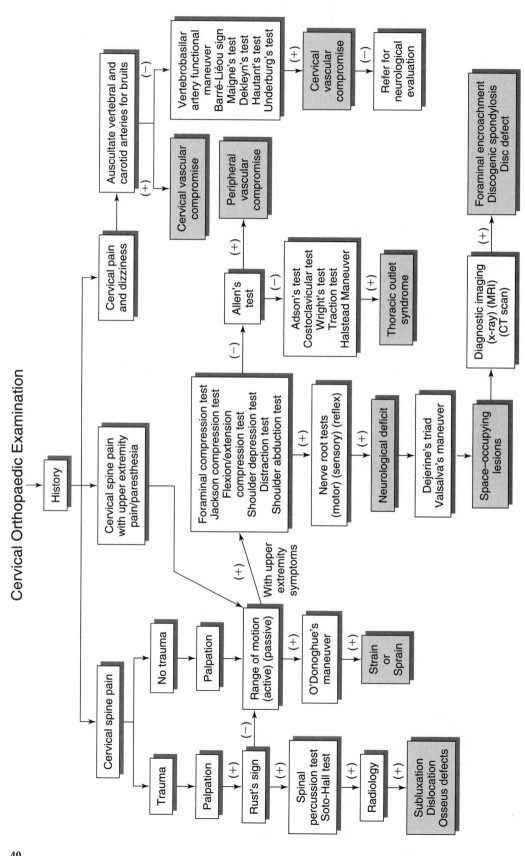

3

CERVICAL PALPATION

Anterior Aspect

Sternocleidomastoid Muscle

DESCRIPTIVE ANATOMY

The sternocleidomastoid muscle extends from the mastoid process of the temporal bone down to the clavicle and sternum (Fig. 3-1). It divides the neck into anterior and posterior triangles. Its action is to flex the head to the same side and rotate it to the opposite side. Both muscles acting together flex the neck forward.

PROCEDURE

Instruct the patient to turn the head to one side. Pinch the muscle on the side of head rotation between your thumb and forefinger, traveling from the clavicle upward to the mastoid (Fig. 3-2). Compare each muscle bilaterally, noting any inflammation, tenderness, and palpable bands. Palpable bands are hyperirritable spots within a taut band of skeletal muscle or fascia. Rate tenderness based on tenderness rating scale (Box 3-1).

Inflammation and tenderness secondary to trauma usually are associated with cervical acceleration and deceleration (CAD) types of injuries. Torticollis may also cause local inflammation and tenderness. Palpable bands may indicate a myofascial trigger point. These trigger points may be caused by overuse, trauma, or chilling. They may also indicate arthritic joints or emotional distress.

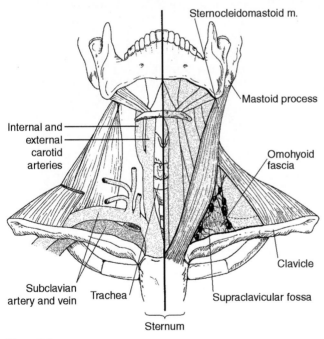

Sternocleidomastoid m.

Mastoid process

Internal and external carotid arteries

Omohyoid fascia

Clavicle

Subclavian artery and vein   Trachea

Supraclavicular fossa

Sternum

Figure 3-1

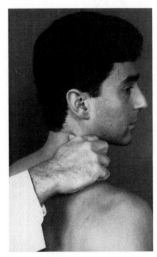

Figure 3-2

Box 3-1	**Tenderness Grading Scale**
Grade I	Mild tenderness to moderate palpation
Grade II	Mild tenderness with grimace and flinch to moderate palpation
Grade III	Severe tenderness with withdrawal
Grade IV	Severe tenderness with withdrawal from nonnoxious stimuli

Carotid Arteries

DESCRIPTIVE ANATOMY

The carotid arteries lie lateral to the trachea and medial to the sternocleidomastoid muscle. These arteries branch to form the internal and external carotid arteries, which supply blood to the brain (see Fig. 3-1).

PROCEDURE

With your first and second digits, lightly press on the carotid artery against the transverse process of the cervical vertebra (Fig. 3-3). Palpate each artery individually and assess amplitude equality. A difference in the strength of the pulses may indicate carotid artery stenosis or compression. If carotid artery stenosis or compression is suspected, auscultate the carotid arteries for bruits and evaluate the vertebrobasilar circulation.

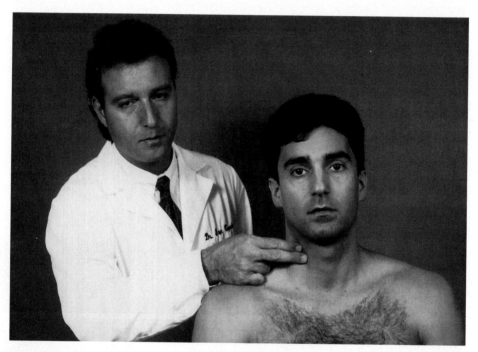

Figure 3-3

Supraclavicular Fossa

DESCRIPTIVE ANATOMY

The supraclavicular fossa is superior to the clavicle. It contains the omohyoid fascia, the lymph nodes, and the pressure point for the subclavian artery. It is usually a smooth, contoured depression (Fig. 3-1).

3

PROCEDURE

Palpate each fossa for swelling, tenderness, and any abnormal bony or soft tissue masses (Fig. 3-4). Pain and tenderness associated with swelling secondary to trauma may indicate a fractured clavicle or a separated acromioclavicular joint. Abnormal bony tissue may indicate a cervical rib, which may cause neurological or vascular symptoms in the upper extremity. If an extra rib is suspected, evaluate for thoracic outlet syndrome (see Chapter 5). An abnormal soft tissue mass may indicate lymph adenopathy or a tumor.

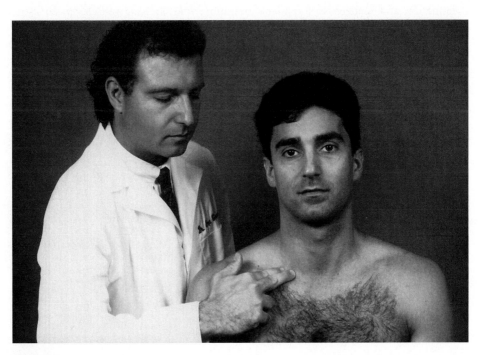

Figure 3-4

Posterior Aspect

Trapezius Muscle

DESCRIPTIVE ANATOMY

The trapezius muscle is a large, triangular muscle that extends from the occiput and spinous processes of the cervical and thoracic vertebra to the acromion process of the clavicle and spine of the scapula (Fig. 3-5). Its superior fibers elevate the shoulders; the middle fibers retract the scapula; and the inferior fibers depress the scapula and lower the shoulders.

PROCEDURE

Palpate each muscle from the superior aspect just below the occiput downward, continuing to the superior aspect of the spine of the scapula, then lateral to the acromion process (Fig. 3-6). From the inferior, palpate from the spinous processes of the thoracic vertebra lateral and superior toward the acromion process (Fig. 3-7).

Inflammation and tenderness secondary to trauma may indicate muscle spasm caused by torn muscle fibers associated with edema. Inflammation and tenderness that are not trauma related may indicate fibrosis of muscle tissue or fibromyalgia. Assess it according to the tenderness rating scale (see Box 3-1). Palpable bands indicate myofascial trigger points that may be caused by overuse, overload, trauma, or chilling. These palpable bands may also indicate arthritic joints or emotional distress.

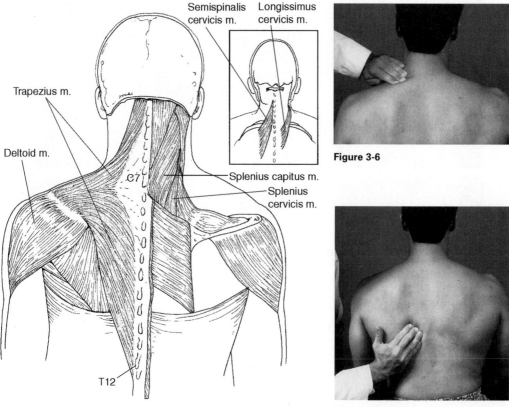

Figure 3-5

Figure 3-6

Figure 3-7

Cervical Intrinsic Musculature

DESCRIPTIVE ANATOMY

The palpable intrinsic spinal muscles in the cervical spine consist of splenius capitis and cervicis, longissimus cervicis, and semispinalis cervicis. These layered muscles are used for the maintenance of posture and movements of the cervical spine. The superficial layer consists of the splenius capitis and cervicis, and the intermediate layer consists of the longissimus and semispinalis cervicis. These muscles stretch from the base of the occiput to the upper aspect of the thoracic spine (Fig. 3-5). The deep muscles on the cervical spine at best are difficult to palpate and are not discussed here.

PROCEDURE

Palpate the superficial layer by moving the fingers in a transverse fashion over the belly of the muscle with the cervical spine in slight extension (Fig. 3-8). Note any abnormal tone, tenderness, or palpable bands. Palpate the intermediate layer with the fingertips directly adjacent to the spinous processes, also with the cervical spine in slight extension (Fig. 3-9). Note any abnormal tone, tenderness, or palpable bands. Rate the layers according to the tenderness rating scale (Box 3-1). Any abnormal tone or tenderness may indicate an inflammatory process in the muscle, such as muscle strain, myofascitis, or fibromyalgia. Palpable bands indicate myofascial trigger points, which may be caused by overuse, overload, trauma, or chilling. They may also indicate arthritic joints or emotional distress.

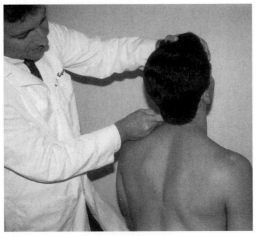

Figure 3-8

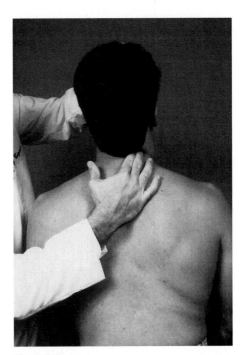

Figure 3-9

Spinous Process/Facet Joints

DESCRIPTIVE ANATOMY

The C1, or atlas, vertebra has a posterior arch rather than a spinous process that is difficult at best to palpate. The C2 to C7 vertebrae have relatively prominent spinous processes that are easily palpable. Slightly lateral to the spinous processes lie the facet joints. Each facet joint is composed of a posterior inferior articular process and a posterior superior articular process from congruent vertebra (Fig. 3-10).

PROCEDURE

With the patient seated and head slightly flexed, palpate each spinous process individually with your index and/or middle finger, noting any pain and/or tenderness (Fig. 3-11). Also, evaluate each spinous process as you move the cervical spine in flexion and extension to determine hypomobility versus hypermobility (Fig. 3-12).

Again, with the patient's head slightly flexed, using your thumb and index finger, palpate the facet joints bilaterally both in a static position (Fig. 3-13) and in a flexed position while performing extension movements (Fig. 3-14). Tenderness at the spinous and/or facet joint indicates an inflammatory process at that site. The inflammation is usually secondary to subluxation or trauma, that is, hyperflexion or hyperextension injury. Crepitus on movement may indicate degenerative joint disease.

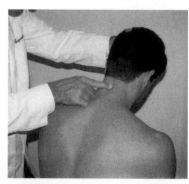

Figure 3-11

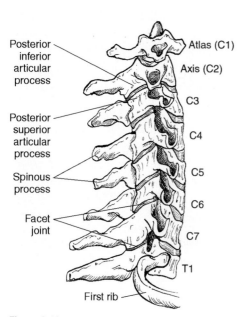

Figure 3-10

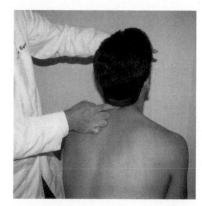

Figure 3-12

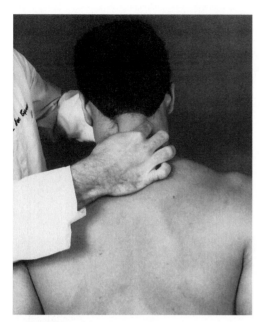

Figure 3-13

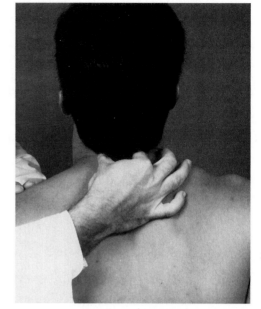

Figure 3-14

CERVICAL RANGE OF MOTION

Cervical range of motion should be evaluated only after taking a proper and thorough history to rule out any indication that these movements will adversely affect the patient. Severe trauma causing a fracture or dislocation or cervical vascular compromise should be ruled out before performing these movements. You should not only note limited motion in the cervical spine but also any pain along with its location and character. The most painful movements should be performed last so that no residual pain is carried over from the previous movement. Crepitus should also be noted upon movement; it may indicate degenerative changes in the cervical spine.

Spinal range of motion is measured using inclinometers, with the patient performing the movements actively and passively. The inclinometer is the preferred instrument for measuring spinal range of motion because it measures angular displacement relative to gravity. For continuity of reporting and for evaluating patient compliance, the movements should be performed three times. The three measurements must be within 5°or 10% of each other for a valid reporting criterion. The full arc of motion is paramount to the evaluation of range of motion in the cervical spine. Adding the opposing measurements to determine the full arc of movement is the most objective way to assess cervical spine movement. For example, the patient carries the head in 10° of flexion, which for this person is the neutral position. When you measure cervical flexion on this individual, cervical flexion may be reduced 10° from average. If you then measure extension, you may possibly have an increase of 10°. This increase may be caused by the 10° flexion angle, which is the neutral position for that patient. If you take each measurement individually, you have a deficit movement in flexion and an increase in movement in extension. If you add both movements, you see that the full arc is within normal limits.

Flexion: Inclinometer Method (1,2)

With the patient seated and the cervical spine in the neutral position, place one inclinometer over the T1 spinous process in the sagittal plane. Place the second inclinometer at the superior aspect of the occiput, also in the sagittal plane (Fig. 3-15). Zero out both inclinometers. Instruct the patient to flex the head forward and record both angles (Fig. 3-16). Subtract the T1 inclination from the occipital inclination to obtain the active *cervical flexion angle.*

NORMAL RANGE

Normal range is 50° or greater from the neutral or 0 position for active movement.

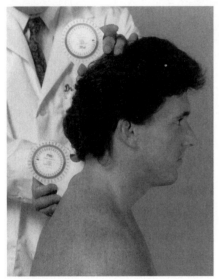

Figure 3-15

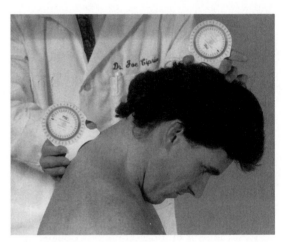

Figure 3-16

Extension: Inclinometer Method (1,2)

With the patient seated and the cervical spine in the neutral position, place one inclinometer slightly lateral to the T1 spinous process in the sagittal plane. Place the second inclinometer at the superior aspect of the occiput, also in the sagittal plane (Fig. 3-17). Zero out both inclinometers. Instruct the patient to extend the head backward and record both inclinations (Fig. 3-18). Subtract the T1 inclination from the occipital inclination to obtain the active *cervical extension angle*.

3

NORMAL RANGE

The normal range is 60° or greater from the neutral or 0 position for active movement and 110°for full arc of active flexion and extension. The normal range of passive flexion and extension varies as follows (3):

Age	Degrees
20–29	151 ± 17
30–49	141 ± 35
> 50	129 ± 14

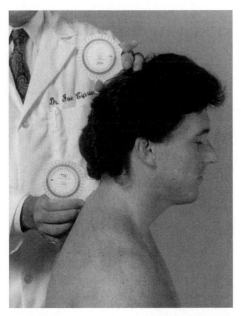

Figure 3-17

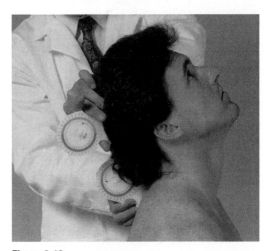

Figure 3-18

Lateral Flexion: Inclinometer Method (1,2)

With the patient seated and the cervical spine in the neutral position, place one inclinometer flat on the T1 spinous process in the coronal plane. Place the second inclinometer at the superior aspect of the occiput, also in the coronal plane (Fig. 3-19). Zero out both inclinometers. Instruct the patient to flex the head to one side and record both inclinations (Fig. 3-20). Subtract the T1 inclination from the occipital inclination to obtain the active *cervical lateral flexion angle.* Repeat with flexion to the opposite side.

NORMAL RANGE

The normal range is 45° or greater from the neutral or 0 position for active movement and 90° for full arc of active right and left lateral flexion. The full arc of passive right and left lateral flexion varies as follows (3):

Age	Degrees
20–29	101 ± 11
30–49	93 ± 13
> 50	80 ± 17

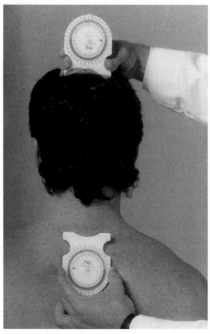

Figure 3-19

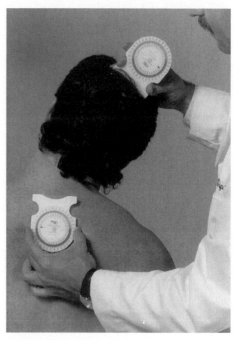

Figure 3-20

Rotation: Inclinometer Method (1,2)

With the patient supine, place the inclinometer at the crown of the head in the transverse plane (Fig. 3-21). Zero out the inclinometer. Instruct the patient to rotate the head to one side, and then record your findings (Fig. 3-22). Repeat the procedure with the patient's head rotated to the opposite side.

NORMAL RANGE

Normal range is 80° or greater from the neutral or 0 position for active movement. The full arc of active right and left rotation is 160°. The full arc of passive right and left rotation varies as follows (3):

Age	Degrees
20–29	183 ± 11
30–49	172 ± 13
> 50	155 ± 15

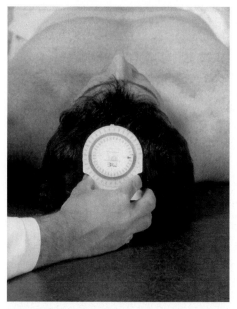

Figure 3-21

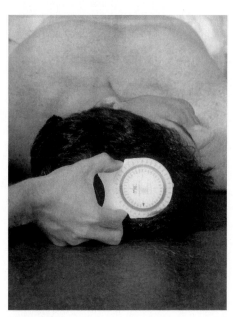

Figure 3-22

CERVICAL RESISTIVE ISOMETRIC MUSCLE TESTING

The same movements can also be tested for resistive strength. Contraindications such as fracture, dislocation, and cervical vascular compromise must be considered before testing for resistive strength.

Resistive isometric muscle testing is performed to evaluate muscle strength or muscle state. Weakness of a particular muscle or muscle group may indicate neurological dysfunction in the nerves supplying the affected muscles. Pain of a particular muscle or muscle group during resistive isometric muscle testing may indicate muscle dysfunction, such as a muscle strain.

Each of the following movements includes a chart that indicates the muscles that make the movement and the nerve supply to each muscle. The clinician evaluates each movement according to muscle strength; grade is based on the muscle grading scale adopted by the American Academy of Orthopaedic Surgeons (Box 3-2).

Box 3-2	Muscle Grading Scale
5	Complete range of motion against gravity with full resistance
4	Complete range of motion against gravity with some resistance
3	Complete range of motion against gravity
2	Complete range of motion with the gravity eliminated
1	Evidence of slight contractility; no joint motion
0	No evidence of contractility

Flexion

With the patient seated and in the neutral position, instruct him or her to flex the head forward against your resistance, making sure that there is no patient movement and only muscle contraction (Fig. 3-23).

Muscles	Nerve Supply
1. Longus colli	C2–C5
2. Scalenus anterior	C4–C5
3. Scalenus medius	C3–C8
4. Scalenus posterior	C6–C8
5. Sternocleidomastoid	Accessory, C2

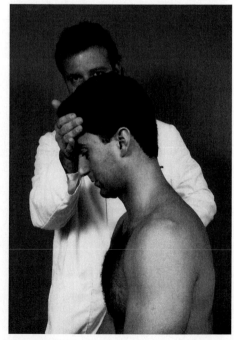

Figure 3-23

Extension

With the patient seated and in the neutral position, instruct him or her to extend the head backward against your resistance, making sure that there is no patient movement and only muscle contraction (Fig. 3-24).

Muscles	*Nerve Supply*
1. Splenius cervicis	C6, C7, C8
2. Semispinalis cervicis	C1–C6, C7, C8
3. Longissimus cervicis	C6–C8
4. Levator scapulae	C3–C4
5. Iliocostalis cervicis	C6, C7, C8
6. Spinalis cervicis	C6, C8
7. Multifidus	C1–C6, C7, C8
8. Interspinalis cervicis	C1–C8
9. Trapezius (Upper)	C3, C4
10. Rectus capitis posterior major	C1
11. Rotatores breves	C1–C8
12. Rotatores longi	C1–C8

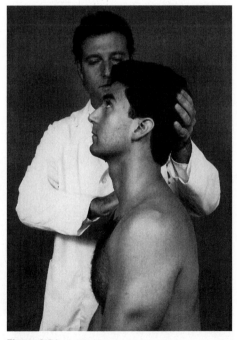

Figure 3-24

Lateral Flexion

With the patient seated and in the neutral position, instruct him or her to bend the head to one side against your resistance, making sure that there is no patient movement and only muscle contraction (Fig. 3-25). This action should be performed bilaterally.

Muscles	_Nerve Supply_
1. Levator scapulae	C3–C4
2. Splenius cervicis	C4–C6
3. Iliocostalis cervicis	C6–C8
4. Longissimus cervicis	C6–C8
5. Semispinalis cervicis	C1–C8
6. Multifidus	C1–C8
7. Intertransversarii	C1–C8
8. Scaleni	C3–C8
9. Sternocleidomastoideus	C2
10. Obliquus capitis inferior	C1
11. Rotatores breves	C1–C8
12. Rotatores longi	C1–C8
13. Longus colli	C2–C6
14. Trapezius	C3–C4

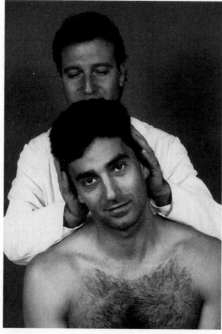

Figure 3-25

Rotation

With the patient seated and in the neutral position, instruct him or her to rotate the head to one side against your resistance, making sure that there is no patient movement and only muscle contraction (Fig. 3-26). This action should be performed bilaterally.

Muscles	*Nerve Supply*
Moves Face to Same Side	
1. Levator scapulae	C3–C4
2. Splenius cervicis	C4–C6
3. Iliocostalis cervicis	C6–C8
4. Longissimus cervicis	C6–C8
5. Intertransversarii	C1–C8
6. Obliquus capitis inferior	C1
7. Rotatores breves	C1–C8
8. Rotatores longi	C1–C8
Moves Face to Opposite Side	
1. Multifidus	C1–C8
2. Scaleni	C3–C8
3. Sternocleidomastoideus	C2

RATIONALE

Pain on resistive isometric contraction may indicate a musculotendinous strain of one or more of the muscles involved in the action. Weakness may indicate a neurological disruption to the muscle or muscles involved in the action.

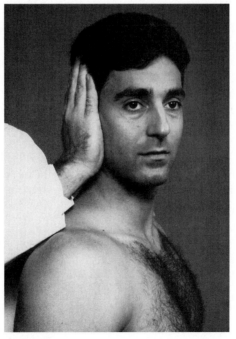

Figure 3-26

VERTEBROBASILAR CIRCULATION ASSESSMENT

CLINICAL DESCRIPTION

Vascular insufficiency may be aggravated by positional change in the cervical spine. Assessment of vertebrobasilar circulation must be done if cervical adjustment or manipulation is to be performed. Absolute contraindications and risks of cervical adjustment or manipulation can be minimized significantly, even though reportedly small, with proper diagnostic evaluation. These risks and contraindications may be predicted in some cases by functional or provocative testing and by adequate history (familial history of stroke or cardiovascular disease, hypertension, smoking, cervical spondylosis or arthrosis, bleeding disorders, medication, and/or anatomic anomaly or pathology). Vascular accidents may still occur with no evidence of vascular insufficiency, deficit, and negative provocative procedures. Box 3-3 lists the eight most common predispositions associated with cerebrovascular accidents.

Box 3-3	**Predispositions to Cerebrovascular Accidents**
• Headaches, migraine	
• Dizziness	
• Sudden severe head or neck pain	
• Hypertensive	
• Cigarette smoking	
• Oral contraceptives	
• Obesity	
• Diabetes	

All of the following tests incorporate a positional change in the cervical spine. The rotation aspect of this change is the common denominator of all the following tests. Rotation of C1 on C2 between 30° and 45° compresses the vertebral artery at the atlantoaxial junction on the opposite side of head rotation, reducing blood flow to the basilar artery (Fig. 3-27) (4,5). In the normal patient, this diminution of blood flow caused by positional change of the cervical spine does not cause any neurological symptoms, such as dizziness, nausea, tinnitus, faintness, or nystagmus. This lack of symptoms is a result of the normal flow of collateral circulation by the opposite vertebral artery, common carotid arteries, and a communicating cerebral arterial circle (Circle of Willis) (Fig. 3-28).

Rotational instability in the upper cervical spine caused by trauma, arterial artery disease, and/or degenerative joint disease in the cervical spine may lead to a mechanical reduction of blood flow to an area, causing neurological symptoms. This reduction of blood flow may be such that the collateral circulation is not sufficient to sustain normal function to the brain. Therefore, when you positionally stress a vessel in the cervical spine, you are testing the integrity of the collateral circulation supplied to the area, which is normally supplied by the vessel being stressed.

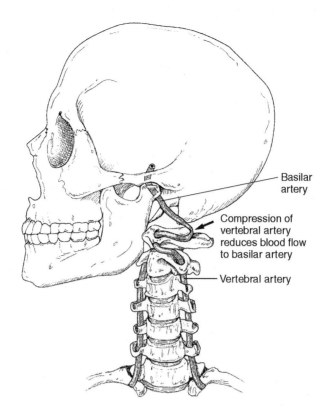

Figure 3-27

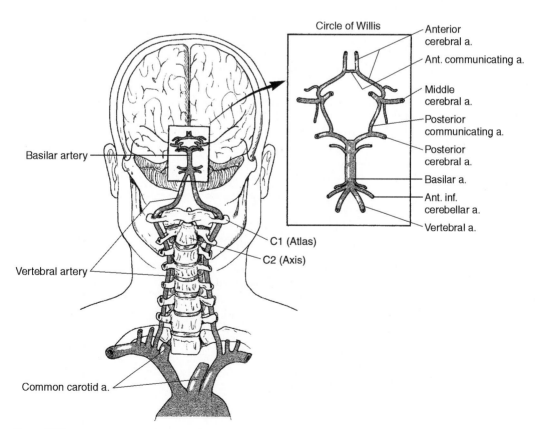

Figure 3-28

Assessment of the vertebrobasilar circulation by provocative or functional testing stresses seven areas of possible compression. These areas are as follows (Fig. 3-29):

1. Between C1 and C2 transverse processes, where the vertebral arteries are relatively fixed at the C1 and C2 transverse foramina
2. C2 to C3 at the level of the superior articular facet of C3 on the ipsilateral side to head rotation
3. The C1 transverse process and the internal carotid artery
4. The atlanto-occipital aperture by the posterior arch of Atlas and the rim of foramen magnum or anteriorly at the atlanto-occipital joint capsule and posteriorly at atlanto-occipital membrane.
5. C4 to C5 or C5 to C6 levels because of arthrosis of the joints of the uncovertebral joints with compression on the ipsilateral side to head rotation
6. At the transverse foramina of the atlas or axis between the obliquus capitis inferior and intertransversarii during rotatory movements
7. Before entering the C6 transverse process by the longus colli muscle or by tissue communicating between the longus colli and scalenus anterior muscles

Most compression and/or damage is reported at the first four sites.

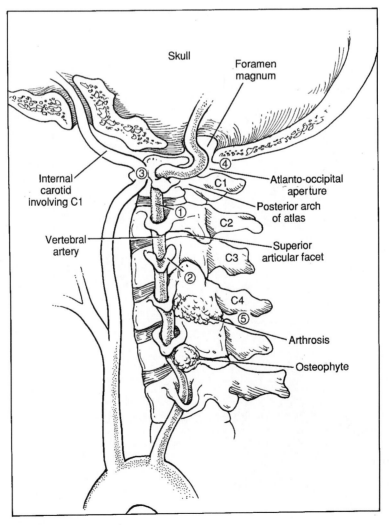

Figure 3-29

Allow a 10-second interval between tests to ensure that there are no latent symptoms. If symptoms are reproduced, there is no need to progress to any other cervical vascular provocative tests. The most common clinical signs and symptoms exhibited in cerebrovascular episodes are presented in the box below.

3

Clinical Signs and Symptoms of Cerebrovascular Episodes

- Vertigo, dizziness, giddiness, light-headedness
- Drop attacks, loss of consciousness
- Diplopia
- Dysarthria
- Dysphagia
- Ataxia of gait
- Nausea, vomiting
- Numbness on one side of the face
- Nystagmus

Barré-Liéou Sign (6)

Sensitivity/Reliability Scale

0   1   2   3   4

PROCEDURE

With the patient seated, instruct him or her to rotate the head to one side and then the other (Fig. 3-30).

RATIONALE

Rotating the head causes compression of the vertebral artery opposite the side of head rotation (Fig. 3-27). Therefore, you are testing the patency of the vertebral artery on the same side of head rotation. Vertigo, dizziness, visual blurring, nausea, faintness, and nystagmus are all signs of a positive test. This sign indicates buckling vertebral artery syndrome. Also, consideration must be given to the patency of the carotid arteries and a communicating cerebral arterial circle.

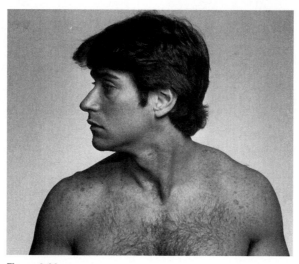

Figure 3-30

Vertebrobasilar Artery Functional Maneuver (7)

Sensitivity/Reliability Scale

0   1   2   3   4

PROCEDURE

With the patient seated, palpate and auscultate the carotid (Fig. 3-31)and subclavian arteries (Fig. 3-32) for pulsations or bruits. When auscultating, instruct the patient to hold his or her breath. If neither artery is palpable, instruct the patient to rotate and hyperextend the head to one side and then the other (Fig. 3-33). If pulsations or bruits are present, **do not perform** the rotation and hyperextension portion of the test.

RATIONALE

If pulsations or bruits are present at the carotid or subclavian arteries, this test is considered positive. It may indicate a compression or stenosing of the carotid or subclavian arteries. The rotation and hyperextension portion of the test places a motion-induced compression on the vertebral artery opposite the side of head rotation (Fig. 3-27). Vertigo, dizziness, visual blurring, nausea, faintness, and nystagmus are all signs of a positive test. A positive result indicates vertebral or basilar artery stenosis or compression at one of the seven sites discussed earlier in the chapter. Consideration must also be given to the patency of the carotid arteries and a communicating cerebral arterial circle.

NOTE

Vertebrobasilar artery functional maneuver and George's screening procedure are both subsections of George's Cerebrovascular Craniocervical Functional Test.

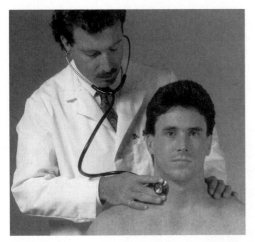

Figure 3-31

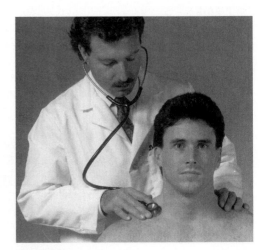

Figure 3-32

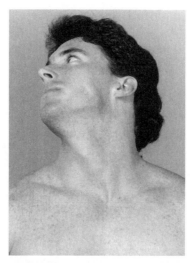

Figure 3-33

Maigne's Test (8)

Sensitivity/Reliability Scale
0   1   2   3   4

PROCEDURE

With the patient seated, instruct the patient to extend and rotate the head and hold that position for 15 to 40 seconds (Fig. 3-34). Repeat the test with the patient's head rotated to the opposite side.

RATIONALE

Rotation and extension of the head place a motion-induced compression on the vertebral artery on the opposite side of head rotation (Fig. 3-27). Vertigo, dizziness, visual blurring, nausea, faintness, and nystagmus are all signs of a positive test. This test indicates vertebral, basilar, or carotid artery stenosis or compression at one of the seven sites discussed at the beginning of this section. Consideration must also be given to the patency of the carotid arteries and a communicating cerebral arterial circle.

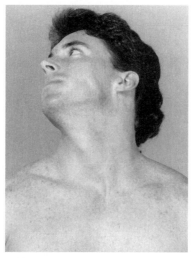

Figure 3-34

Vertebral Artery (Cervical Quadrant) Test (9)

Sensitivity/Reliability Scale

0   1   2   3   4

PROCEDURE

With the patient supine and the patient's head off the table, the examiner passively hyperextends and laterally flexes the head and holds this position for 30 seconds (Fig. 3-35). Repeat with the head laterally flexed to the opposite side.

RATIONALE

Lateral flexion and hyperextension of the head place a slight motion-induced compression on the vertebral artery on the same side of lateral head flexion. Vertigo, dizziness, visual blurring, nausea, faintness, and nystagmus are all signs of a positive test. This test indicates vertebral, basilar, or carotid artery stenosis or compression at one of the seven sites discussed at the beginning of this section. Consideration must also be given to the patency of the carotid arteries and a communicating cerebral arterial circle.

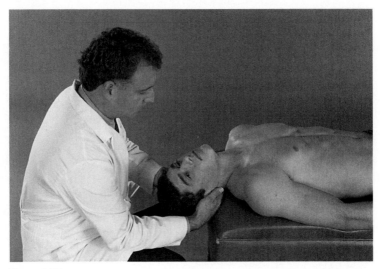

Figure 3-35

Dekleyn's Test (10,11)

Sensitivity/Reliability Scale

0   1   2   3   4

PROCEDURE

With the patient supine and the patient's head off the table, instruct the patient to hyperextend and rotate the head and hold for 15 to 40 seconds (Fig. 3-36). Repeat with the head rotated and extended to the opposite side.

RATIONALE

Rotation and hyperextension of the head place a motion-induced compression on the vertebral arteries on the opposite side of head rotation (Fig. 3-27). Vertigo, dizziness, visual blurring, nausea, faintness, and nystagmus are all signs of a positive test. This test indicates vertebral, basilar, or carotid artery stenosis or compression at one of the seven sites discussed at the beginning of this section. Consideration must also be given to the patency of the carotid arteries and a communicating cerebral arterial circle.

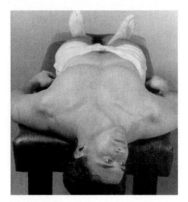

Figure 3-36

Hautant's Test (12)

Sensitivity/Reliability Scale

0   1   2   3   4

PROCEDURE

With the patient seated and the patient's eyes closed, instruct the patient to extend the arms to the front with palms up. Instruct the patient to extend and rotate the head to one side (Fig. 3-37). Repeat with the head rotated and extended to the opposite side.

RATIONALE

A patient with stenosis or compression to the vertebral, basilar, or subclavian arteries without sufficient collateral circulation will tend to lose balance, drop the arms, and pronate the hands. If this occurs, suspect a vertebral, basilar, or carotid artery stenosis or compression at one of the seven sites discussed at the beginning of this section.

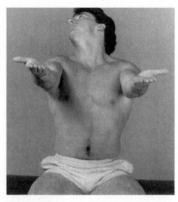

Figure 3-37

Underburg's Test

Sensitivity/Reliability Scale

0   1   2   3   4

PROCEDURE

With the patient standing, instruct him or her to close the eyes and look for difficulty in equilibrium (Fig. 3-38). Next, instruct the patient to stretch out the arms and supinate the hands (Fig. 3-39). Look for difficulty in equilibrium and drifting or pronating of the arms. Then instruct the patient to march in place (Fig. 3-40). Next, instruct the patient to extend and rotate the head while continuing to march in place (Fig. 3-41). Repeat with the patient's head rotated and extended to the opposite side.

RATIONALE

Marching in place increases the heart rate, which increases the rate of blood flow through the suspected vessels. Extension and rotation of the head place a motion-induced compression on the vertebral arteries on the opposite side of head rotation (see Fig. 3-27). Vertigo, dizziness, visual blurring, nausea, faintness, and nystagmus are all signs of a positive test. This test indicates vertebral, basilar, or carotid artery stenosis or compression at one of the seven sites discussed at the beginning of this section. Consideration must also be given to the patency of the carotid arteries and a communicating cerebral arterial circle.

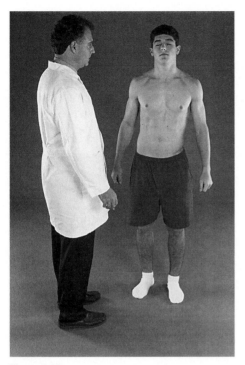

Figure 3-38

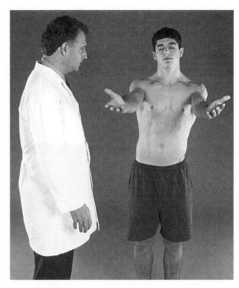

Figure 3-39

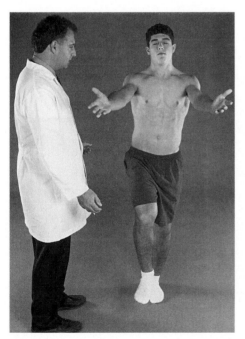

Figure 3-40

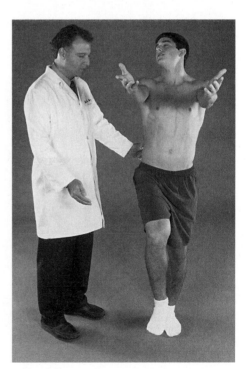

Figure 3-41

Hallpike's Maneuver

Sensitivity/Reliability Scale

0   1   2   3   4

PROCEDURE

Have the patient lie supine with the head extending off the examination table. Support the patient's head and move it into extension (Fig. 3-42). Then rotate and laterally flex the head to one side (Fig. 3-43) and hold for 15 to 45 seconds looking for nystagmus or other neurological signs. Repeat the test to the opposite side. Finally, slowly release the head and allow it to hang free in hyperextension (Fig. 3-44).

RATIONALE

Rotation hyperextension and lateral flexion of the head place a motion-induced compression on the vertebral arteries on the opposite side of head rotation (see Fig. 3-27). Vertigo, dizziness, visual blurring, nausea, faintness, and nystagmus are all signs of a positive test. This test indicates vertebral, basilar, or carotid artery stenosis or compression at one of the seven sites discussed at the beginning of this section. Consideration must also be given to the patency of the carotid arteries and a communicating cerebral arterial circle.

> **SUGGESTED DIAGNOSTIC IMAGING**
> - Plain film cervical radiography
>   AP open mouth
>   AP lower cervical, upper thoracic
>   Neutral lateral cervical
>   Oblique views
> - Vertebral and carotid ultrasound
> - Magnetic resonance angiogram
> - Cerebral angiogram

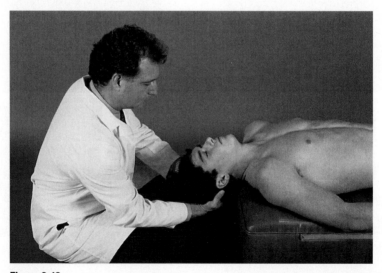

Figure 3-42

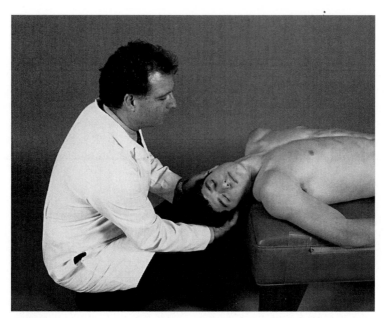

Figure 3-43

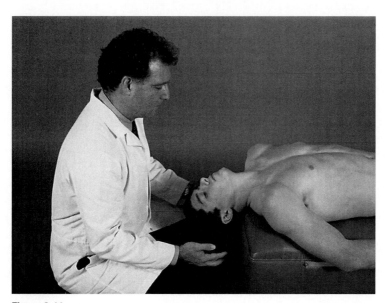

Figure 3-44

SUBCLAVIAN ARTERY COMPROMISE

DESCRIPTION

The subclavian arteries arch superiorly and posteriorly, grooving the pleura and the lungs. They then pass inferiorly behind the midpoint of the clavicle. They are crossed anteriorly by the scalenus anterior muscles (Fig. 3-45). Compromise of the subclavian artery may be produced by atherosclerosis, muscle dysfunction, or a space-occupying lesion. The following conditions may compromise the subclavian artery: (*a*) sclerotic plaque on the walls of the artery, (*b*) spasm of the scalenus anterior muscle, and (*c*) superior pulmonary sulcus tumor (Pancoast's tumor).

CLINICAL SIGNS AND SYMPTOMS

- Upper extremity pain
- Cold upper extremity
- Upper extremity claudication
- Supraclavicular pain

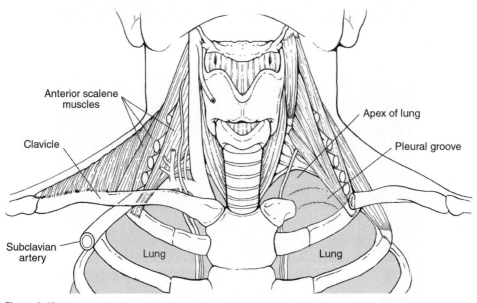

Figure 3-45

George's Screening Procedure (7)

Sensitivity/Reliability Scale

0   1   2   3   4

PROCEDURE

With the patient seated, take the patient's blood pressure bilaterally and record the findings (Fig. 3-46). Determine the character of the patient's radial pulse bilaterally (Fig. 3-47).

RATIONALE

A difference of 10 mm Hg between the two systolic blood pressures and a feeble or absent radial pulse suggests subclavian artery stenosis on the side of the feeble or absent pulse.

3

NOTE

If the test is negative, place a stethoscope over the supraclavicular fossa and auscultate the subclavian artery for bruits (Fig. 3-48). If bruits are present, suspect subclavian artery stenosis or compression.

SUGGESTED DIAGNOSTIC IMAGING

- Plain film radiography
    AP Lower cervical, thoracic
    AP open mouth
    Neutral lateral cervical
    PA chest
    Apical lordotic view
    AP shoulder
- Vascular ultrasound
- Magnetic resonance angiogram

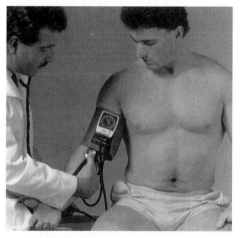

Figure 3-46

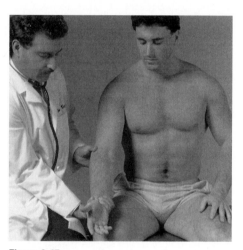

Figure 3-47

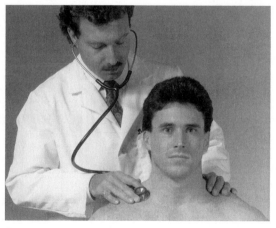

Figure 3-48

DIFFERENTIAL DIAGNOSIS: STRAIN VERSUS SPRAIN

CLINICAL DESCRIPTION

Cervical strain is an irritation and spasm of the muscles of the cervical spine with or without partial muscle fiber tearing (see Cervical Resistive Isometric Muscle Testing, earlier in the chapter). Cervical sprain is a wrenching of the joints of the cervical spine with partial tearing of its ligaments. Traumatic injuries such as cervical acceleration–deceleration injuries produce strain and sprain injuries. Other traumatic and nontraumatic conditions, such as athletic injuries, overuse, overstretching, overcontraction against resistance, and a direct blow, usually produce a muscular condition that may indicate sprain. Strains are categorized by degree of muscle tissue damage (Box 3-4). Sprains are categorized by degree of ligament damage (Box 3-4).

CLINICAL SIGNS AND SYMPTOMS OF STRAIN VERSUS SPRAIN

- Cervical and upper back pain
- Cervical and upper back stiffness
- Cervical and upper trapezius tightness
- Reduced cervical range of motion
- Cervical and upper trapezius spasm

Box 3-4	Categories of Strains and Sprains

Degree of Strain

1. Mild: Slight disruption of muscle fibers with no appreciable hemorrhage and minimal amounts of swelling and edema
2. Moderate: Laceration of muscle fibers with an appreciable amount of hemorrhage into the surrounding tissues and a moderate amount of swelling and edema
3. Severe: Complete disruption of the muscle tendon unit, possibly with tearing of the tendon from the bone or a rupture of the muscle through its belly

Degree of Sprain

1. Mild: Slight tears of a few ligamentous fibers
2. Moderate: More severe tearing of ligamentous fibers but not complete separation of the ligament
3. Severe: Complete tearing of a ligament from its attachments
4. Avulsion: A ligament that attaches to a bone is pulled loose with a fragment of that bone

---

O'Donoghue's Maneuver (13)

Sensitivity/Reliability Scale

0   1   2   3   4

PROCEDURE

With the patient seated, put the cervical spine through resisted range of motion (Fig. 3-49), then through passive range of motion (Fig. 3-50). See sections on Cervical Range of Motion and Cervical Resistive Isometric Muscle Testing in this chapter.

RATIONALE

Pain during resisted range of motion or isometric muscle contraction signifies muscle strain (see resistive range of motion for muscles involved). Pain during passive range of motion may indicate a sprain of any of these ligaments: alar ligaments, transverse ligament, supraspinous ligament, interspinous ligament, ligamentum flavum, articular capsule, intertransverse ligaments, posterior longitudinal ligament, and anterior longitudinal ligament (Fig. 3-51).

3

NOTE

This maneuver can be applied to any joint or series of joints to determine ligamentous or muscular involvement. Since resistive range of motion mainly stresses muscles and passive range of motion mainly stresses ligaments, you should be able to determine between strain and sprain or a combination thereof.

> **SUGGESTED DIAGNOSTIC IMAGING**
> - Plain film radiography
>   - AP lower cervical, upper thoracic
> - AP open mouth
> - Neutral lateral cervical
> - Cervical flexion/extension views[a]
> - Cervical lateral flexion views[a]

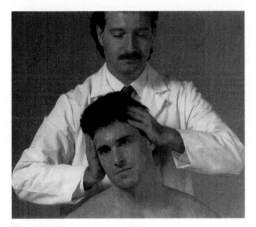

Figure 3-49

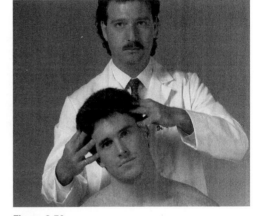

Figure 3-50

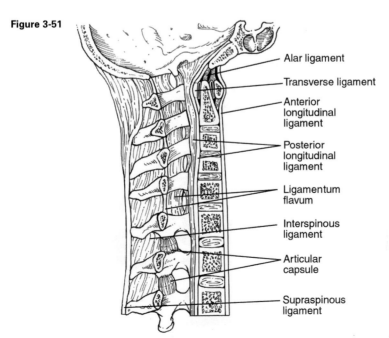

Figure 3-51

Alar ligament

Transverse ligament

Anterior longitudinal ligament

Posterior longitudinal ligament

Ligamentum flavum

Interspinous ligament

Articular capsule

Supraspinous ligament

---

[a]Based on outcome of the cervical AP, open-mouth, and neutral lateral radiographs and if movement will not adversely affect the patient.

CERVICAL FRACTURES

CLINICAL DESCRIPTION

Cervical fractures due to trauma are classified as either disrupting or not disrupting the spinal canal and as either stable or unstable. Fractures, dislocations, and fracture dislocations of the cervical spine are often the result of either a sudden and forceful flexion of the head and neck or a severe axial force, such as an object falling on the top of the head. The main concern with cervical fractures is compression or transection of the spinal cord. Compression of any part of the central nervous system for 3 to 5 minutes results in death of nervous tissue, particularly nerve cells.

Care must be taken if you suspect a cervical fracture. Radiographs of the affected area should be performed prior to any cervical movement. Fractures may be caused by a motor vehicle accident, falling, athletic injuries, or falling objects. Some of the common cervical fractures are spinous process fracture, vertebral body compression fracture, posterior arch of Atlas fracture, odontoid fractures, and burst fracture, a compound fracture anterior and posterior to the lateral masses. Most cervical fractures that cause severe disability are most likely evaluated in an emergency situation.

CLINICAL SIGNS AND SYMPTOMS
- Severe cervical pain
- Patient stabilizing the head
- Little or no cervical motion
- Severe cervical muscle spasm
- Upper extremity neurological dysfunction (see Chapter 4)
- Lower extremity neurological dysfunction (see Chapter 11)

Spinal Percussion Test (13,14)

PROCEDURE

With the patient sitting and the head slightly flexed, percuss the spinous process (Fig. 3-52) and associated musculature (Fig. 3-53) of each of the cervical vertebrae with a neurological reflex hammer.

Rationale

Evidence of local pain may indicate a fractured vertebra with no neurological compromise. Evidence of radicular pain may indicate a fractured vertebra with neurological compromise or a disc lesion with neurological compromise. If a fracture is suspected, a full cervical radiography series is indicated. If radicular pain is elicited, assess which neurological level is affected (see Chapter 4).

NOTE

This test is not specific; other conditions also elicit a positive pain response. A ligamentous sprain elicits a positive sign on percussion of the spinous processes. Percussing the paraspinal musculature elicits a positive sign for muscular strain.

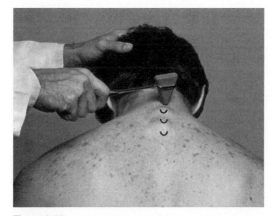

Figure 3-52

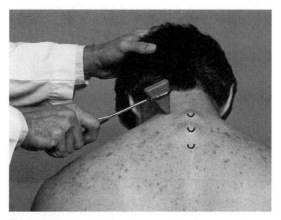

Figure 3-53

Soto-Hall Test (15)

Sensitivity/Reliability Scale
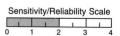
0   1   2   3   4

Procedure

With the patient supine, press on the patient's sternum with one hand. With the other hand, passively flex the patient's neck to the chest (Fig. 3-54).

Rationale

Evidence of local pain may indicate ligament, muscular, osseous pathology or injury, or cervical cord disease. This test is nonspecific; it merely isolates the cervical spine in passive flexion. If the patient reports radicular symptoms in the upper extremity on passive flexion, suspect a disc defect. When the cervical spine is flexed forward, the intervertebral disc is compressed at the anterior and stretched at the posterior (Fig. 3-55). The dura is also in traction at the posterior. If the patient has a posterior disc defect, this movement may exacerbate the defect, resulting in spinal cord or nerve root compression.

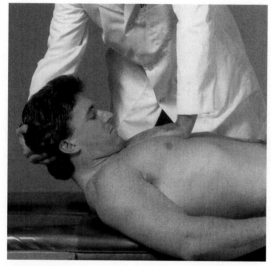

Figure 3-54

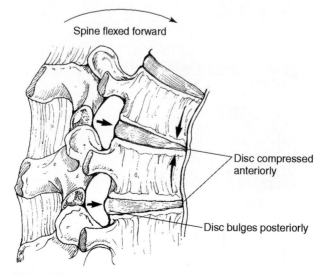

Spine flexed forward

Disc compressed anteriorly

Disc bulges posteriorly

Figure 3-55

Rust's Sign

PROCEDURE

A patient with severe injury to the upper cervical spine will grasp the head with both hands to support the weight of the head on the cervical spine (Fig. 3-56). The supine patient will support the head while attempting to rise.

3

RATIONALE

The patient with a severe upper cervical injury, such as severe muscular strain, ligamentous instability, posterior disc defect, upper cervical fracture, or dislocation, is subject to guarded movements, including stabilization of the head with slight traction to reduce the pain.

> **SUGGESTED DIAGNOSTIC IMAGING**
> - Plain film radiography
>   AP lower cervical, upper thoracic
>   AP open mouth
>   Neutral lateral cervical
>   Cervical flexion/extension views[b]
> - Computed tomography
> - Myelography

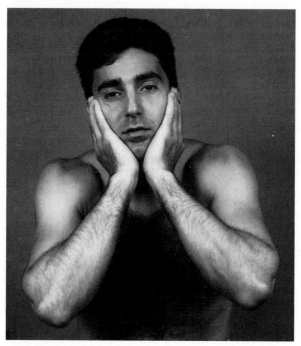

Figure 3-56

---

[b]Based on outcome of the cervical AP, open-mouth, and neutral lateral radiographs and if movement will not adversely affect the patient.

CERVICAL INSTABILITY

CLINICAL DESCRIPTION

Cervical instability, like fracture, is usually associated with trauma to the head and cervical spine. If the instability is not to due to a fracture, it may be due to a torn or stretched ligament of the atlanto-occipital joint and/or the atlantoaxial joints (Fig. 3-57), which may cause a subluxation or dislocation of either of those joints. If cervical instability is suspected, the main concern is compression or transection of the cervical spinal cord. Cervical spinal cord compression may lead to severe neurological problems, and cervical spinal cord transection may lead to death. Most severe cervical spinal cord injuries are evaluated in an emergency department.

The following tests attempt to evaluate stability of the atlanto-occipital and atlantoaxial joints and their associated ligaments. The ligaments being tested are the alar and the transverse. Radiographs of the cervical spine should be obtained before these tests are performed because of the possibility of cervical instability, which may lead to neurological deficit. Because of the nature of unstable cervical injuries, the following tests must be performed with extreme caution.

> ### CLINICAL SIGNS AND SYMPTOMS
> - Severe cervical pain
> - Patient stabilizing the head
> - Little or no cervical motion
> - Severe cervical muscle spasm
> - Upper extremity neurological dysfunction (see Chapter 4)
> - Lower extremity neurological dysfunction (see Chapter 11)

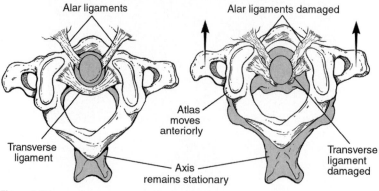

Figure 3-57

Sharp-Purser Test (16)

Sensitivity/Reliability Scale
0   1   2   3   4

PROCEDURE

With a patient seated, the examiner places one hand over the patient's forehead and the thumb of the opposite hand over the spinous process of C2 for stabilization (Fig. 3-58). Instruct the patient to flex the head slowly as you apply a posterior pressure with the palm of your hand (Fig. 3-59). A positive test is indicated if you feel the head slide backward during the movement.

RATIONALE

In an anterior Atlas subluxation due to severe trauma the Atlas is anterior to the axis with alar or transverse ligament damage. A backward slide indicates that the subluxation of the Atlas on axis has been reduced, and the slide may be accompanied by a "clunk." The subluxation may be caused by a stretched or torn alar or transverse ligament (Fig. 3-60).

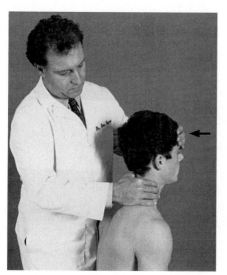

Figure 3-58

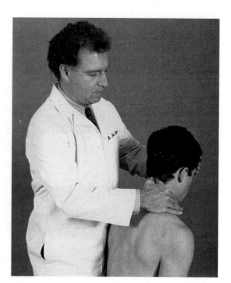

Figure 3-59

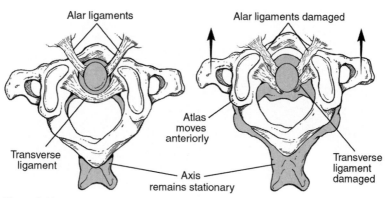

Figure 3-60

Transverse Ligament Stress Test (17,18)

PROCEDURE

With the patient supine, support the occiput with the palms of both hands and the third, fourth, and fifth fingers. Place the index fingers of both hands between the occiput and C2 at the posterior arch or Atlas, which is not palpable (Fig. 3-61). Carefully lift the head and C1 off the table, not allowing any flexion or extension of the cervical spine. (Fig. 3-62). Hold this position for 10 to 20 seconds.

RATIONALE

Lifting the head and C1 off the table places motion-induced posterior traction on the transverse ligament by the odontoid process. This movement should be limited by a transverse ligament. If the transverse ligament is torn or stretched, compression of the spinal cord by this anterior shear may occur. Possible signs include a soft end feel, muscle spasm, dizziness, nausea, paresthesia of the lip, face or limbs, nystagmus or a lump sensation in the throat. This indicates a hypermobile atlantoaxial articulation.

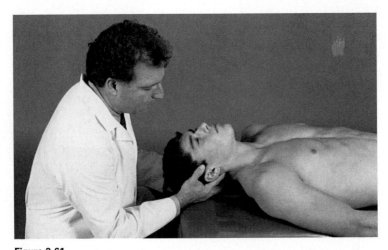

Figure 3-61

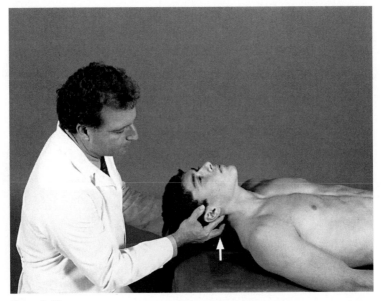

Figure 3-62

Alar Ligament Stress Test (17,18)

Sensitivity/Reliability Scale

0   1   2   3   4

PROCEDURE

With the patient supine, grasp the head with one hand. With the opposite hand grasp C2 with a pinch grip around the spinous process and lamina (Fig. 3-63). Attempt a shear side-to-side movement of the head against the axis (Fig. 3-64). There should be a minimal amount of lateral motion with a strong capsular end feel.

3

RATIONALE

The alar ligaments extend from the odontoid process to the lateral margins of the foramen magnum. These ligaments limit side-to-side movement of the skull on the axis. Excessive side-to-side movement indicates a stretched or torn alar ligament or ligaments.

SUGGESTED DIAGNOSTIC IMAGING

- Plain film radiography
  - AP lower cervical, upper thoracic
    AP open mouth
    Neutral lateral cervical
    Cervical flexion/extension views[c]
    Cervical lateral flexion views[c]
    AP open-mouth rotational views[c]
- Computed tomography
- Myelography
- Magnetic resonance imaging

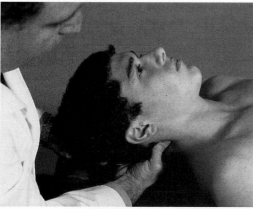

Figure 3-63

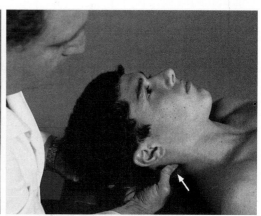

Figure 3-64

---

[c]Based on outcome of the cervical AP, open-mouth, and neutral lateral radiographs and if movement will not adversely affect the patient.

SPACE-OCCUPYING LESIONS

CLINICAL DESCRIPTION

Space-occupying lesions in and around the cervical spine may have any of various origins. Some masses, such as posterior disc defects, posterior osteophytes, tumors, and displaced fractures, are within the spinal canal. The same types of masses outside of the spinal canal include anterior disc defects, anterior osteophytes, tumors, and displaced fractures. Space-occupying lesions within the spinal canal may cause neurological deficit. Most of these masses are identified by various imaging studies. The following tests attempt to distinguish between masses within and outside of the spinal canal. If the suspected mass is within the spinal canal and is causing neurological dysfunction, the examiner should evaluate for neurological deficit based on the outcome of the tests in this section. The diagnostic imaging studies listed at the end of this section are imperative for determining the location and type of mass.

> ### CLINICAL SIGNS AND SYMPTOMS
> - Cervical pain
> - Upper extremity neurological symptoms
> - Lower extremity neurological symptoms

Valsalva's maneuver (19)

Sensitivity/Reliability Scale

0   1   2   3   4

PROCEDURE

With the patient seated, instruct him or her to bear down as if defecating but concentrating the bulk of the stress at the cervical region (Fig. 3-65). Ask the patient if he or she feels any increased pain, and if so, have the patient point to its location. This test is subjective and requires an accurate response from the patient.

RATIONALE

This test increases intrathecal pressure in the entire spine, but the patient should be able to localize the stress to the cervical spine. Local pain secondary to the increased pressure may indicate a space-occupying lesion (e.g., disc defect, mass, osteophyte) in the cervical canal or foramen.

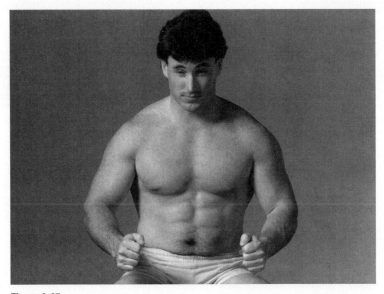

Figure 3-65

Déjérine's Sign

Sensitivity/Reliability Scale
0 1 2 3 4

PROCEDURE

With the patient seated, instruct the patient to cough, sneeze, and bear down as if defecating (Valsalva's maneuver).

RATIONALE

Pain, either local or radiating to the shoulders or upper extremities after either of these actions, indicates an increase in the intrathecal pressure. This pain may be caused by a space-occupying lesion, such as a disc defect, osteophyte, or mass.

Swallowing Test (19)

Sensitivity/Reliability Scale
0 1 2 3 4

PROCEDURE

Instruct the seated patient to swallow (Fig. 3-66).

RATIONALE

Pain upon swallowing usually indicates esophageal or pharyngeal injury, dysfunction, or pathology. Pain upon swallowing has orthopaedic significance. Because of the proximity of the esophagus to the anterior longitudinal ligament in the cervical spine, anterior pathology of the cervical spine, such as anterior disc defect, osteophyte, mass, or muscle spasm, may compress or irritate the esophagus and cause pain upon swallowing.

> SUGGESTED DIAGNOSTIC IMAGING
> - Plain film radiography
>   AP lower cervical, upper thoracic
>   AP open mouth
>   Neutral lateral cervical
>   Cervical oblique views
>   Lateral extension view (for retropharyngeal mass)
> - Computed tomography
> - Cervical magnetic resonance imaging

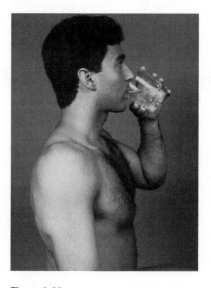

Figure 3-66

CERVICAL NEUROLOGICAL COMPRESSION AND IRRITATION

CLINICAL DESCRIPTION

Compression and irritation of the neurological structures in the cervical spine involve mainly the spinal cord and nerve roots. Compression of these structures may be caused by disc defects, osteophytes, degenerative joint disease, tumors, or fractures. Most of the tests in this section are provocative, that is, they aggravate the compression if present. If neurological compression is suspected, the examiner should evaluate for neurological deficit as described in Chapter 4. After performing these tests and evaluating for neurological deficit, select the appropriate imaging procedures for the suspected condition.

> ### CLINICAL SIGNS AND SYMPTOMS
> - Cervical pain
> - Upper extremity radicular pain
> - Loss of upper extremity sensation
> - Loss of upper extremity reflexes
> - Loss of upper extremity muscle strength

Foraminal Compression Test (20–22)

Sensitivity/Reliability Scale

0   1   2   3   4

PROCEDURE

With the patient seated and the patient's head in the neural position, exert strong downward pressure on the head (Fig. 3-67). Repeat the test with the head rotated bilaterally (Fig. 3-68).

RATIONALE

When downward pressure is applied to the head, the following biomechanical actions take place: (*a*) narrowing of the intervertebral foramina, (*b*) compression of the apophyseal joints in the cervical spine, and (*c*) compression of the intervertebral discs in the cervical spine. Local pain may indicate foraminal encroachment without nerve root pressure or apophyseal capsulitis. Radicular pain may indicate pressure on a nerve root by a decrease in the foraminal interval (foraminal encroachment) or by a disc defect. If nerve root involvement is suspected, evaluate the neurological level (see Chapter 4).

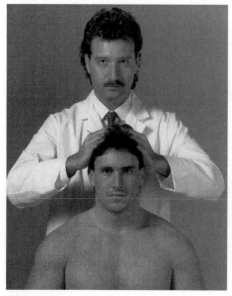

Figure 3-67

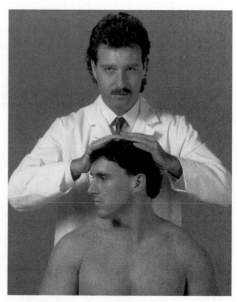

Figure 3-68

Jackson's Compression Test (23)

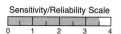

PROCEDURE

With the patient seated, laterally flex the neck and exert strong downward pressure on the head. Perform this test bilaterally (Fig. 3-69).

RATIONALE

With the neck laterally flexed and downward pressure applied, the following biomechanical actions take place: (*a*) narrowing of the intervertebral foramina on the side of lateral bending, (*b*) compression of the facet joints on the side of lateral bending, and (*c*) compression of the intervertebral discs in the cervical spine.

Local pain may indicate foraminal encroachment without nerve root pressure or apophyseal joint pathology. Radicular pain may indicate pressure on a nerve root by a decrease in the foraminal interval (foraminal encroachment) or a disc defect. If nerve root involvement is suspected, evaluate the neurological level (see Chapter 4).

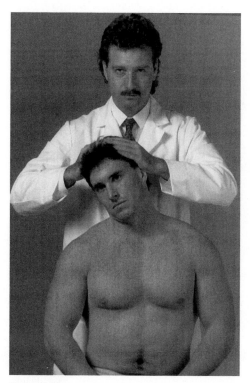

Figure 3-69

Extension Compression Test (24)

Sensitivity/Reliability Scale

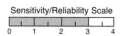

0   1   2   3   4

PROCEDURE

With the patient seated, instruct the patient to extend the head approximately 30°. Then place downward pressure on the patient's head (Fig. 3-70).

RATIONALE

When pressure is applied to the patient's head with the cervical spine in extension, the cervical intervertebral disc space is decreased posteriorly and increased vertically and anteriorly, with an increased load on the posterior apophyseal joints (Fig. 3-71). If the patient's symptoms decrease, suspect a posterolateral disc defect because of the anterior and vertical displacement of discal material away from the nerve root or spinal cord. Downward pressure on the head also compresses the posterior apophyseal joints, which, if irritated, can cause local cervical pain.

An increase in upper extremity radicular symptoms may indicate pathology in the intervertebral foramina, such as an osteophyte or mass or a degenerating cervical intervertebral disc. This is possible because the pressure on the head decreases the intervertebral foraminal interval.

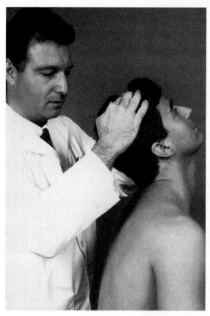

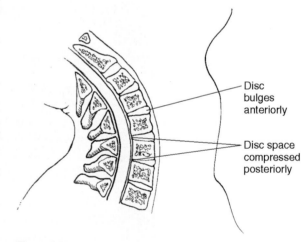

Disc bulges anteriorly

Disc space compressed posteriorly

Figure 3-70   **Figure 3-71**

Flexion Compression Test (24)

PROCEDURE

With the patient seated, instruct the patient to flex the head forward. Then place downward pressure on the patient's head (Fig. 3-72).

RATIONALE

When the patient flexes the head forward under pressure, the intervertebral disc is compressed anteriorly and the load is placed on the intervertebral disc. This pressure also causes the posterior aspect of the disc to bulge posteriorly (Fig. 3-73). An increase in cervical and/or radicular symptoms may indicate a discal defect. Flexion of the cervical spine and compression on the head also reduces the load on the posterior apophyseal joints. A decrease in localized scleratogenous pain may indicate apophyseal joint injury or pathology.

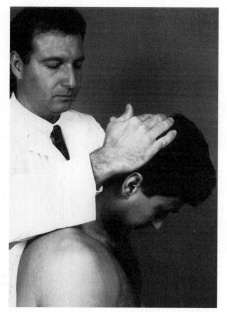

Figure 3-72

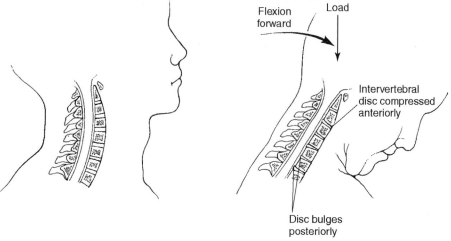

Flexion forward

Load

Intervertebral disc compressed anteriorly

Disc bulges posteriorly

Figure 3-73

Spurling's Test (20)

Sensitivity/Reliability Scale

0   1   2   3   4

PROCEDURE

Laterally flex the seated patient's head and gradually apply strong downward pressure (Fig. 3-74). If pain is elicited, the test is considered positive; *do not continue* with the next procedure. If no pain is elicited, put the patient's head to a neutral position and deliver a vertical blow to the uppermost portion of the patient's head (Fig. 3-75).

RATIONALE

Local pain may indicate facet joint involvement, either from the strong downward pressure on the head or from the vertical blow to the head. Radicular pain may indicate foraminal encroachment, degenerating cervical intervertebral disc, or disc defect with nerve root pressure. This test may also indicate a lateral disc defect.

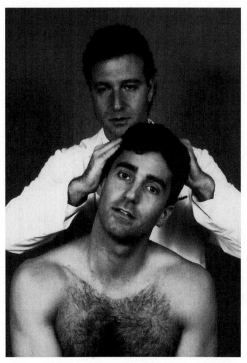

Figure 3-74

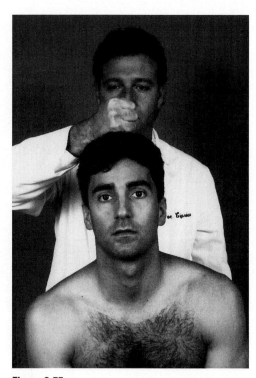

Figure 3-75

Maximal Foraminal Compression Test

PROCEDURE

Instruct the seated patient to approximate the chin to the shoulder and extend the neck. Perform this test bilaterally (Fig. 3-76).

RATIONALE

Rotation of the head and hyperextension of the neck causes the following biomechanical actions: (*a*) narrowing of the intervertebral foramina on the side of head rotation; (*b*) compression of the facet joints on the side of head rotation; and (*c*) compression of the intervertebral discs in the cervical spine. Pain on the side of head rotation with a radicular component may indicate nerve root compression caused by pathology such as an osteophyte or mass or decreased interval in the foramina,. Local pain with no radicular component may indicate apophyseal joint pathology on the side of head rotation and neck extension. Pain on the opposite side of head rotation indicates muscular strain or ligament sprain.

If nerve root compression is suspected, evaluate the neurological level (see Chapter 4).

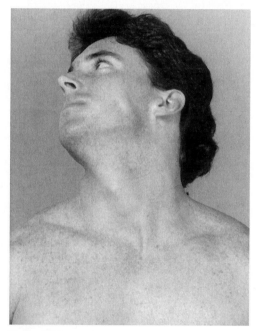

Figure 3-76

L'hermitte's Sign (25,26)

PROCEDURE

With the patient seated, passively flex the patient's chin to the chest (Fig. 3-77).

RATIONALE

When the cervical spine is flexed forward, the spinal cord and its coverings are under traction at the posterior, and the intervertebral disc is compressed at the anterior and bulges at the posterior (Fig. 3-78). If the patient has a posterior disc defect, this movement may exacerbate the defect, resulting in spinal cord or nerve root compression. Cervical cord disease, meningitis, osteophytes, and masses may cause local and/or radicular pain into the upper and/or lower extremities. A sudden electrical tingling felt in the spine and/or extremities during neck flexion may indicate cervical myelopathy or multiple sclerosis.

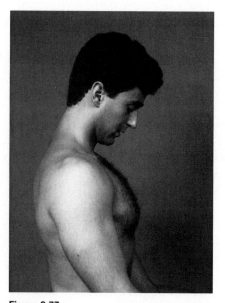

Figure 3-77

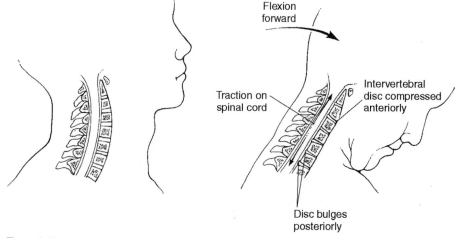

Flexion forward

Traction on spinal cord

Intervertebral disc compressed anteriorly

Disc bulges posteriorly

Figure 3-78

Shoulder Depression Test (23)

PROCEDURE

With the patient seated, place downward pressure on the shoulder while laterally flexing the patient's head to the opposite side (Fig. 3-79).

RATIONALE

3

When pressure is applied to the shoulder and the head is slightly flexed to the opposite side, the muscles, ligaments, nerve roots, nerve root coverings, and brachial plexus are stretched and the clavicle is depressed, approximating the first rib. Local pain on the side being tested indicates shortening of the muscles, muscular adhesions, muscle spasm, or ligamentous injury. Radicular pain may indicate compression of the neurovascular bundle, adhesion of the dural sleeve, or thoracic outlet syndrome. On the opposite side, the foraminal interval is decreased, the apophyseal joints are compressed, and the intervertebral disc is compressed. If pain is elicited on the side opposite the one being tested, it may indicate a pathological decrease in the foraminal interval, facet pathology, or disc defect.

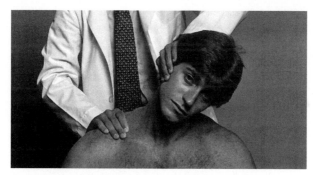

Figure 3-79

Distraction Test (19)

PROCEDURE

With the patient seated, grasp beneath the mastoid processes and press up on the patient's head. This removes the weight of the patient's head on the neck (Fig. 3-80).

RATIONALE

When the head is pulled upward, the cervical muscles, ligaments, and apophyseal joint capsules are stretched. If local pain increases, suspect muscle strain, spasm, ligamentous sprain, or facet capsulitis. Also, when the head is pulled upward, the interforaminal and intervertebral interval increase. Relief of local or radicular pain indicates either foraminal encroachment or a disc defect.

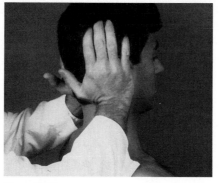

Figure 3-80

Shoulder Abduction Test (Bakody's Sign) (27)

PROCEDURE

Instruct the seated patient to abduct the arm and place the hand on top of the head (Fig. 3-81).

RATIONALE

Placing the hand above the head elevates the suprascapular nerve, reducing the traction on the lower trunk of the brachial plexus. This procedure reduces the traction on a compressed nerve. A decrease in or relief of the patient's symptoms indicates a cervical extradural compression problem, such as a herniated disc, epidural vein compression, or nerve root compression, usually in the C5–C6 area.

> **SUGGESTED DIAGNOSTIC IMAGING**
> - Plain film radiography
>   AP lower cervical, upper thoracic
>   AP open mouth
>   Neutral lateral cervical
>   Cervical oblique views
> - Cervical magnetic resonance imaging
> - Computed tomography
> - Myelography

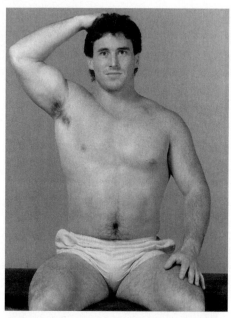

Figure 3-81

References

1. American Medical Association. Guides to the evaluation of permanent impairment. 5th ed. Chicago: American Medical Association, 2000.
2. American Academy of Orthopaedic Surgeons. The clinical measurement of joint motion. Chicago: American Association of Orthopaedic Surgery, 1994.
3. Dvorak J, Antinnes JA, Panjabi M, et al. Age and gender normal motion of the cervical spine. Spine 1992;17(suppl 10):S393–S398.
4. Okawara S, Nibbelink D. Vertebral artery occlusion following hyperextension and rotation of the head. Stroke 1974;5;640–643.
5. White AA, Panjabi MM. Clinical biomechanics of the spine, 2nd ed. Philadelphia: JB Lippincott, 1990.
6. Barré JA. Le syndrome sympathique cervical postérieur. Rev Neurol 1926;33:248–249.
7. George PE, Silverstein HT, Wallace H, et al. Identification of the high risk pre-stroke patient. J Chiropractic 1981;15:26–28.
8. Maigne R. Orthopaedic medicine. A new approach to vertebral manipulations. Springfield, IL: Charles C Thomas, 1972:155.
9. Maitland GD. Vertebral Manipulation. London, Butterworths, 1973.
10. deKleyn A, Versteegh C. Über verschiendene Formen von Méniére's Syndrom. Deutsche Ztschr 1933;132:157.
11. deKleyn A, Nieuwenhuyse P. Schwindelandfaelle und Nystagmus bei einer bestimmten Stellung des Kopfes. Acta Otolaryng 1927;11:555.
12. Lewis CB, Knotz NA. Orthopedic Assessment and Treatment of the Geriatric Patient. St. Louis: Mosby, 1993.
13. O'Donoghue D. Treatment of injuries to athletes. 4th ed. Philadelphia: WB Saunders, 1984.
14. Turek SL. Orthopaedics. 3rd ed. Philadelphia: JB Lippincott, 1977.
15. Soto-Hall R, Haldeman K. A useful diagnostic sign in vertebral injuries. Surg Gynecol Obstet 827–831.
16. Magee DJ. Orthopedic Physical Assessment. 3rd ed. Philadelphia: WB Saunders, 1997.
17. Pettman E. Stress test of the craniovertebral joints. In Boyling JD, Palastanga N, eds. Grieve's Modern Manual Therapy: The Vertebral Column. 2nd ed. Edinburgh: Churchill Livingstone, 1994.
18. Meadows JJ, Magee DJ. An overview of dizziness and vertigo for the orthopedic manual therapist. In Boyling JD, Palastanga N, eds. Grieve's Modern Manual Therapy: The Vertebral Column. 2nd ed. Edinburgh: Churchill Livingstone, 1994.
19. Hoppenfeld S. Physical examination of the spine and extremities. New York: Appleton-Century-Crofts, 1976:127.
20. Spurling RG, Scoville WB. Lateral rupture of the cervical IVDs–a common cause of shoulder and arm pain. Surg Gynecol Obstet 1944;78:350–358.
21. Harris NM. Cervical spine dysfunction. GP 1967;32(4):78–88.
22. Depalma A, Rothman RH. The Intervertebral Disc. Philadelphia: WB Saunders, 1970:88.
23. Jackson R. The Cervical Syndrome. 3rd ed. St. Louis: Mosby, 1985.
24. Gerard J, Kleinfeld S. Orthopaedic testing. New York: Churchill Livingstone, 1993.
25. L'hermitte J. Étude de la commotion de la moella. Rev Neurol (Paris), 1:210, 1933.
26. L'hermitte J, Bollak P, Nicholas M. Les douleurs a type de décharge électrique dans la sclérose en plaques. Un cas forme sensitive de la sclérose multiple. Rev Neurol (Paris).
27. Davidson RI, Dunn EJ, Metzmater JN. The shoulder abduction test in the diagnosis of radicular pain in cervical extradural compressive monoradiculopathies. Spine 1981;6:441.

General References

Clarkson HM. Musculoskeletal Assessment: Joint Range of Motiond Manual Muscle Strength. 2nd ed. Baltimore: Lippincott Williams & Wilkins, 2000.

Cyriax J. Textbook of Orthopaedic Medicine. Vol. 1. Diagnosis of Soft Tissue Lesions. London: Bailliere Tindall, 1983.

Edwards BC. Combined movements in the cervical spine (C2-C7): their value in examination and technique choice. Aust J Physiother 1980;26:165.

Foreman SM, Croft AC. Whiplash Injuries: The Cervical Acceleration/Deceleration Syndrome. 3rd ed. Baltimore: Lippincott Williams & Wilkins, 2002.

Kapandji IA. The Physiology of Joints. Vol. 3. The Trunk and the Vertebral Column. New York: Churchill Livingstone, 1974.

Naffzinger HC, Grant WT. Neuritis of the brachial plexus mechanical in origin: the scalenus syndrome. Clin Orthop 1967;51:7.

Neviaser JS. Musculoskeletal disorders of the shoulder region causing cervicobrachial pain: differential diagnosis and treatment. Surg Clin North Am 1963;43:1703.

Nichols HM. Anatomic structures of the thoracic outlet. Clin Orthop 1967;51:17.

Norkin CC, Levangie PK. Joint Structure and Function: A Comprehensive Analysis. Philadelphia: FA Davis, 1983.

Terrett AGJ. Importance and interpretation of tests designed to predict susceptibility to neurocirculatory accidents from manipulation. J Aust Chiropr Assoc 1983;13(2):29–34.

4

CERVICAL NERVE ROOT LESIONS

The cervical spine consists of eight pairs of spinal nerves. Each spinal nerve consists of a dorsal root (sensory component) and a ventral root (motor component). These nerve roots emerge from the spinal column through lateral intervertebral foramina. The first four cervical nerves collectively form the cervical plexus. The second four nerves, together with the first thoracic nerve, form the brachial plexus (Fig. 4-1).

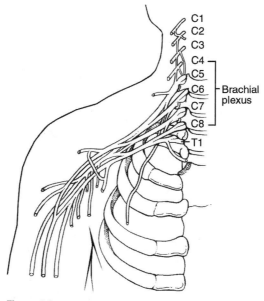

Figure 4-1

If a nerve root lesion is suspected, you must evaluate three clinical aspects of the neurological examination: sensory, motor, and reflex dysfunction. Sensory testing attempts to delineate the segmental cutaneous innervation to the skin. It is done with a sterile or disposable Neurotip or pinwheel in specific dermatomal patterns.

Two dermatomal maps are provided. Figure 4-2 is based on the body areas of intact sensation when roots above and below an isolated root were interrupted; sensation loss when one or more continuous roots were interrupted; or the pattern of herpetic rash and hypersensitivity when there is isolated root involvement. Figure 4-3 is based on the hyposensitivity to pin scratch in various root lesions and is consistent with electrical skin resistance studies showing axial dermatomes extending to the distal extremities. This pattern is useful in evaluating paresthesias and hyperesthesias secondary to root irritation. This is the pattern this chapter delineates to evaluate sensory root dysfunction. A fair amount of segmental overlap exists; therefore, a single unilateral lesion may affect more than one dermatomal level.

Motor function is evaluated by testing the muscle strength of specific muscles innervated by a particular nerve root or roots using the muscle grading chart adopted by the American Academy of Orthopaedic Surgeons (Box 4-1). The reflex arc is tested by evaluating the superficial stretch reflex associated with the particular nerve root. These arcs are graded by the Wexler Scale (Box 4-2).

The clinical presentation of nerve root lesions depends on two important factors: location and severity of the injury or pathology. These two factors together determine the injury's clinical presentation. The possibilities are endless, ranging from no clinical presentation or slight clinical manifestation, such as slight loss of sensation and pain, to total denervation with loss of total function to the structures innervated by that nerve root (motor, reflex, and sensory).

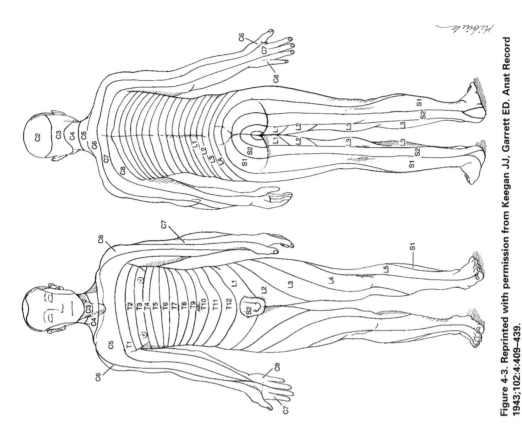

Figure 4-3. Reprinted with permission from Keegan JJ, Garrett ED. Anat Record 1943;102:4:409–439.

Figure 4-2. Adapted with permission from Haymaker and Woodall. Peripheral Nerve Injuries. 2nd ed. Philadelphia: WB Saunders, 1954.

Box 4-1	Muscle Grading Chart
5	Complete range of motion against gravity with full resistance
4	Complete range of motion against gravity with some resistance
3	Complete range of motion against gravity
2	Complete range of motion with gravity eliminated
1	Evidence of slight contractility, no joint motion
0	No evidence of contractility

4

Box 4-2	Wexler Scale
0	No response
+1	Hyporeflexia
+2	Normal
+3	Hyperreflexia
+4	Hyperreflexia with transient clonus
+5	Hyperreflexia with sustained clonus

Each nerve root has its own sensory distribution, muscle test or tests, and a stretch reflex; these are grouped to facilitate the identification of the suspected level.

The clinical evaluation is not made solely on one aspect of the neurological package but is instead determined by the combination of history, inspection, palpation, the three individual tests (motor, reflex, and sensory) and appropriate diagnostic imaging and/or functional neurological testing, such as electromyography. Furthermore, the injury or pathology under evaluation may not necessarily be affecting a nerve root, but it may be affecting the brachial plexus, a trunk of that plexus, or a named nerve. Depending on the severity and location of the injury or pathology, various combinations of neurological dysfunction may be elicited.

CLINICAL SIGNS AND SYMPTOMS
- Cervical pain
- Upper extremity paresthesia
- Diminution or loss of upper extremity sensation
- Diminution or loss of upper extremity reflexes
- Decrease or loss of muscle strength
- Atrophic upper extremity lesions

C5

The C5 nerve root exits the spinal canal between the C4 and C5 vertebrae and may be affected by the C4 intervertebral disc (Fig. 4-4).

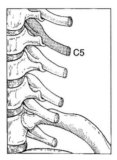

Figure 4-4

Motor

Deltoid Muscle (C5 Axillary Nerve Innervation)

Sensitivity/Reliability Scale

0   1   2   3   4

PROCEDURE

Stand behind the seated patient and place your hand at the lateral aspect of the elbow. Instruct the patient to abduct the arm against resistance (Fig. 4-5). Grade the strength according to the muscle grading chart. Perform this test bilaterally and compare each side.

RATIONALE

A grade of 0 to 4 unilaterally may indicate a neurological deficit of the C5 nerve root, upper trunk of the brachial plexus, or the axillary nerve. A weak or strained deltoid muscle may be suspected if the sensory and reflex portions of the C5 neurological package are intact.

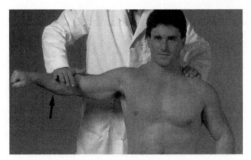

Figure 4-5

Biceps Muscle (C5, C6 Musculocutaneous Nerve Innervation)

PROCEDURE

With the patient in the seated position and the forearm flexed, stabilize the patient's elbow with one hand and grasp the anterior aspect of the patient's wrist with your opposite hand. Instruct the patient to flex the forearm against resistance (Fig. 4-6). Grade the strength according to the muscle grading chart and compare each side.

RATIONALE

A grade of 0 to 4 unilaterally may indicate a neurological deficit of the C5 or C6 nerve roots, upper trunk of the brachial plexus, or musculocutaneous nerve. A weak or strained biceps muscle may be suspected if the sensory and reflex portions of the C5 neurological package are intact.

4

Figure 4-6

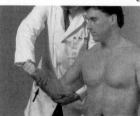

Reflex

Sensitivity/Reliability Scale

0   1   2   3   4

Biceps Reflex (C5, C6 Musculocutaneous Nerve Innervation)

PROCEDURE

Place the patient's arm across your opposite arm with your thumb on the biceps tendon. Strike your thumb with the narrow end of the reflex hammer (Fig. 4-7). The biceps muscle should contract slightly under your thumb. Grade your response according to the reflex chart and evaluate bilaterally.

RATIONALE

Hyporeflexia may indicate a C5, C6 nerve root deficit. Loss of reflex may indicate an interruption of the reflex arc (lower motor neuron lesion). Hyperreflexia may indicate an upper motor neuron lesion.

Figure 4-7

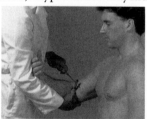

Sensory

Sensitivity/Reliability Scale

0   1   2   3   4

PROCEDURE

With a pin, stroke the lateral aspect of the arm (Fig. 4-8).

RATIONALE

Unilateral hypoesthesia may indicate a neurological deficit of the C5 nerve root or the axillary nerve.

Figure 4-8

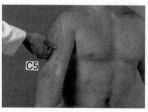

C6

The C6 nerve root exits the spinal canal between the C5 and C6 vertebrae and may be affected by the C5 intervertebral disc (Fig. 4-9).

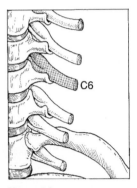

Figure 4-9

Motor

Sensitivity/Reliability Scale

0   1   2   3   4

Biceps Muscle (C5, C6 Musculocutaneous Nerve Innervation)

See Figure 4-6 and accompanying text.

Wrist Extensor Group: Extensor Carpi Radialis, Longus, and Brevis (C6, C7 Radial Nerve Innervation)

PROCEDURE

With the patient seated, stabilize the patient's forearm by grasping the elbow with your hand. Instruct the patient to make a fist, and dorsiflex the wrist (Fig. 4-10). With your opposite hand, grasp the patient's fist and attempt to force the wrist into flexion as the patient resists (Fig. 4-11). Evaluate according to the muscle grading chart and compare bilaterally.

RATIONALE

A grade of 0 to 4 unilaterally may indicate a neurological deficit of the C6 or C7 nerve root. A weak or strained wrist extensor may be suspected if the sensory and reflex portions of the C6 and C7 neurological packages are intact.

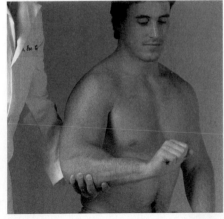

Figure 4-10

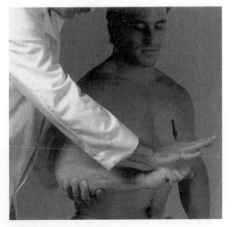

Figure 4-11

Reflex

Sensitivity/Reliability Scale

0   1   2   3   4

Brachioradialis Reflex (C5, C6 Radial Nerve Innervation)

PROCEDURE

Place the patient's arm across your opposite arm and tap the brachioradialis tendon at the distal aspect of the forearm with the neurological reflex hammer (Fig. 4-12). The brachioradialis muscle should contract slightly on your arm. Grade the response according to the reflex chart and evaluate bilaterally.

RATIONALE

Hyporeflexia may indicate a nerve root deficit. Loss of reflex may indicate an interruption of the reflex arc (lower motor neuron lesion). Hyperreflexia may indicate an upper motor neuron lesion.

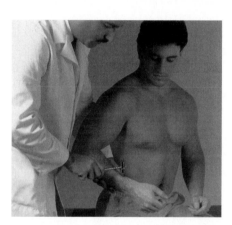

Figure 4-12

Sensory

PROCEDURE

With a pin, stroke the lateral aspect of the forearm, thumb, and index finger (Fig. 4-13).

RATIONALE

Unilateral hypoesthesia may indicate a neurological deficit of the C6 nerve root or the musculocutaneous nerve.

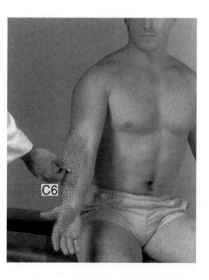

Figure 4-13

C7

The C7 nerve root exits the spinal canal between the C6 and C7 vertebrae and may be affected by the C6 intervertebral disc (Fig. 4-14).

Figure 4-14

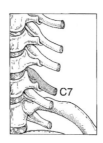

Motor

Triceps Muscle (C7 Radial Nerve Innervation)

PROCEDURE

With the patient supine, flex the shoulder and elbow to 90°. Grasp the proximal aspect of the arm to stabilize the extremity. With your opposite hand, grasp the patient's wrist and ask the patient to extend the forearm against your resistance (Fig. 4-15). Grade the strength according to the muscle grading chart and compare bilaterally.

RATIONALE

A grade of 0 to 4 unilaterally may indicate a neurological deficit of the C7 nerve root or radial nerve. A weak or strained triceps muscle may be suspected if the sensory and reflex portions of the C7 neurological package are intact.

Figure 4-15

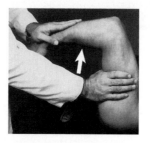

Wrist Flexor Group: Flexor Carpi Radialis (C7 Median Nerve Innervation) and Flexor Carpi Ulnaris (C8 Ulnar Nerve Innervation)

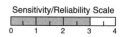

PROCEDURE

With the patient seated, stabilize the patient's forearm by grasping the forearm with your hand. Instruct the patient to make a fist and flex the wrist. With your opposite hand, grasp the patient's fist and attempt to force the wrist into extension as the patient resists (Fig. 4-16). Grade according to the muscle grading chart and compare bilaterally.

RATIONALE

A grade of 0 to 4 unilaterally may indicate a neurological deficit of the C7 or C8 nerve root. A weak or strained wrist flexor may be suspected if the sensory and reflex portions of the C7 and C8 neurological packages are intact.

Figure 4-16

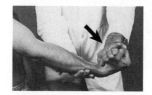

Finger Extensor Group: Extensor Digitorum Communis, Extensor Digiti Indicis, Extensor Digiti Minimi (C7 Radial Nerve Innervation)

Procedure

With the patient's wrist in the neutral position, grasp the wrist with your hand. Have the patient extend the metacarpophalangeal joints and flex the proximal and distal interphalangeal joints (Fig. 4-17). Place your hand on the distal aspect of the proximal phalanges and attempt to force the metacarpophalangeal joints into flexion as the patient resists (Fig. 4-18). Grade according to the muscle grading chart and evaluate bilaterally.

Rationale

A grade of 0 to 4 unilaterally may indicate a neurological deficit of the C7 or C8 nerve root. A weak or strained finger extensor may be suspected if the sensory and reflex portions of the C7 and C8 neurological packages are intact.

Figure 4-17

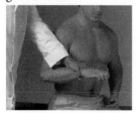
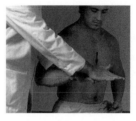

Figure 4-18

Reflex

Triceps Reflex (C7 Radial Nerve Innervation)

Procedure

Flex the patient's arm across your opposite arm and tap the triceps tendon at the olecranon fossa with the neurological reflex hammer (Fig. 4-19). The triceps muscle should contract slightly. Grade your response according to the reflex chart and evaluate bilaterally.

Rationale

Unilateral hyporeflexia may indicate a nerve root deficit. Loss of reflex unilaterally may indicate an interruption of the reflex arc (lower motor neuron lesion). Unilateral hyperreflexia may indicate an upper motor neuron lesion.

Figure 4-19

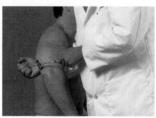

Sensory

Procedure

With a pin, stroke the palmar surface of the middle finger (Fig. 4-20).

Rationale

Unilateral hypoesthesia may indicate a neurological deficit of the C7 nerve root or the radial nerve.

Figure 4-20

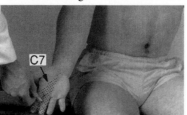

C8

The C8 nerve root exits the spinal canal between the C7 and T1 vertebrae and may be affected by the C7 intervertebral disc (Fig. 4-21).

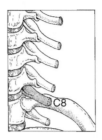

Figure 4-21

Motor

Sensitivity/Reliability Scale

0   1   2   3   4

Finger Flexor Group: Flexor Digitorum Superficialis (C7, C8 Median Nerve Innervation) and Flexor Digitorum Profundus (C7, C8 Median and Ulnar Nerve Innervation)

PROCEDURE

Grasp the seated patient's wrist with one hand to stabilize the hand. Curl your fingers into the patient's fist and attempt to pull the fingers out of flexion as the patient resists (Fig. 4-22). Grade according to the muscle grading chart and compare bilaterally.

RATIONALE

A grade of 0 to 4 unilaterally may indicate a neurological deficit of the C8 nerve root. A weak or strained finger flexor group muscle may be suspected if the sensory portion of the C8 neurological package is intact.

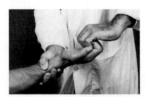

Figure 4-22

Finger Abductor Group: Dorsal Interossei, Abductor Digiti Minimi (C8, T1 Ulnar Nerve Innervation)

PROCEDURE

Instruct the patient to pronate the hand and abduct the fingers. Take each pair of fingers and pinch them together as the patient resists (Fig. 4-23). Grade your findings according to the muscle grading chart and compare bilaterally.

RATIONALE

A grade of 0 to 4 unilaterally may indicate a neurological deficit of the C8 or T1 nerve root. A weak or strained finger abductor may be suspected if the sensory portion of the C8 and T1 neurological packages is intact.

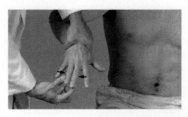

Figure 4-23

Palmar Interossei (C8, T1 Ulnar Nerve Innervation)

PROCEDURE

With the patient's hand pronated, have the patient adduct all the fingers. The examiner is to grasp each pair of the patient's fingers and attempt to pull them apart against patient resistance (Fig. 4-24). Grade according to the muscle grading chart and compare bilaterally.

RATIONALE

A grade of 0 to 4 unilaterally may indicate a neurological deficit of the C8 or T1 nerve root. A weak or strained finger adductor may be suspected if the sensory portion of the C8 and T1 neurological packages is intact.

4

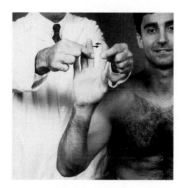

Figure 4-24

Reflex

None

Sensory

Sensitivity/Reliability Scale

0   1   2   3   4

PROCEDURE

With a pin, stroke the palmar surface of the last two digits and the ulnar aspect of the forearm (Fig. 4-25).

RATIONALE

Unilateral hypoesthesia may indicate a neurological deficit of the C8 nerve root or the ulnar nerve.

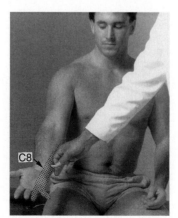

Figure 4-25

T1

The T1 nerve root exits the spinal canal between the T1 and T2 vertebrae and may be affected by the T1 intervertebral disc (Fig. 4-26).

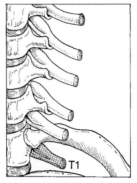

Figure 4-26

Motor

Finger Abductor and Adductor Groups

See C8 Neurological Level

Sensitivity/Reliability Scale
0   1   2   3   4

Reflex

None

Sensory

Sensitivity/Reliability Scale
0   1   2   3   4

PROCEDURE

With a pin, stroke the medial proximal aspect of the arm and forearm (Fig. 4-27).

RATIONALE

Unilateral hypoesthesia may indicate a neurological deficit of the T1 nerve root or the medial brachial cutaneous nerve.

SUGGESTED IMAGING AND FUNCTIONAL TESTING
- Cervical magnetic resonance imaging
- Electromyography
- Somatosensory evoked potential

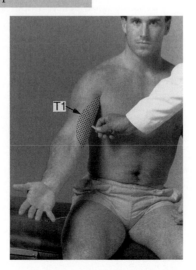

Figure 4-27

General References

Bronisch FW. The Clinically Important Reflexes. New York: Grune & Stratton, 1952.

Chusid JG. Correlative Neuroanatomy and Functional Neurology. 17th ed. Los Altos, CA: Lange, 1976.

DeJong RN. The Neurologic Examination. 4th ed. Hagerstown, MD: Harper & Row, 1979.

Hoppenfeld S. Physical Examination of the Spine and Extremities. New York: Appleton-Century-Croft, 1976:127.

Kendall FP, McCreary EK, Provance PG. Muscles: Testing and Function. 4th ed. Baltimore: Williams & Wilkins, 1994.

Mancall E. Essentials of the Neurologic Examination. 2nd ed. Philadelphia: FA Davis, 1981.

Parsons N. Color Atlas of Clinical Neurology. Chicago: Year Book, 1989.

VanAllen MW, Rodnitzky RL. Pictorial Manual of Neurologic Tests. 2nd ed. Chicago: Year Book, 1981.

4

SHOULDER ORTHOPAEDIC TESTS

Shoulder Orthopaedic Examination

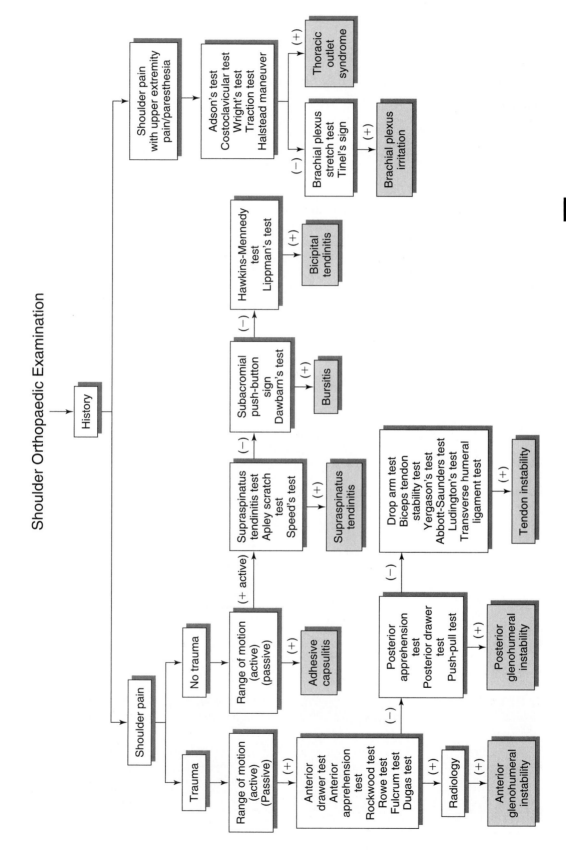

SHOULDER PALPATION

Anterior Aspect

Clavicle and Sternoclavicular and Acromioclavicular Joints

DESCRIPTIVE ANATOMY

The clavicle is slightly anterior and inferior to the top of the shoulder. The sternoclavicular joint, which attaches the clavicle to the sternum, lies at the medial end of the clavicle. The acromioclavicular joint, which is lateral, attaches the clavicle to the acromion process of the scapula (Fig. 5-1).

PROCEDURE

With your fingertips, palpate the length of the clavicle from the medial aspect at the sternoclavicular joint to the lateral aspect at the acromioclavicular joint (Fig. 5-2). Note any abnormal tenderness or bumps along the length of the clavicle that indicate a fracture secondary to recent trauma or a healed fracture with callus formation. Compare the clavicles for symmetry and placement. Next, palpate the sternoclavicular joint (Fig. 5-3) and acromioclavicular joint (Fig. 5-4) for tenderness with your index and middle fingers. If the affected clavicle and associated joint are more anterior, posterior, or superior than the other, suspect a subluxation or dislocation of the clavicle at the affected joint. Flexing and extending the shoulder during acromioclavicular joint palpation may reveal crepitus (Fig. 5-5). Crepitus is secondary to joint inflammation, such as osteoarthritis.

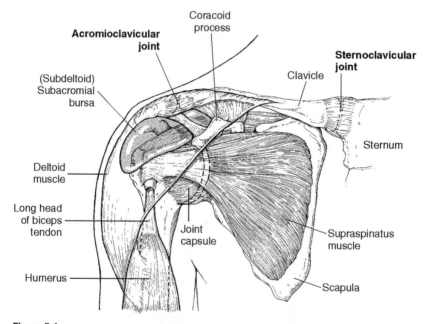

Figure 5-1

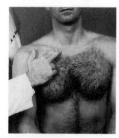

Figure 5-2

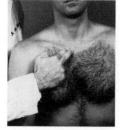

Figure 5-3

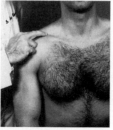

Figure 5-4

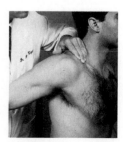

Figure 5-5

Subacromial (Subdeltoid) Bursa

DESCRIPTIVE ANATOMY

The subacromial portion of the bursa is a fluid-filled sac that extends over the supraspinatus tendon and beneath the acromion process. The subdeltoid portion, beneath the deltoid muscle, (Fig. 5-6) separates the deltoid muscle from the rotator cuff.

PROCEDURE

With one hand, extend the patient's arm. With your opposite hand, palpate for tenderness, masses, and thickening of both subacromial (Fig. 5-7) and subdeltoid (Fig. 5-8) portions of the bursa. Suspect subacromial or subdeltoid bursitis if the bursa is tender. Tenderness may also be associated with restriction of motion and crepitus of the shoulder, especially in abduction and forward flexion.

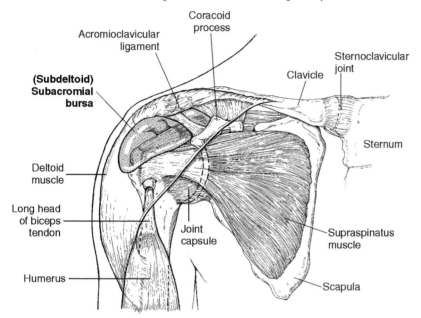

Figure 5-6

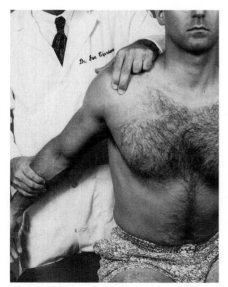

Figure 5-7

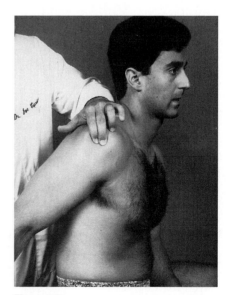

Figure 5-8

Rotator Cuff

Descriptive Anatomy

The rotator cuff is composed of four muscles, three that are palpable and one that is not. The three palpable muscles are the supraspinatus, which lies above the spine of the scapula and whose tendon lies under the acromion process; the infraspinatus, which lies inferior to the supraspinatus; and the teres minor, which is inferior to the infraspinatus (Figs. 5-9 and 5-10) The fourth muscle is the subscapularis, which is under the scapula and is difficult to palpate. The rotator cuff holds the humerus in the glenoid cavity and blends with the articular capsule to provide dynamic stabilization.

Procedure

Sitting behind the patient, grasp the patient's arm and extend it backward 20°. With your other hand, palpate inferior to the anterior border of the acromion process (Fig. 5-11). Note any tenderness, swelling, nodular masses, or gaps in the cuff. Tendinitis, tears, abnormal calcium deposits, and degeneration in the cuff may elicit tenderness and pain upon palpation. A palpable gap may indicate a ruptured tendon.

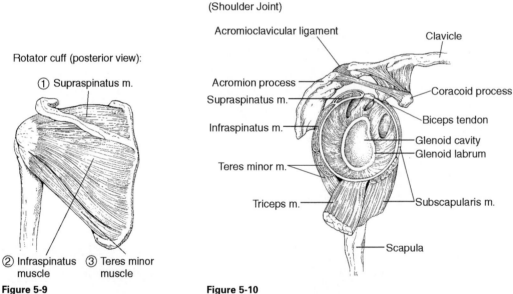

Rotator cuff (posterior view):

① Supraspinatus m.

② Infraspinatus muscle ③ Teres minor muscle

Figure 5-9

(Shoulder Joint)

Acromioclavicular ligament

Clavicle

Acromion process

Supraspinatus m.

Coracoid process

Infraspinatus m.

Biceps tendon

Glenoid cavity
Glenoid labrum

Teres minor m.

Triceps m.

Subscapularis m.

Scapula

Figure 5-10

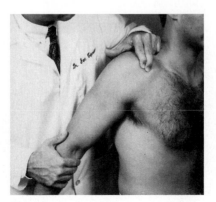

Figure 5-11

Bicipital Groove

DESCRIPTIVE ANATOMY

The bicipital groove is anterior and medial to the greater tuberosity of the humerus. The tendon of the long head of the biceps muscle and its synovial sheath lie in its groove. The transverse humeral ligament holds the tendon in place (Fig. 5-12).

PROCEDURE

With one hand, locate the inferior tip of the acromion process, then move inferiorly to the greater tuberosity of the humerus. With your other hand, grasp the patient's arm and externally rotate it (Fig. 5-13). You will feel the bicipital groove slip under your fingers. Note any tenderness, which may indicate tenosynovitis of the bicipital tendon and its sheath. Also note any excessive movement of the tendon in its groove; it may indicate a predisposition of the tendon to dislocate out of the bicipital groove or a torn or ruptured transverse humeral ligament.

5

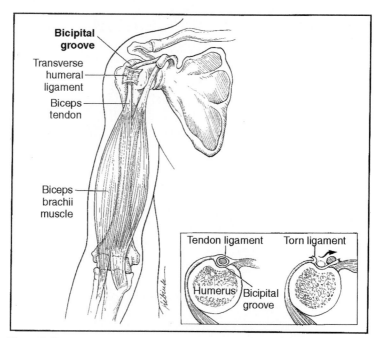

Figure 5-12

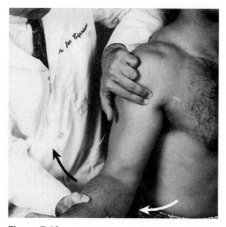

Figure 5-13

Biceps Muscle

Descriptive Anatomy

The biceps muscle has two heads that originate from different areas. The long head originates from the tuberosity above the glenoid cavity, and the short head originates from the coracoid process of the scapula. They both insert into the bicipital tuberosity of the radius (Fig. 5-12).

Procedure

With the patient's elbow flexed to 90°, begin palpating distally from the bicipital tuberosity of the radius upward to the bicipital groove (Fig. 5-14). Note any tenderness, spasm, or muscle mass. Tenderness at the proximal end may indicate tenosynovitis of the biceps tendon. Tenderness at the belly of the muscle may indicate muscle strain or an active trigger point. If a curling of the muscle secondary to overload is evident at the mid arm, suspect a rupture of the biceps tendon from its origin.

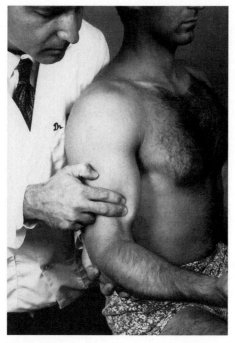

Figure 5-14

Deltoid Muscle

DESCRIPTIVE ANATOMY

The deltoid muscle originates from the clavicle and acromion process of the scapula and inserts into the deltoid tuberosity of the humerus (Fig. 5-15). The three parts of the fibers are the anterior, middle, and posterior. This muscle is capable of acting in parts or as a whole. The anterior part flexes and medially rotates the humerus. The middle part abducts the humerus. The posterior part extends and laterally rotates the humerus.

PROCEDURE

Begin palpation of the anterior portion of the deltoid muscle from the acromion process inferiorly (Fig. 5-16), then from the lateral aspect of the shoulder (again inferiorly) for the middle part of the deltoid muscle (Fig. 5-17). Finally, palpate the posterior aspect of the deltoid muscle from the superior aspect to the inferior aspect with the patient's shoulder extended (Fig. 5-18). Note any tenderness or taut muscle fibers. Tenderness at the lateral aspect of the deltoid is associated with subdeltoid bursitis. Tenderness at the anterior aspect of the deltoid may be associated with pathology or injury in the bicipital groove, because the anterior aspect of the deltoid muscle covers the groove and its tendon. General tenderness may indicate a strain or active trigger point of the deltoid muscle secondary to overuse, overload, trauma, or chilling.

Figure 5-15

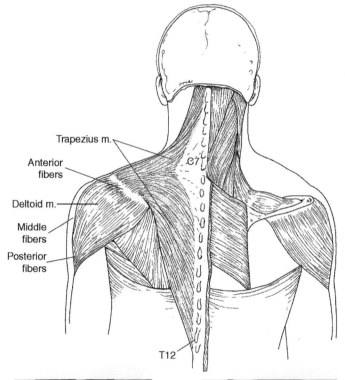

Trapezius m.

Anterior fibers

Deltoid m.

Middle fibers

Posterior fibers

C7

T12

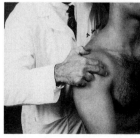

Figure 5-16

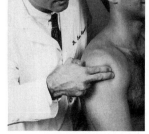

Figure 5-17

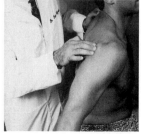

Figure 5-18

Posterior Aspect

Scapula

Descriptive Anatomy

The scapula lies between T2 and T7. It has three borders, medial, lateral, and superior. It also has a sharp ridge that extends from the acromion process, which is the spine of the scapula (Fig. 5-19).

Procedure

Starting with the medial border of the scapula, palpate all three borders, noting any tenderness (Figs. 5-20–5-22). Next, palpate the spine of the scapula, noting any tenderness and/or abnormality (Fig. 5-23). Finally, palpate the posterior surfaces above the spine of the scapula for the supraspinatus muscle (Fig. 5-24) and below the spine for the infraspinatus muscle (Fig. 5-25). Note any tenderness, palpable bands, atrophy, or spasm. Palpable bands in the supraspinatus and infraspinatus muscle may indicate a myofascial syndrome caused by overuse, overload trauma, or chilling. Atrophy may indicate a disruption of the nerve supply to the suspected muscle.

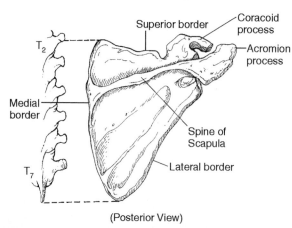

(Posterior View)

Figure 5-19

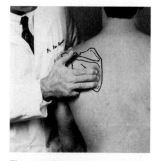

Figure 5-20

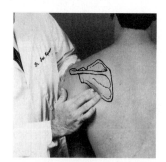

Figure 5-21

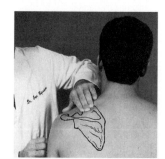

Figure 5-22

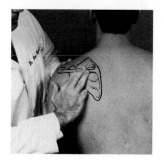

Figure 5-23

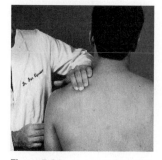

Figure 5-24

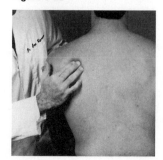

Figure 5-25

Trapezius Muscle

DESCRIPTIVE ANATOMY

The trapezius muscle originates from the occiput, ligamentum nuchae, and spine of C7 to T12 vertebra. It inserts into the acromion process and spine of the scapula (Fig. 5-26). The trapezius contains three sets of fibers that perform different actions. The superior fibers elevate the shoulders; the middle fibers retract the scapula; and the inferior fibers depress the scapula and lower the shoulders.

PROCEDURE

Begin at the origin at the base of the occiput, palpating superior fibers inferior toward the spine of the scapula (Fig. 5-27). Then, from the spine of the scapula, palpate the middle (Fig. 5-28) and inferior (Fig. 5-29) fibers down toward the T12 spinous process. Note any tenderness, spasm, palpable bands, or asymmetry of the muscles. Tenderness and spasm may be present secondary to hyperextension or hyperflexion injuries. Tight palpable bands may be secondary to active myofascial trigger points. According to Travell, myofascial trigger points in muscle are activated directly by trauma, overuse, overload, or chilling. They are activated indirectly by visceral disease, arthritis, and emotional distress.

Figure 5-26

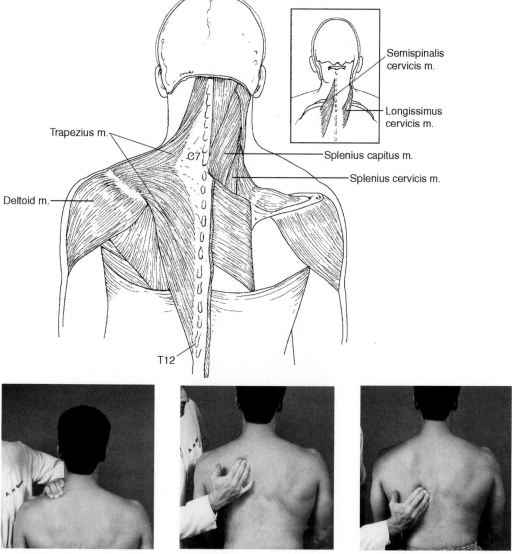

Figure 5-27   **Figure 5-28**   **Figure 5-29**

SHOULDER RANGE OF MOTION

Flexion (1,2)

With the patient seated, place the goniometer in the sagittal plane at the level of the glenohumeral joint (Fig. 5-30). Instruct the patient to elevate the arm forward while following it with one arm of the goniometer (Fig. 5-31).

NORMAL RANGE

Normal range is 167° ± 5.7° from the 0 or neutral position.

Note: This expressed degree of motion probably did not permit enough external rotation and abduction to achieve 180° of flexion described by others.

Muscles	*Nerve Supply*
1. Anterior deltoid	Axillary
2. Pectoralis major	Lateral pectoral
3. Coracobrachialis	Musculocutaneous
4. Biceps	Musculocutaneous

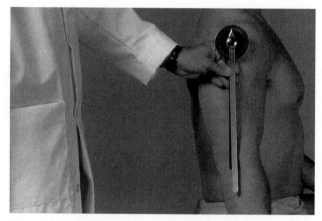

Figure 5-30

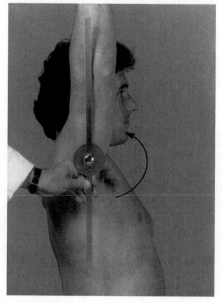

Figure 5-31

Extension (1,2)

With the patient seated, place the goniometer in the sagittal plane at the level of the glenohumeral joint (Fig. 5-32). Instruct the patient to elevate the arm backward while following it with one arm of the goniometer (Fig. 5-33).

NORMAL RANGE

Normal range is 62° ± 9.5° from the 0 or neutral position.

Muscles	*Nerve Supply*
1. Posterior Deltoid	Axillary
2. Teres major, minor	Subscapular
3. Latissimus dorsi	Thoracodorsal
4. Pectoralis major	Lateral Pectoral
5. Triceps	Radial

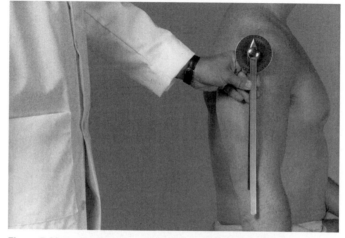

Figure 5-32

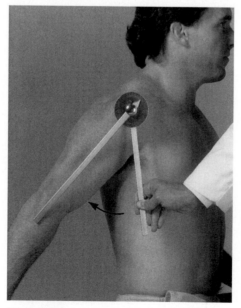

Figure 5-33

Internal Rotation (1,2)

Have the seated patient abduct the arm to 90° and flex the elbow to 90°. This is the 0 or neutral position for rotation of the shoulder. Place the goniometer in the sagittal plane with the center at the lateral aspect of the elbow (Fig. 5-34). Instruct the patient to rotate the shoulder inward by moving the forearm so that the palm of the hand faces posteriorly, and follow the forearm with one arm of the goniometer (Fig. 5-35).

NORMAL RANGE

Normal range is 69° ± 5.6° from the 0 or neutral position.

Muscles	*Nerve Supply*
1. Pectoralis major	Lateral Pectoral
2. Anterior deltoid	Axillary
3. Latissimus dorsi	Thoracodorsal
4. Teres major	Subscapular
5. Subscapularis	Subscapular

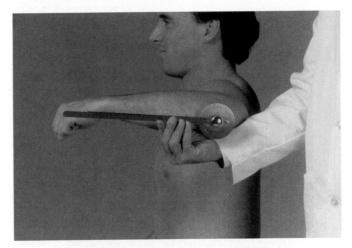

Figure 5-34

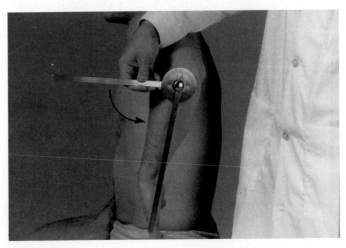

Figure 5-35

External Rotation (1,2)

Have the seated patient abduct the arm to 90° and flex the elbow to 90°. This is the 0 or neutral position for rotation of the shoulder. Place the goniometer in the sagittal plane with the center at the lateral aspect of the elbow (Fig. 5-36). Instruct the patient to rotate the shoulder outward by moving the forearm so that the palm of the hand faces anteriorly, and follow the forearm with one arm of the goniometer (Fig. 5-37).

NORMAL RANGE

Normal range is 104° ± 8.5° from the 0 or neutral position.

Muscles	*Nerve Supply*
1. Infraspinatus	Suprascapular
2. Posterior deltoid	Axillary
3. Teres minor	Axillary

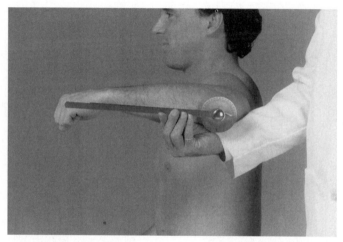

Figure 5-36

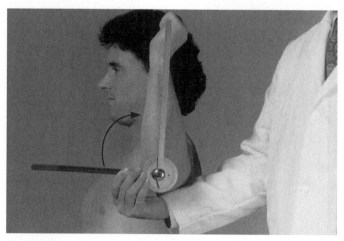

Figure 5-37

Abduction (1,2)

With the patient seated, place the goniometer in the coronal plane with the center at the level of the glenohumeral joint (Fig. 5-38). Instruct the patient to raise the arm laterally. Follow it with one arm of the goniometer (Fig. 5-39).

NORMAL RANGE

Normal range is $184° \pm 7°$ from the 0 or neutral position.

Muscles	Nerve Supply
1. Deltoid	Axillary
2. Supraspinatus	Suprascapular
3. Infraspinatus	Suprascapular
4. Subscapularis	Suprascapular
5. Teres minor	Axillary
6. Biceps brachii, long head	Musculocutaneous

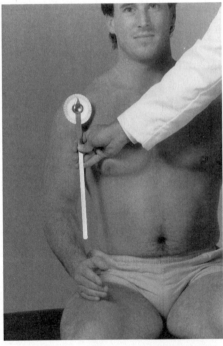

Figure 5-38

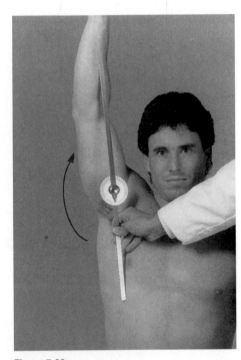

Figure 5-39

Adduction

With the patient seated, place the goniometer in the coronal plane with the center at the level of the glenohumeral joint (Fig. 5-40). Instruct the patient to raise the arm medially. Follow it with one arm of the goniometer (Fig. 5-41).

NORMAL RANGE

Normal range is 75° or greater from the 0 or neutral position.

NOTE

Adduction is a composite movement of flexion and adduction. Most sources do not measure composite movements. I consider it a clinically important movement and think it should be measured.

Muscles	*Nerve Supply*
1. Pectoralis major	Lateral pectoral
2. Latissimus dorsi	Thoracodorsal
3. Teres major	Subscapular
4. Subscapularis	Subscapular

5

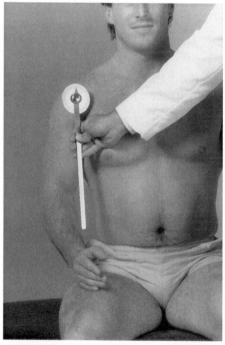

Figure 5-40

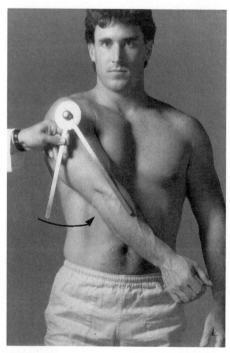

Figure 5-41

TENDINITIS (SUPRASPINATUS)

CLINICAL DESCRIPTION

Supraspinatus tendinitis is a common inflammatory condition of the shoulder that causes anterior shoulder pain. This inflammatory condition may be caused by trauma, overuse (especially overhead movements), or faulty body mechanics during athletic activity, such as pitching or bowling.

Especially in abduction, the patient has painful passive range of motion and limited active range of motion and is apprehensive while performing these movements. The painful arc is usually between 60° and 90° of abduction. During this range the greater tuberosity passes under the acromion and the coracoacromial ligament. Pain and anterior spasm of the shoulder may indicate a moderately inflamed swollen tendon. If the irritation of the tendon continues, calcific deposits may develop and lead to calcific tendinitis.

> ### CLINICAL SIGNS AND SYMPTOMS
> - Anterolateral shoulder pain
> - Pain sleeping on the affected side
> - Stiffness
> - Catching of the shoulder during use
> - Pain on active and passive range of motion
> - Local tenderness

Supraspinatus Tendinitis Test

Sensitivity/Reliability Scale

0   1   2   3   4

PROCEDURE

With the patient seated, instruct him to abduct the arm to 90° with the arm between abduction and forward flexion. Instruct the patient to abduct the arm against resistance (Fig. 5-42).

RATIONALE

Resisting shoulder abduction stresses mainly the deltoid muscle and the supraspinatus muscle and tendon. Pain and/or weakness over the insertion of the supraspinatus tendon may indicate degenerative tendinitis or a tear of the supraspinatus tendon. Pain over the deltoid muscle may indicate a strained deltoid muscle.

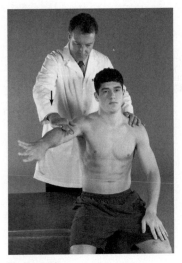

Figure 5-42

Apley Scratch Test (3)

Sensitivity/Reliability Scale

0   1   2   3   4

PROCEDURE

Instruct the seated patient to place the hand on the side of the affected shoulder behind the head and touch the opposite superior angle of the scapula (Fig. 5-43). Then instruct the patient to place the hand behind the back and attempt to touch the opposite inferior angle of the scapula (Fig. 5-44).

RATIONALE

Actively attempting to touch the opposite superior and inferior aspect of the scapula places stress on the tendons of the rotator cuff. Exacerbation of the patient's pain indicates degenerative tendinitis of one of the tendons of the rotator cuff, usually the supraspinatus tendon.

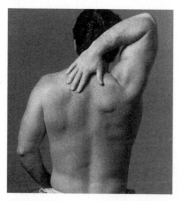

Figure 5-43

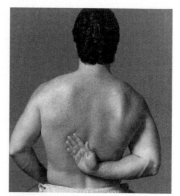

Figure 5-44

Hawkins-Kennedy Impingement Test (4)

Sensitivity/Reliability Scale

0   1   2   3   4

PROCEDURE

With the patient standing, flex the shoulder forward to 90°, then force the shoulder in an internal rotation without resistance by the patient (Fig. 5-45).

RATIONALE

This movement pushes the supraspinatus tendon against the anterior surface of the coracoacromial ligament. Local pain indicates supraspinatus tendinitis.

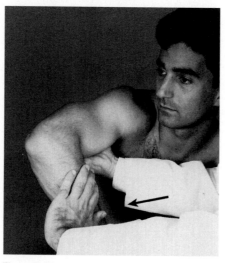

Figure 5-45

Neer Impingement Sign (5)

Sensitivity/Reliability Scale

0   1   2   3   4

PROCEDURE

With the patient seated, grasp the patient's wrist and passively move the shoulder through forward flexion (Fig. 5-46).

RATIONALE

Moving the shoulder through forward flexion jams the greater tuberosity of the humerus against the anterior inferior border of the acromion. Shoulder pain and a look of apprehension on the patient's face indicate a positive sign. This indicates an overuse injury to the supraspinatus muscle or sometimes to the biceps tendon.

> **SUGGESTED DIAGNOSTIC IMAGING**
> - Anteroposterior shoulder radiographs
>   Neutral position
>   Internal rotation
>   External rotation
> - Ultrasonography
> - Magnetic resonance imaging

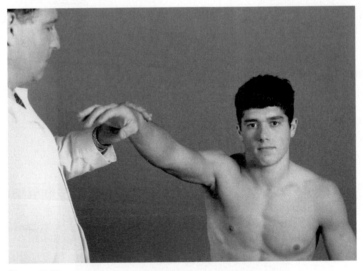

Figure 5-46

TENDINITIS (BICIPITAL)

CLINICAL DESCRIPTION

The biceps brachii has two heads, the long and the short. The long head originates from the superior lip of the glenoid fossa, proceeds laterally, and angles 90° at the bicipital groove on the superior aspect of the humeral head. It is the affected tendon in bicipital tendinitis (Fig. 5-47). Bicipital tendinitis is a chronic condition of shoulder pain with tenderness over the bicipital groove (see Fig. 5-51). Most cases are associated with lesions such as synovitis of the surrounding capsule, adhesive capsulitis, osteophytes in the area of the bicipital groove, or rotator cuff tears. True isolated bicipital tendinitis allows a full free range of passive movement.

CLINICAL SIGNS AND SYMPTOMS

- Anterior shoulder pain
- Pain on palpation of the bicipital groove
- Pain on active and passive elbow flexion and extension

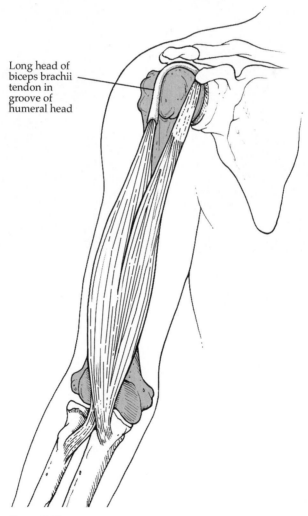

Long head of biceps brachii tendon in groove of humeral head

Figure 5-47

Speed's Test (3,6)

Sensitivity/Reliability Scale

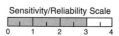

0   1   2   3   4

PROCEDURE

With the patient's elbow completely extended, supinated, and the shoulder flexed forward to 45°, place your fingers on the bicipital groove and your opposite hand on the patient's wrist (Fig. 5-48). Instruct the patient to elevate the arm forward against your resistance (Fig. 5-49).

RATIONALE

This test stresses the biceps tendon in the bicipital groove. Pain or tenderness in the bicipital groove indicates bicipital tendinitis.

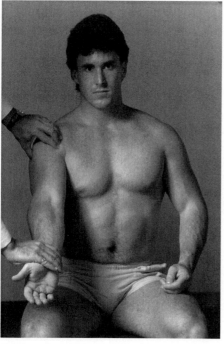

Figure 5-48

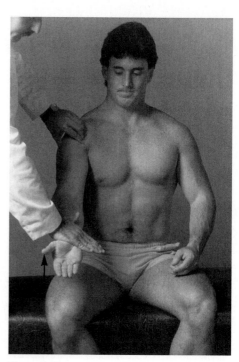

Figure 5-49

Lippman's Test (6)

PROCEDURE

Instruct the sitting patient to flex the elbow to 90°. Stabilize the elbow with one hand, and with your other hand palpate the biceps tendon and move it from side to side in the bicipital groove (Fig. 5-50).

RATIONALE

Moving the biceps tendon manually in the bicipital groove stresses the tendon and transverse humeral ligament. Pain indicates bicipital tendinitis. Apprehension may indicate a propensity for subluxation or dislocation of the biceps tendon out of the bicipital groove or a ruptured transverse humeral ligament (Fig. 5-51).

5

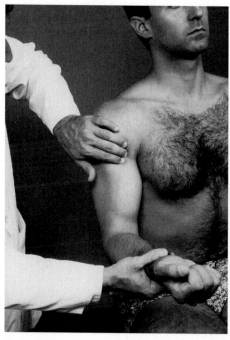

Figure 5-50

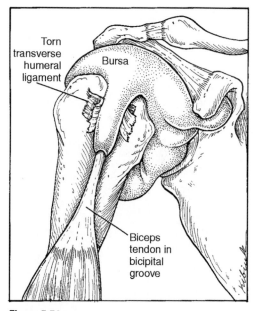

Torn transverse humeral ligament

Bursa

Biceps tendon in bicipital groove

Figure 5-51

Gilchrest's Sign (7)

Sensitivity/Reliability Scale

0   1   2   3   4

PROCEDURE

Instruct the standing patient to grasp a 5- to 7-lb weight and lift it overhead (Fig. 5-52). Next, instruct the patient to rotate the shoulder externally and the lower the arm slowly to the side (Fig. 5-53).

RATIONALE

This test is similar to the Abbott-Saunders test, but it is not passive, and it requires the use of a weight. Abduction and external rotation of the shoulder stress the biceps tendon against the transverse humeral ligament. Pain and/or discomfort in the bicipital groove indicates bicipital tendinitis. An audible snap may indicate a subluxation or dislocation of the biceps tendon out of the bicipital groove, which may be due to a lax or ruptured transverse humeral ligament or a congenitally shallow bicipital groove.

> SUGGESTED DIAGNOSTIC IMAGING
> * Anteroposterior shoulder radiographs
>   Neutral position
>   Internal rotation
>   External rotation
> * Ultrasonography
> * Magnetic resonance imaging

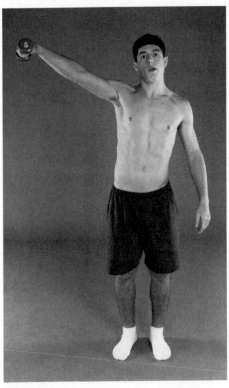

Figure 5-52

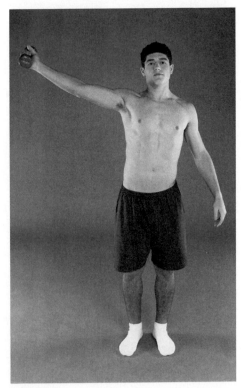

Figure 5-53

BURSITIS

CLINICAL DESCRIPTION

The subacromial bursa overlies the rotator cuff tendons and is continuous with the subdeltoid bursa (see Fig. 5-55). Isolated subacromial or subdeltoid bursitis is rare. Usually the bursitis is associated with tendinitis of the adjacent supraspinatus tendon. Anatomically the inner synovial wall of the subdeltoid bursa is the outer wall of the supraspinatus tendon, so if there is inflammation in one of those structures, there is inflammation of the other. Some of the most common causes of bursitis are trauma, overuse, repeated multiple minor traumas, and improper executed activity.

> ### CLINICAL SIGNS AND SYMPTOMS
> - Anterolateral shoulder pain
> - Pain sleeping on the affected side
> - Stiffness
> - "Catching" of the shoulder during use
> - Pain on active and passive range of motion
> - Local tenderness

Subacromial Push-Button Sign

PROCEDURE

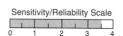

Sensitivity/Reliability Scale

0   1   2   3   4

With the patient seated, apply pressure to the subacromial bursa (Fig. 5-54).

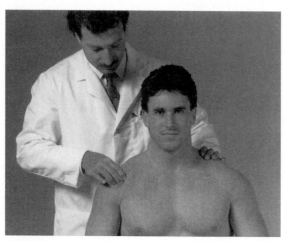

Figure 5-54

RATIONALE

Pressure to the subacromial bursa will irritate an already inflamed bursa. Local pain suggests inflammation of the subacromial bursa or bursitis (Fig. 5-55).

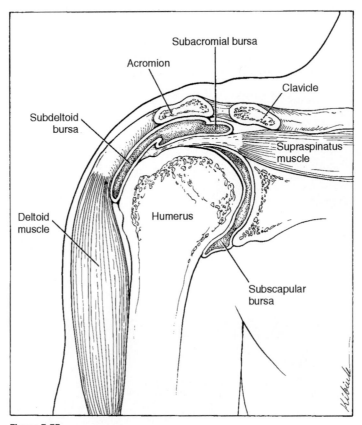

Figure 5-55

Dawbarn's Test (6)

Sensitivity/Reliability Scale
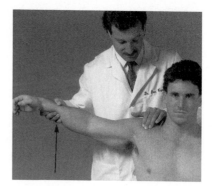
0   1   2   3   4

PROCEDURE

With the patient seated, apply pressure just below the acromion process on the side being tested. Note any pain or tenderness (Fig. 5-56). Then, abduct the patient's arm past 90°, maintaining pressure on the spot below the acromion (Fig. 5-57).

RATIONALE

The spot below the acromion is the palpable portion of the subacromial bursa. Pain and/or tenderness at that location may indicate inflammation of the bursa or bursitis. When the arm is abducted, the deltoid muscle will cover that spot below the acromion. Covering that spot reduces pressure on the bursa, decreasing the tenderness if the bursa is inflamed. A decrease in the tenderness to that point indicates subacromial bursitis (Fig. 5-58).

5

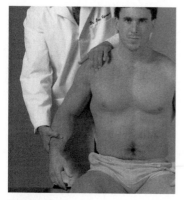

Figure 5-56

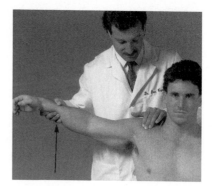

Figure 5-57

SUGGESTED DIAGNOSTIC IMAGING

- Anteroposterior shoulder radiographs
    Neutral position
    Internal rotation
    External rotation
- Ultrasonography
- Magnetic resonance imaging

Figure 5-58

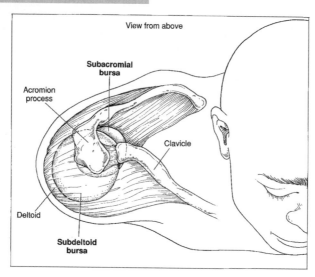

ANTERIOR GLENOHUMERAL INSTABILITY

CLINICAL DESCRIPTION

Anterior shoulder instability is the major cause of shoulder dislocations. This is attributed to anatomic weakness on the anterior structures of the glenohumeral joint: the anterior capsule, glenohumeral ligaments, rotator cuff tendons, and glenoid labrum. There are three types of anterior dislocations, based on the direction of dislocation: subclavicular, subcoracoid and subglenoid. The subcoracoid is the most common. The most common cause of shoulder dislocation is a fall on an outstretched arm.

CLINICAL SIGNS AND SYMPTOMS

- Painful arc (if dislocated)
- Feeling of shoulder slippage
- Apprehension on movement
- Crepitus on movement
- Increased shoulder girth (if dislocated)

Anterior Drawer Test (8)

Sensitivity/Reliability Scale

0   1   2   3   4

PROCEDURE

With the patient supine, place his or her hand in your axilla. With your opposite hand, grasp the posterior scapula with your fingers and place your thumb over the coracoid process (Fig. 5-59). Using the arm that is holding the patient's hand, grasp the posterior aspect of the patient's arm and draw the humerus forward (Fig. 5-60).

RATIONALE

Attempting to move the humerus forward while stabilizing the scapula tests the integrity of the anterior portion of the rotator cuff, which holds the humerus into the glenoid cavity. A click and/or an abnormal amount of movement compared with the normal side indicates anterior instability of the glenohumeral joint.

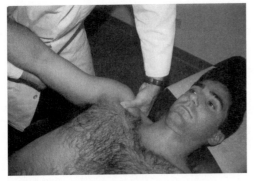

Figure 5-59

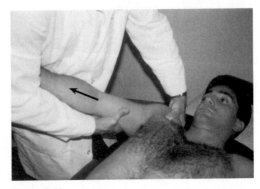

Figure 5-60

Anterior Apprehension Test (3)

Sensitivity/Reliability Scale

0   1   2   3   4

PROCEDURE

Stand behind the seated patient. Abduct the affected arm to 90° and externally rotate it slowly while stabilizing the posterior aspect of the shoulder with the opposite hand (Fig. 5-61).

RATIONALE

Local pain indicates a chronic anterior shoulder dislocation. This test is called apprehension because it is intended to elicit a look of apprehension on the patient's face. The patient may also state that the test feels the same as when the shoulder was dislocated.

External rotation of the arm predisposes the humerus to dislocate anteriorly. This test forces external rotation to dislocate the humerus anteriorly from the glenoid fossa. If the rotator cuff muscles, joint capsule, and glenoid fossa are sound, the patient should have no pain or apprehension when this test is performed. It tests the integrity of the inferior glenohumeral ligament, anterior capsule, rotator cuff tendons, and glenoid labrum.

5

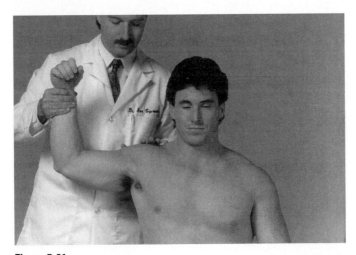

Figure 5-61

Prone Anterior Instability Test (9)

Sensitivity/Reliability Scale

0   1   2   3   4

PROCEDURE

With the patient prone, grasp the patient's forearm, abduct the arm to 90°, with the elbow flexed to 90° (Fig.5-62). Place your other hand over the humeral head and push it forward (Fig. 5-63).

RATIONALE

This is an attempt to dislocate the head of the humerus anteriorly. Anterior shoulder pain or a reproduction of the patient's symptoms indicate a positive test. This procedure tests the integrity of the inferior glenohumeral ligament, anterior capsule, rotator cuff tendons, and glenoid labrum.

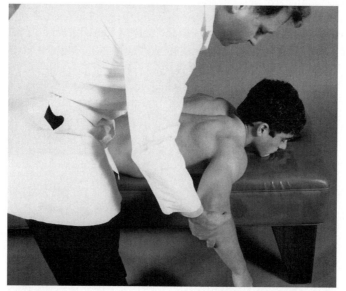

Figure 5-62

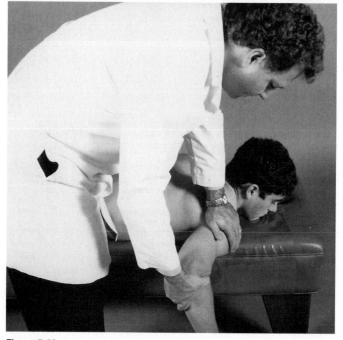

Figure 5-63

Andrews Anterior Instability Test (9)

PROCEDURE

With the patient supine, grasp the patient's distal humerus, abduct the shoulder to 130°, and externally rotate it to 90° (Fig. 5-64). With your opposite hand grasp the humeral head from the posterior and push it anterior (Fig. 5-65).

RATIONALE

This is an attempt to dislocate the head of the humerus anteriorly. Anterior shoulder pain or a reproduction of the patient's symptoms indicate a positive test. This procedure tests the integrity of the inferior glenohumeral ligament, anterior capsule, rotator cuff tendons, and glenoid labrum. If a labral tear is present, a clunk may be heard.

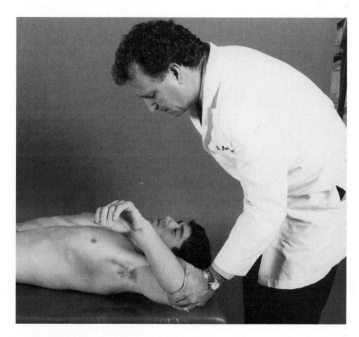

Figure 5-64

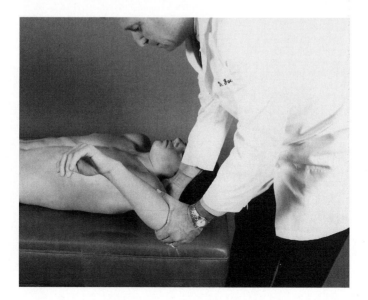

Figure 5-65

Rockwood Test (10)

PROCEDURE

This test is a variation of the anterior apprehension test. With the patient seated, externally rotate the shoulder with the arm in the neutral position (Fig. 5-66). Repeat the test with the arm at 45° of abduction (Fig. 5-67), then at 90° of abduction (Fig. 5-68), then at 120° of abduction (Fig. 5-69).

RATIONALE

The patient must show marked apprehension at 90° with pain. At 0° there is rarely any apprehension. At 45° and 120° there should be more pain with slight apprehension. The patient may say that it felt the same as when the shoulder was previously dislocated. This procedure tests the integrity of the inferior glenohumeral ligament, anterior capsule, rotator cuff tendons, and glenoid labrum.

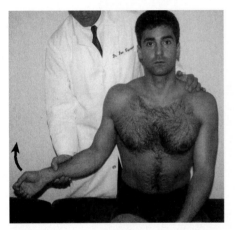

Figure 5-66

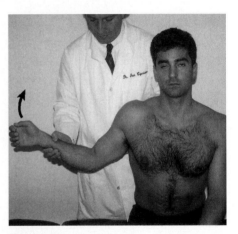

Figure 5-67

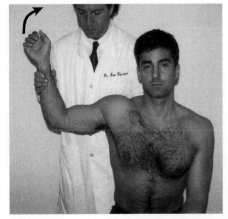

Figure 5-68

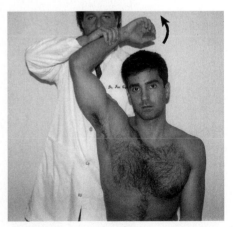

Figure 5-69

Rowe Test for Anterior Instability (11)

PROCEDURE

Instruct the seated patient to place the hand on the side of the affected shoulder behind the head. Then, place your clenched fist against the posterior humeral head and push anteriorly, using your opposite hand to extend the patient's arm (Fig. 5-70).

RATIONALE

The examiner is attempting to dislocate the patient's glenohumeral joint anteriorly. A look of apprehension indicates a positive test. The patient may also may say that it felt the same as when the shoulder was previously dislocated. This procedure tests the integrity of the inferior glenohumeral ligament, anterior capsule, rotator cuff tendons, and glenoid labrum.

5

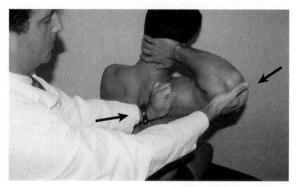

Figure 5-70

Fulcrum Test (12)

PROCEDURE

With the patient supine and the arm abducted to 90°, place your hand under the glenohumeral joint and externally rotate the patient's arm over the hand (Fig. 5-71).

RATIONALE

This is an attempt to dislocate the head of the humerus anteriorly. A look of apprehension with pain is a positive sign. The patient may say that it felt the same as when the shoulder was previously dislocated. This procedure also tests the integrity of the inferior glenohumeral ligament, anterior capsule, rotator cuff tendons, and glenoid labrum. A congenitally shallow glenoid fossa may also predispose the shoulder to dislocation.

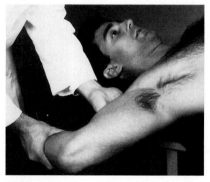

Figure 5-71

Dugas Test (13,14)

Sensitivity/Reliability Scale

0   1   2   3   4

PROCEDURE

With the patient seated, instruct him or her to touch the opposite shoulder and bring the elbow to the chest wall (Fig. 5-72).

RATIONALE

Inability to touch the opposite shoulder because of pain indicates an anterior dislocation of the humeral head out of the glenoid cavity. This dislocation is usually caused by forced external rotation when the arm is abducted. When the humerus is dislocated anteriorly, a characteristic sign is a prominent acromion process.

> **SUGGESTED DIAGNOSTIC IMAGING**
> - Anteroposterior shoulder radiographs
>   Neutral position
>   Internal rotation
>   External rotation
> - Axillary shoulder radiograph
> - Tangential shoulder radiograph
> - Computed tomographic (CT) arthrography

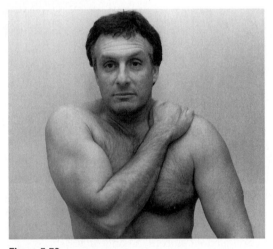

Figure 5-72

POSTERIOR GLENOHUMERAL INSTABILITY

CLINICAL DESCRIPTION

Posterior glenohumeral dislocation is seen in only 5% to 10% of shoulder dislocations. In this type of dislocation the head of the humerus dislocates posteriorly and is found behind the scapula. This is usually caused by trauma to the anterior aspect of the shoulder that drives a forceful backward movement of the humeral head. Instability of the rotator cuff and/or the posterior joint capsule may predispose the joint to posterior dislocation.

> ### CLINICAL SIGNS AND SYMPTOMS
> - Painful arc (if dislocated)
> - Feeling of shoulder slippage
> - Apprehension on movement
> - Crepitus on movement
> - Increased shoulder girth (if dislocated)

Posterior Apprehension Test (6)

Sensitivity/Reliability Scale

0   1   2   3   4

PROCEDURE

With the patient supine, forwardly flex and internally rotate his or her shoulder. With your hand, apply posterior pressure on the elbow (Fig. 5-73).

RATIONALE

This test attempts to dislocate the shoulder posteriorly and stresses the rotator cuff and posterior joint capsule. Local pain or discomfort and a look of apprehension on the patient's face indicates chronic posterior shoulder instability. The patient may say that it felt the same as when the shoulder was previously dislocated. The mechanism of injury is commonly a position of forced adduction with internal rotation in some degree of elevation.

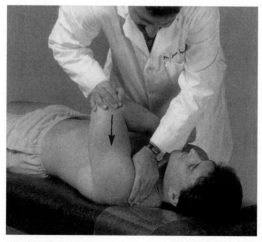

Figure 5-73

Posterior Drawer Test (15)

Sensitivity/Reliability Scale

0   1   2   3   4

PROCEDURE

With the patient supine, grasp the patient's forearm, flex the patient's elbow, and abduct and flex the shoulder. With your opposite hand, stabilize the scapula with your index and middle finger on the spine of the scapula and your thumb on the coracoid process (Fig. 5-74). Rotate the forearm internally and flex the shoulder forward, taking the thumb of your other hand off the coracoid and forcing the humerus posteriorly (Fig. 5-75).

RATIONALE

This is an attempt to dislocate the shoulder posteriorly, stressing the rotator cuff and joint capsule. Local pain and a look of apprehension are the signs of a positive test. This test stresses the rotator cuff and the posterior joint capsule.

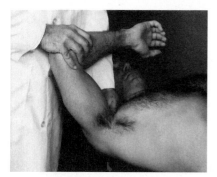

Figure 5-74

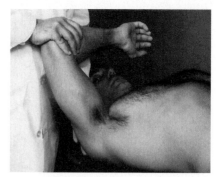

Figure 5-75

Norwood Stress Test (16,17)

Sensitivity/Reliability Scale

0   1   2   3   4

PROCEDURE

With the patient supine, instruct the patient to abduct the shoulder to 90°, externally rotate it to 90°, and flex the elbow to 90°. With one hand, stabilize the scapula while palpating the posterior aspect of the humeral head (Fig. 5-76). With your opposite hand, grasp the elbow, bringing the shoulder into forward flexion and forcing the elbow posteriorly (Fig. 5-77).

RATIONALE

This test is an attempt to dislocate the shoulder posteriorly, stressing the rotator cuff and the posterior joint capsule. A positive test is indicated by the humeral head slipping posteriorly out of the glenoid fossa. When the arm is returned to the starting position, the humeral head should reduce. A clicking sound may accompany the reduction.

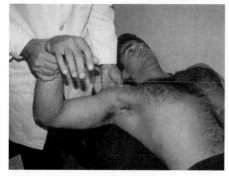

Figure 5-76

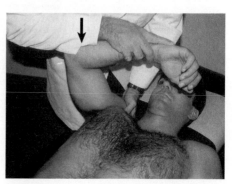

Figure 5-77

Push-Pull Test (12)

Sensitivity/Reliability Scale

0   1   2   3   4

PROCEDURE

With the patient supine, grasp the patient's wrist and abduct the arm to 90° and forward flex it to 30° forward (Fig. 5-78). With your opposite hand, grasp the arm near the humeral head, pull up on the wrist, and push down on the arm (Fig. 5-79).

RATIONALE

In the normal patient, up to 50% of translation is considered a negative test. More than 50% translation and a look of apprehension indicate a positive test. This test is also an attempt to dislocate the shoulder posteriorly. It stresses the rotator cuff and posterior joint capsule.

5

> **SUGGESTED DIAGNOSTIC IMAGING**
>
> - Anteroposterior shoulder radiographs
>   Neutral position
>   Internal rotation
>   External rotation
> - Axillary shoulder radiograph
> - Tangential shoulder radiograph
> - CT arthrography

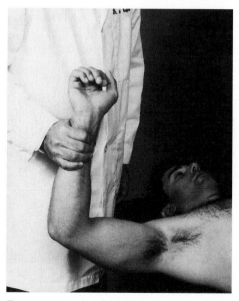

Figure 5-78

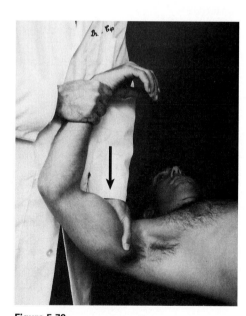

Figure 5-79

MULTIDIRECTIONAL SHOULDER INSTABILITY

CLINICAL DESCRIPTION

Multidirectional shoulder instability is a combination of anterior and posterior shoulder instability. The following tests are attempts to dislocate the shoulder in multiple directions. The different instabilities are described in the sections on the anterior and posterior shoulder instabilities.

> **CLINICAL SIGNS AND SYMPTOMS**
> - Painful arc (if dislocated)
> - Feeling of shoulder slippage
> - Apprehension on movement
> - Crepitus on movement
> - Increased shoulder girth (if dislocated)

Feagin Test (10)

Sensitivity/Reliability Scale

0   1   2   3   4

PROCEDURE

With the patient standing, instruct the patient to abduct the arm and place the hand on your shoulder (Fig. 5-80). With both hands, grasp the patient's humerus next to the humeral head and exert downward and forward pressure (Fig. 5-81).

RATIONALE

A look of apprehension on the patient's face signifies a positive test. This indicates an anterior inferior shoulder instability. This test is an attempt to dislocate the shoulder anteriorly and inferiorly. It tests the integrity of the inferior glenohumeral ligament, anterior capsule, rotator cuff tendons, and glenoid labrum.

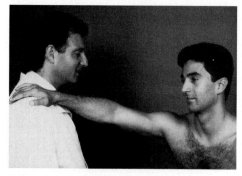

Figure 5-80

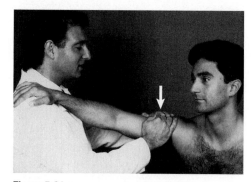

Figure 5-81

Rowe Test for Multidirectional Instability (11)

Sensitivity/Reliability Scale

0   1   2   3   4

PROCEDURE

To test for inferior instability, have the patient stand bending forward 45°. Grasp the shoulder with the index and middle finger over the posterior humeral head and the thumb at the anterior humeral head. With your opposite hand, grasp the patient's elbow and pull down on the arm (Fig. 5-82). To test for anterior instability, push the humeral head forward from behind with your thumb and extend the patient's arm 20° to 30° (Fig. 5-83). To test for posterior instability, push the humeral head posteriorly from the anterior with your index and middle fingers with the patient's shoulder flexed 20° to 30° (Fig. 5-84).

RATIONALE

This test is an attempt to dislocate the humeral head out of the glenoid fossa in various directions. A look of apprehension and/or local discomfort on the patient's face is a positive sign. This test stresses the glenohumeral ligament, rotator cuff tendons, and the joint capsule.

5

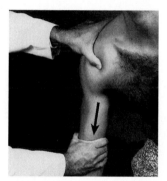

Figure 5-82

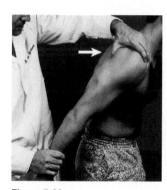

Figure 5-83

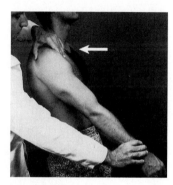

Figure 5-84

Sulcus Sign (18)

Sensitivity/Reliability Scale

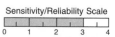

0   1   2   3   4

PROCEDURE

With the patient seated, instruct the patient to flex the elbow to 90° with the shoulder in the neutral position for rotation (Fig. 5-85). Grasp the patient's wrist with one hand, pressing down on the forearm with the other hand (Fig. 5-86).

RATIONALE

Pressing down on the forearm with the patient's shoulder in the neutral position is an attempt to dislocate the shoulder inferiorly. A sulcus at the anterolateral aspect of the shoulder indicates an inferior shoulder instability. The sulcus is graded according to its size. A +1 sulcus indicates less than 1cm. A +2 sulcus indicates 1 to 2 cm. A +3 sulcus indicates more than 2 cm.

SUGGESTED DIAGNOSTIC IMAGING
- Anteroposterior shoulder radiographs
  Neutral position
  Internal rotation
  External rotation
- Axillary shoulder radiograph
- Tangential shoulder radiograph
- CT arthrography

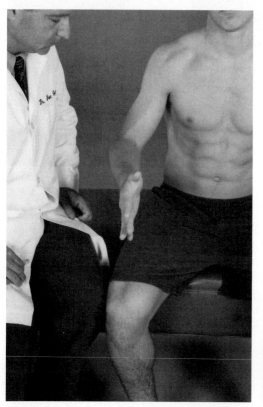

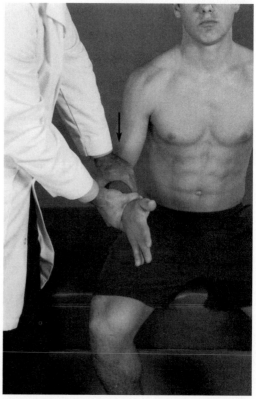

Figure 5-85   **Figure 5-86**

LABRAL TEARS

CLINICAL DESCRIPTION

The edge of the glenoid fossa is surrounded by a fibrocartilage rim called the glenoid labrum. The superior portion of the labrum blends with the tendon of the long head of the biceps muscle (Fig. 5-87). This fibrocartilage rim adds depth to the glenoid fossa and helps to hold the humerus in place. Tearing of any part of the labrum predisposes dislocation of the humerus out of the glenoid cavity in the direction of the tear. These tears are relatively common to throwing athletes.

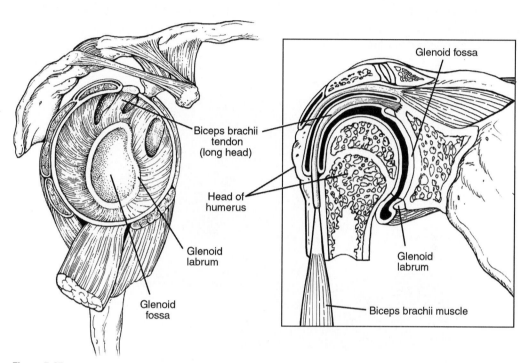

Figure 5-87

Clunk Test (6)

Sensitivity/Reliability Scale

0   1   2   3   4

PROCEDURE

With the patient supine the examiner places one hand over the posterior aspect of the humeral head. With the opposite hand the examiner grasps the elbow and fully abducts the shoulder (Fig. 5-88). The examiner then pushes anteriorly with the hand over the humeral head and externally rotates the shoulder with the opposite hand (Fig. 5-89).

RATIONALE

Anterior pressure to the humeral head with external rotation of the shoulder attempts to dislocate the shoulder anteriorly. A clunk or grinding sound indicates a positive test which suggests an anterior tear of the glenoid labrum.

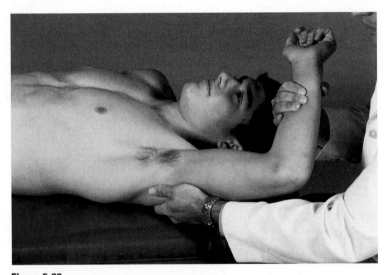

Figure 5-88

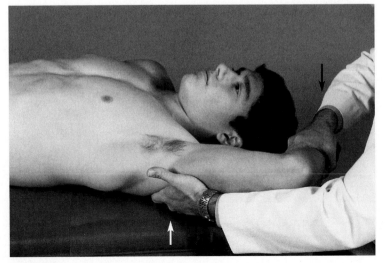

Figure 5-89

Anterior Slide Test (18,19)

PROCEDURE

With the patient seated, instruct the patient to place the hands on the waist with the thumbs posterior (Fig. 5-90). With one hand, stabilize the scapula and clavicle. With the opposite hand, grasp the humerus and place anterior superior force to the shoulder (Fig. 5-91).

RATIONALE

Anterior and superior force to the shoulder may dislocate the shoulder anteriorly and superiorly. If a pop or crack is noted and the patient complains of pain to the anterosuperior aspect of the shoulder, this indicates a superior or anterior tear of the glenoid labrum.

5

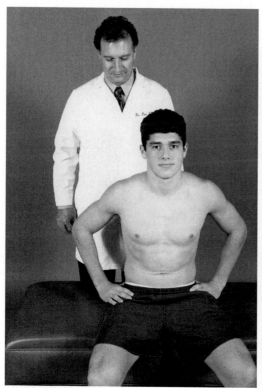

Figure 5-90

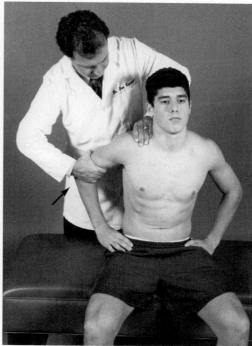

Figure 5-91

ROTATOR CUFF INSTABILITY

CLINICAL DESCRIPTION

Rotator cuff instability involves partial or complete tearing of one of the tendons of the rotator cuff. Usually the supraspinatus tendon is involved, but it may involve the adjacent subscapularis or infraspinatus tendon. Incomplete tears in younger adults are usually due to microtrauma. In older adults, diminishing blood supply may cause the tendons to become frail and tear. Complete tears are usually due to sudden severe strain caused by a fall or overexertion. Incomplete tears usually clinically resemble supraspinatus tendinitis. In complete tears the patient cannot abduct the arm, and any attempt to do so is followed by severe pain.

CLINICAL SIGNS AND SYMPTOMS

- Severe anterior lateral shoulder pain
- Pain when sleeping on the affected side
- Stiffness
- "Catching" of the shoulder during use
- Pain on active and passive range of motion
- Localized tenderness
- Unable to abduct shoulder

Drop Arm Test (2)

Sensitivity/Reliability Scale

| | | | | |
|0|1|2|3|4|

PROCEDURE

With the patient seated, abduct the arm past 90° (Fig. 5-92). Instruct the patient to lower the arm slowly (Fig. 5-93).

RATIONALE

If the patient cannot lower the arm slowly or if it drops suddenly, this indicates a rotator cuff tear, usually of the supraspinatus. The supraspinatus muscle acts as an abductor of the arm and holds the head of the humerus in place. A tear of the supraspinatus tendon causes unsteadiness of the humerus in abduction, causing it to drop suddenly.

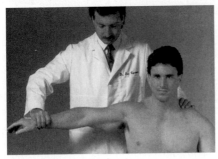

Figure 5-92

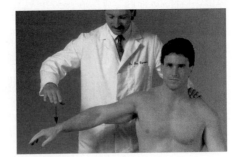

Figure 5-93

Supraspinatus Test (20)

Sensitivity/Reliability Scale

0   1   2   3   4

PROCEDURE

With the patient either sitting or standing, instruct the patient to abduct the shoulder to 90°. Grasp the patient's arm and press down against resistance by the patient (Fig. 5-94). Next, instruct the patient to rotate the shoulders internally so that the thumb faces downward. Again, press down on the arm against resistance by the patient (Fig. 5-95).

RATIONALE

Resistance to abduction stresses the supraspinatus muscle and tendon. Weakness or pain may indicate a tear of the supraspinatus muscle or tendon. Weakness may also indicate suprascapular neuropathy.

5

> **SUGGESTED DIAGNOSTIC IMAGING**
>
> - Anteroposterior shoulder radiographs
>   Neutral position
>   Internal rotation
>   External rotation
> - Axillary shoulder radiograph
> - CT arthrography
> - Magnetic resonance imaging (MRI)

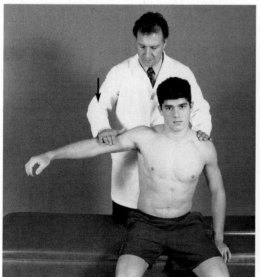

Figure 5-94

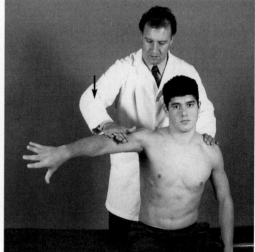

Figure 5-95

BICEPS TENDON INSTABILITY

CLINICAL DESCRIPTION

The biceps brachii has two heads: long and short. The long head originates from the superior lip of the glenoid fossa and proceeds laterally and angles 90° at the bicipital groove. It is held in the bicipital groove by the transverse humeral ligament (see Fig. 5-98). A shallow bicipital groove or lax or ruptured transverse humeral ligament may snap the biceps tendon into and out of the bicipital groove, causing anterior shoulder pain with point tenderness at the bicipital groove. This painful snap may also indicate a tear of the biceps tendon. A bicipital tendon tear is followed by swelling and ecchymosis near the bicipital groove and a characteristic bulging of the belly of the biceps muscle near the antecubital fossa (Popeye sign).

> **CLINICAL SIGNS AND SYMPTOMS**
> - Anterior shoulder pain
> - Stiffness
> - Pain on active and passive range of motion
> - Localized tenderness
> - Bulging of bicep muscle (complete tear)

Yergason's Test (21)

Sensitivity/Reliability Scale

0   1   2   3   4

PROCEDURE

With the patient seated and the elbow flexed to 90°, stabilize the patient's elbow with one hand (Fig. 5-96). With your opposite hand, grasp the patient's wrist and have the patient externally rotate the shoulder and supinate the forearm against your resistance (Fig. 5-97).

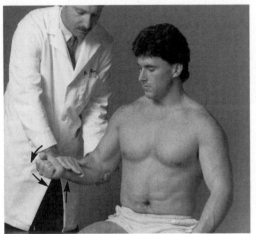

Figure 5-96

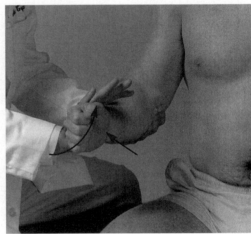

Figure 5-97

RATIONALE

Resisted supination of the forearm and external rotation of the shoulder stress the bicipital tendon and the transverse humeral ligament. Local pain and/or tenderness in the bicipital tendon indicates an inflammation of the biceps tendon or tendinitis. If the tendon pops out of the bicipital groove, suspect a lax or ruptured transverse humeral ligament or a congenital shallow bicipital groove causing the tendon to subluxate (Fig. 5-98).

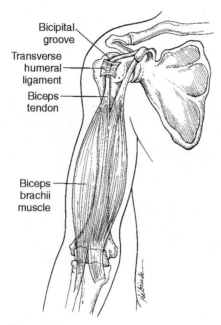

Figure 5-98

Abbott-Saunders Test (22)

Sensitivity/Reliability Scale

0 1 2 3 4

PROCEDURE

With the patient seated, abduct and maximally rotate the patient's arm externally (Fig. 5-99), then lower the arm to the patient's side while palpating the bicipital groove with your opposite hand (Fig. 5-100).

RATIONALE

Abduction and external rotation of the shoulder stress the biceps tendon against the transverse humeral ligament. A palpable or audible click at the bicipital groove indicates a subluxation or dislocation of the biceps tendon out of the groove caused by a lax or ruptured transverse humeral ligament or congenitally shallow bicipital groove.

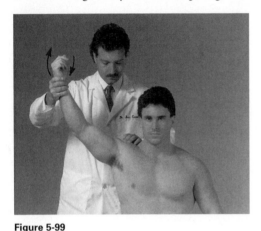

Figure 5-99

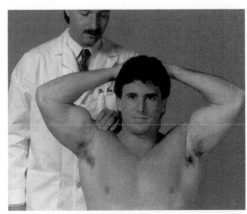

Figure 5-100

Ludington's Test (6)

Sensitivity/Reliability Scale

0 1 2 3 4

PROCEDURE

Instruct the patient to clasp both hands on top of the head, interlocking the fingers, (Fig. 5-101) and alternately contract and relax the biceps muscle while you palpate the biceps tendon (Fig. 5-102).

RATIONALE

Placing the hands on the head supports the upper limb and allows relaxation of the biceps muscle. If the biceps tendon on the affected side is not contracting and palpable, suspect a rupture of the long head of the biceps tendon.

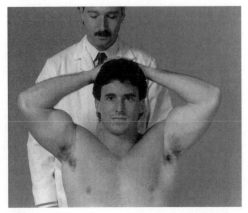

Figure 5-101

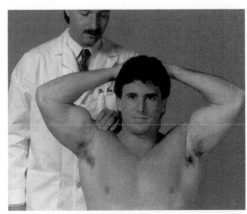

Figure 5-102

Transverse Humeral Ligament Test (6)

PROCEDURE

With the patient seated, grasp the patient's wrist. Abduct the shoulder to 90° and internally rotate it with one hand. With your opposite hand, palpate the bicipital groove (Fig. 5-103). Then externally rotate the shoulder (Fig. 5-104).

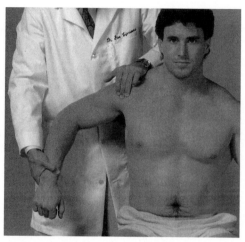

Figure 5-103

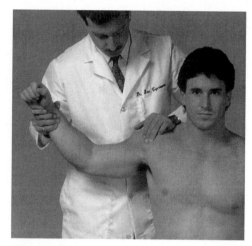

Figure 5-104

5

RATIONALE

External rotation of the shoulder moves the biceps tendon in the bicipital groove. If you feel the bicipital tendon snap in and out of the bicipital groove, suspect a torn or lax transverse humeral ligament or shallow bicipital groove (Fig. 5-105).

SUGGESTED DIAGNOSTIC IMAGING

- Anteroposterior shoulder radiographs
  - Neutral position
  - Internal rotation
  - External rotation
  - Axillary
- CT arthrography
- MRI

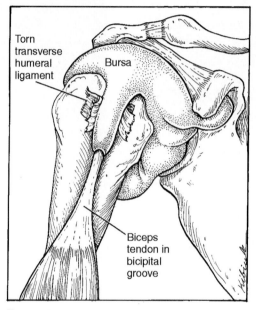

Figure 5-105

THORACIC OUTLET SYNDROME

CLINICAL DESCRIPTION

Thoracic outlet syndrome is a group of signs and symptoms that result from compression of the subclavian vessels and brachial plexus at the superior aperture of the thorax. It may be caused by trauma, repetitive motions, overuse, and some systemic diseases, such as diabetes and thyroid disease. Patients may complain of neck and shoulder pain with numbness and tingling affecting the entire upper extremity. The ulnar side of the limb is predominantly involved. Using the affected extremity in an overhead or elevated position is difficult.

> ### CLINICAL SIGNS AND SYMPTOMS
> - Upper extremity pain
> - Upper extremity paresthesias
> - Grip weakness
> - Upper extremity edema
> - Upper extremity coldness
> - Excessive dryness of arm or hand
> - Excessive sweating of arm or hand

Adson's Test (23–25)

Sensitivity/Reliability Scale

0   1   2   3   4

PROCEDURE

With the patient seated, establish the amplitude of the radial pulse (Fig. 5-106). Compare the amplitude bilaterally. Instruct the patient to take a deep breath and sustain it while he or she rotates the head and elevates the chin to the side being tested (Fig. 5-107). If the test is negative, have the patient rotate and elevate the chin to the opposite side (Fig. 5-108).

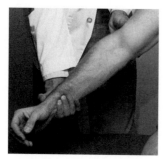

Figure 5-106

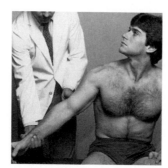

Figure 5-107

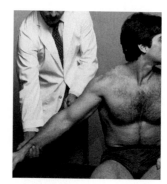

Figure 5-108

RATIONALE

Rotation and extension of the head compress the subclavian artery and brachial plexus. A decrease or absence of the amplitude of the radial pulse indicates a compression of the vascular component of the neurovascular bundle (subclavian artery) by a spastic or hypertrophied scalenus anterior muscle, on a cervical rib, or a mass, such as a Pancoast tumor. Paresthesias or radiculopathy in the upper extremity indicates compression of the neural component of the neurovascular bundle (brachial plexus) (Fig. 5-109).

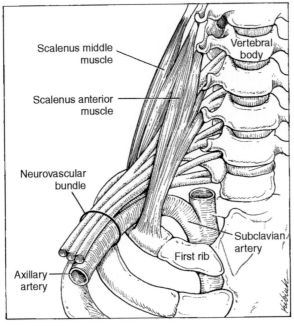

Figure 5-109

Costoclavicular Test (26–28)

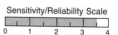
PROCEDURE

With the patient seated, establish a radial pulse (Fig. 5-110). Instruct the patient to force the shoulders posteriorly and have the patient flex the chin to the chest (Fig. 5-111).

RATIONALE

Forcing the shoulders posteriorly decreases the space between the clavicle and first rib. The neurovascular bundle (brachial plexus, axillary artery) and the axillary vein run through a narrow cleft beneath the clavicle and on top of the first rib.

Decrease or absence of the amplitude of the radial pulse indicates a compression to the vascular component of the neurovascular bundle. This compression is caused by a decrease in the space between the clavicle and the first rib. This decrease may be caused by a recent or healed fracture to the clavicle or first rib with or without callus formation, dislocation of the medial aspect of the clavicle, or a spastic or hypertrophied subclavius muscle. Paresthesias or radiculopathy in the upper extremity indicates compression to the brachial plexus or compression of the axillary vein (Fig. 5-112). Compression of the brachial plexus is usually localized to a nerve root or peripheral nerve distribution. Compression of the axillary vein typically presents as diffuse radicular vascular discomfort not localized to a nerve root or peripheral nerve distribution.

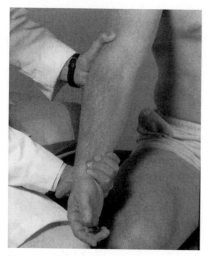

Figure 5-110

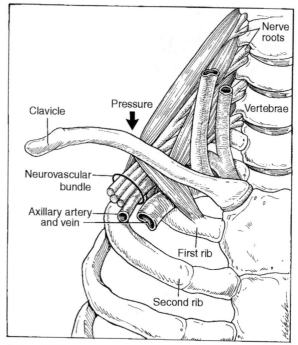

Figure 5-112

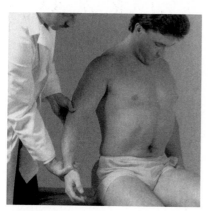

Figure 5-111

Wright's Test (29, 30)

Sensitivity/Reliability Scale
0   1   2   3   4

PROCEDURE

With the patient seated, establish the character of the radial pulse (Fig. 5-113). Hyperabduct the arm and take the pulse again (Fig. 5-114).

RATIONALE

The axillary artery, vein, and three cords of the brachial plexus pass under the pectoralis minor muscle on the coracoid process. Abduction of the arm to 180° stretches these structures around the tendon of the pectoralis minor muscle and the coracoid process. Decrease or absence of the amplitude of the radial pulse indicates compression of the axillary artery either by a spastic or hypertrophied pectoralis minor muscle or by a deformed or hypertrophied coracoid process (Fig. 5-115).

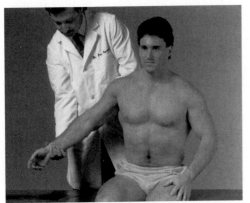

Figure 5-113

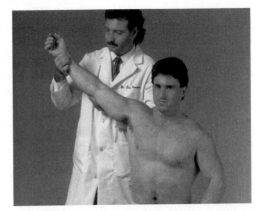

Figure 5-114

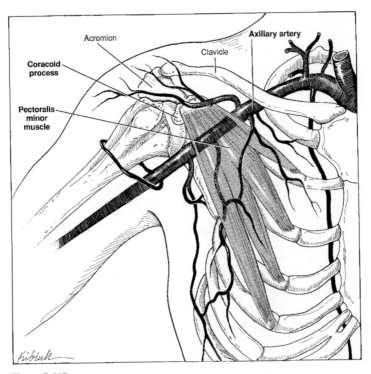

Figure 5-115

Traction Test (31)

Sensitivity/Reliability Scale

0   1   2   3   4

PROCEDURE

With the patient seated, establish a radial pulse (Fig. 5-116). While maintaining the pulse, extend and apply traction to the arm (Fig. 5-117).

RATIONALE

Traction and extension of the arm pulls the subclavian artery over the first rib. A decreased or obliterated pulse is not diagnostic; however, when the test is repeated on the opposite side and reveals no change, the test indicates a subluxated or malpositioned first rib or a cervical rib on the side of the decreased or obliterated pulse.

5

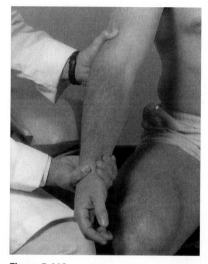

Figure 5-116

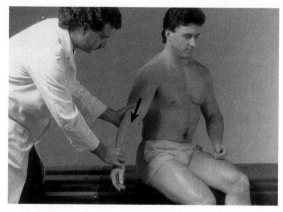

Figure 5-117

Halstead Maneuver (6)

Sensitivity/Reliability Scale

0   1   2   3   4

PROCEDURE

With the patient seated, find the radial pulse and note the amplitude (Fig. 5-118). With your opposite hand, pull on the patient's arm and ask the patient to hyperextend the neck (Fig. 5-119). Repeat the test on opposite arm.

RATIONALE

Traction pressure on the arm pulls the neurovascular bundle (brachial plexus and axillary artery) over the first rib. Extension of the neck tightens the scalene muscles. A decreased or obliterated pulse amplitude indicates a cervical rib, subluxation, or malposition of the first rib. An upper extremity radicular component indicates compression of the brachial plexus by the scalenus anterior muscle (See Fig. 5-109).

> **SUGGESTED DIAGNOSTIC IMAGING**
> - Plain film radiography
>   Posteroanterior chest (if apical mass is suspect)
>   Apical lordotic view
> - Electrodiagnostic study

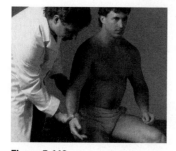

Figure 5-118

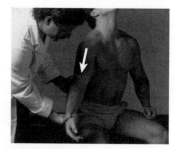

Figure 5-119

BRACHIAL PLEXUS IRRITATION

CLINICAL DESCRIPTION

Irritation of the brachial plexus may be due to various factors, such as a cervical rib, severe upper traction of the arm, fractured clavicle, or pulmonary apical mass. Any of these irritations may cause upper extremity radicular symptoms. Most of the following tests are upper limb tension signs that are equivalent to the straight leg raising test for lumbar radiculopathy. These tests are attempts to stress the neurological structures in the upper limb to determine neurological irritation; they stress all of the structures in the upper extremities but are used here for reproduction of the neurological signs reported by the patient.

> ### CLINICAL SIGNS AND SYMPTOMS
> - Upper extremity radicular pain
> - Upper extremity paresthesias
> - Grip weakness

Brachial Plexus Stretch Test

Sensitivity/Reliability Scale

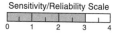

PROCEDURE

With the patient seated, instruct the patient to laterally flex the head opposite the affected side and extend the shoulder and elbow (Fig. 5-120).

RATIONALE

This test is similar to a straight leg raising test for the upper extremity. This test stretches the brachial plexus opposite the side of lateral head flexion. Any damage to the plexus will cause pain and/or paresthesia along the distribution of the brachial plexus. Pain and paresthesia on the side of lateral bending may indicate a nerve root problem. Local cervical pain on the side of lateral bending may indicate a cervical facet joint problem because the facets are compressed on the side of lateral bending.

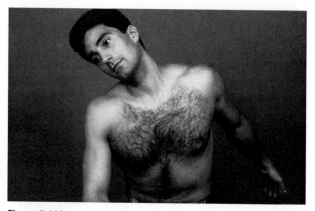

Figure 5-120

Bikele's Sign (32)

Sensitivity/Reliability Scale

0   1   2   3   4

Procedure

With the patient seated, instruct him or her to abduct the shoulder to 90° and extend it as far as possible with the elbow fully flexed (Fig. 5-121). Instruct the patient to extend the elbow fully (Fig. 5-122).

Rationale

Abduction and extension of the shoulder place a motion-induced distraction on the brachial plexus. Adding the motion of elbow extension produces maximum distraction of the brachial plexus. If this movement is met with resistance and/or increases radicular pain to the upper extremity, this may indicate brachial plexus neuritis, nerve root irritation, or meningeal irritation of the covering of the cervical nerve roots.

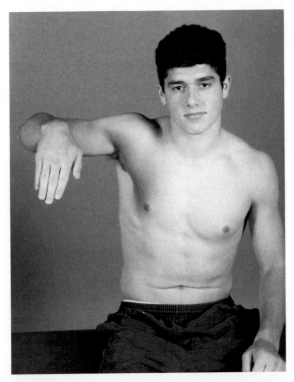

Figure 5-121

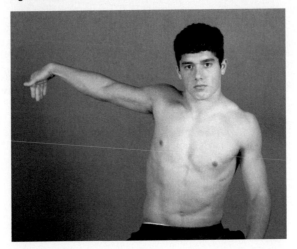

Figure 5-122

Brachial Plexus Tension Test (32)

PROCEDURE

With the patient seated and the arms in the neutral position, grasp the patient's arms and passively abduct it to the end point of joint play or to the point of pain (Fig. 5-123). Tell the patient to rotate the arms externally and maintain that position while you support the arm (Fig. 5-124). Finally, instruct the patient to flex the elbows so that the hand is behind the patient's head (Fig. 5-125).

RATIONALE

Abduction and external rotation of the shoulder with elbow flexion provide maximum stretch to the brachial plexus and the C8 to T1 nerve roots. Reproduction of the patient's symptoms suggests brachial plexus irritation. If the irritation is at the level of the nerve roots, radicular symptoms may also be reproduced.

5

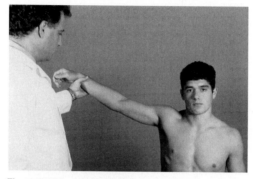

Figure 5-123

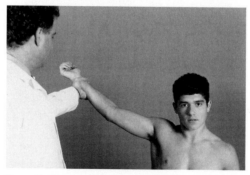

Figure 5-124

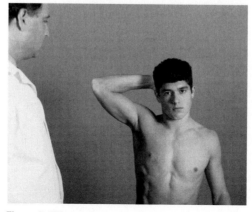

Figure 5-125

Tinnel's Sign (for Brachial Plexus Lesions) (33)

Sensitivity/Reliability Scale

0   1   2   3   4

PROCEDURE

With the patient seated and the head laterally flexed, tap along the trunks of the brachial plexus with your index finger (Fig. 5-126).

RATIONALE

Local pain may indicate a cervical plexus lesion. A tingling sensation in the distribution of one of the trunks may indicate compression or neuroma of one or more of the trunks of the brachial plexus.

SUGGESTED DIAGNOSTIC TESTS
• Electrodiagnostic studies

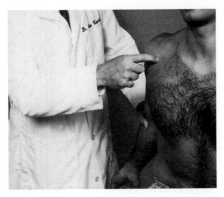

Figure 5-126

References

1. American Academy of Orthopaedic Surgeons. The Clinical Measurement of Joint Motion. Chicago: American Academy of Orthopaedic Surgeons, 1995.
2. Boons DC, Azen SP. Normal range of motion of joints in male subjects. J Bone Joint Surg Am 1979;61:756–759.
3. Hoppenfeld S. Physical Examination of the Spine and Extremities. New York: Appleton-Century-Crofts, 1976;127.
4. Hawkins RJ, Kennedy JC. Impingement syndrome in athletics. Am J Sports Med 1980; 8:151–163.
5. Neer CS, Welsh RP. The shoulder in sports. Orthop Clin North Am 1977;8:583–591.
6. MaGee DJ. Orthopedic Physical Assessment. 2nd ed. Philadelphia: WB Saunders, 1992.
7. Post M. Physical Examination of the Musculoskeletal System. Chicago: Year Book, 1987.
8. Gerber C, Maitland GD. Practical Orthopedic Medicine. London: Butterworths, 1969.
9. Andrews JA, Timmerman LA, Wilks KE. Athletic Injuries of the Shoulder. New York: McGraw-Hill, 1995.
10. Rockwood CA. Subluxations and dislocations about the shoulder. In: Rockwood CA, Green DP, eds. Fractures in adults–1. Philadelphia: JB Lippincott, 1985.
11. Rowe CR. Dislocations of the shoulder. In: Rowe CR, ed. The Shoulder. Vol 1. Edinburgh: Churchill Livingstone, 1988.
12. Matsen FA, Thomas SC, Rockwood CA. Glenohumeral instability. In: Rockwood CA, Matsen FA, eds. The Shoulder. Philadelphia: WB Saunders, 1990.
13. Jahn WT. Standardization of orthopaedic testing of the upper extremity. J Manip Physiol Ther 1981;4(2).
14. Stimson BBA. A Manual of Fractures and Dislocations. 2nd ed. Philadelphia: Lea & Febiger, 1946.
15. Gerber C, Ganz R. Clinical assessment of instability of the shoulder. J Bone Joint Surg 1984;66B:551–556.
16. Norwood LA, Terry GC. Shoulder posterior and subluxation. Am J Sports Med 1984;12:25–30.
17. Cofield RH, Irving JF. Evaluation and classification of shoulder instability. Clin Orthop 1987;223:32–43.
18. Kibler WB. Clinical Examination of the Shoulder. In Pettrone A, ed. Athletic Injuries of the Shoulder. New York: McGraw-Hill, 1995.
19. Kibler WB. Specificity and sensitivity of the anterior slide test in throwing athletes with superior glenoid labral tears. Arthroscopy 1995;11: 296–300.
20. Jobe FW, Moynes DR. Delineation of diagnostic criteria and rehabilitation program for rotator cuff injuries. Am J Sports Med 1982;10: 3336–3339.
21. Yergason RM. Supination sign. J Bone Joint Surg 1931;13:160.
22. Abbott LC, Saunders JB. Acute traumatic dislocation of tendon of long head of biceps brachii: report of cases with operative findings. Surgery 1939;6:817–840.
23. Adson AW. Cervical ribs: symptoms, differential diagnosis and indications for section of the insertion of the scalenus anticus muscle. J Coll Int Surg 1951;106:546.
24. Adson AW, Coffey JR. Cervical rib. Ann Surg 1927;85:839–857.
25. Lord JR, Rosati LM, eds. Thoracic-Outlet Syndromes. New Jersey, CIBA Pharmaceutical, 1971;21(2):9–10.
26. Falconer MA, Li FWP. Resection of first rib in costoclavicular compression of the brachial plexus. Lancet 1962;59(1):63.
27. Falconer MA, Weddel G. Costoclavicular compression of the subclavian artery and vein: relation to scalene anticus syndrome. Lancet 1943;2:542.
28. Devay AD. Costoclavicular compression of brachial plexus and subclavian vessels. Lancet 1945;2:165.
29. Wright JS. The neurovascular syndrome produced by hyperabduction of the arms. Am Heart J 1945;29(1).
30. Wright JS. Vascular diseases in clinical practice. 2nd ed. Chicago: Year Book, 1952.
31. McRae R. Clinical Orthopedic Examination. New York: Churchill Livingstone, 1976.
32. Evans RC. Illustrated Essentials in Orthopedic Physical Assessment. 2nd ed. St. Louis: Mosby 2001.
33. Landi A, Copeland S. Value of the Tinel sign in brachial plexus lesions. Ann Roy Coll Surg Eng 1979;61:470–471.

General References

Cailliet R. Shoulder pain. Philadelphia: FA Davis, 1966.

Cipriano J. Calcific tendinitis vs. chronic bursitis in shoulder joint pathology. Today's Chiropractic 1986;14(4):15–16.

Cyriax J. Textbook of Orthopaedic Medicine. Vol. 1. Diagnosis of Soft Tissue Lesions. London: Bailliéré Tindall, 1982.

De Palma AF, Flannery GF. Acute anterior dislocations of the shoulder. J Sports Med Phys Fitness 1973;1:6–15.

Kapandji IA. The Physiology of the Joints. Vol I. Upper Limb. New York: Churchill Livingstone, 1970.

Neviaser JS. Musculoskeletal disorders of the shoulder region causing cervicobrachial pain: differential diagnosis and treatment. Surg Clin North Am 1963;43:1703.

Post M, Silver R, Singh M. Rotator cuff tear: diagnosis and treatment. Clin Orthop 1983;173:78.

Yocum LA. Assessing the shoulder: history, physical examination, differential diagnosis, special tests used. Clin Sports Med 1983;2:281.

6

ELBOW ORTHOPAEDIC TESTS

Elbow Orthopaedic Examination

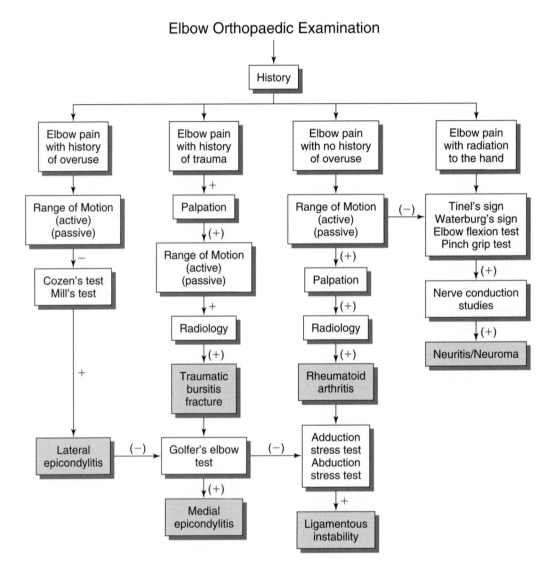

ELBOW PALPATION

Medial Aspect

Ulnar Nerve

DESCRIPTIVE ANATOMY

The ulnar nerve is a branch of the medial cord of the brachial plexus. It passes in the groove between the medial epicondyle and the olecranon fossa (Fig. 6-1).

PROCEDURE

With your index finger, palpate the groove between the medial epicondyle and the olecranon process. Notice whether the nerve is tender to palpation or thickened (Fig. 6-2). This can indicate nerve compression or scar tissue on the nerve leading to paresthesia into the forearm and/or loss of interosseous muscle strength.

6

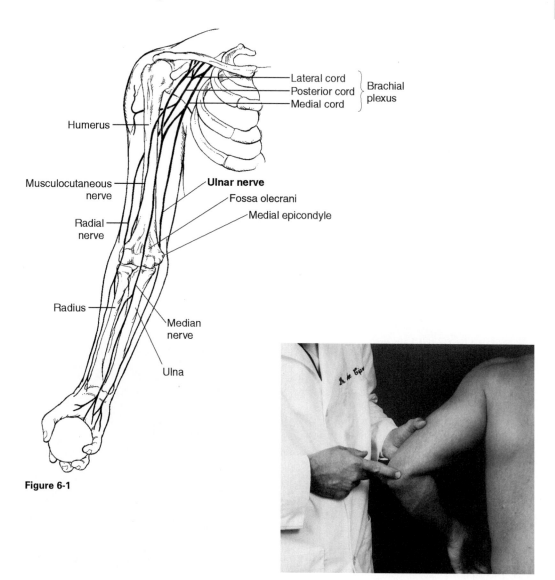

Figure 6-1

Figure 6-2

Medial Epicondyle and Attached Tendons

DESCRIPTIVE ANATOMY

The medial epicondyle is a relatively large protuberance at the medial distal end of the humerus. Attached to the condyle are the wrist flexor and pronator group muscles. This group consists of the pronator teres, flexor carpi radialis, palmaris longus, and flexor carpi ulnaris. All of these muscles originate from the medial epicondyle as a common tendon (Fig. 6-3).

PROCEDURE

With the elbow flexed to 90°, palpate the epicondyle and its tendons with your index finger; look for tenderness, inflammation, and temperature elevation (Fig. 6-4). This may indicate a strain of one or more of the previously mentioned tendons or an inflammation of the medial epicondyle caused by various activities, such as golf or tennis.

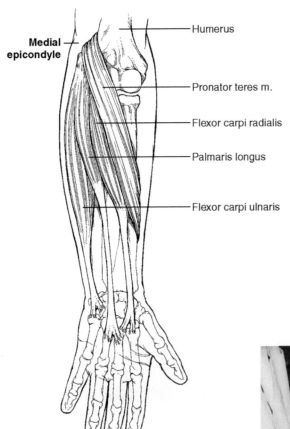

Medial epicondyle

Humerus

Pronator teres m.

Flexor carpi radialis

Palmaris longus

Flexor carpi ulnaris

Figure 6-3

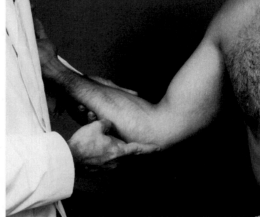

Figure 6-4

Ulnar Collateral Ligament

DESCRIPTIVE ANATOMY

The ulnar collateral ligament attaches the medial epicondyle to the medial aspect of the ulna at the trochanteric notch (Fig. 6-5) and stabilizes the humeroulnar articulation medially.

PROCEDURE

With your index finger, palpate the area of the ulnar collateral ligament (Fig. 6-6). Ordinarily it is not palpable. You should check for tenderness, which may indicate a sprain caused by forced valgus stress.

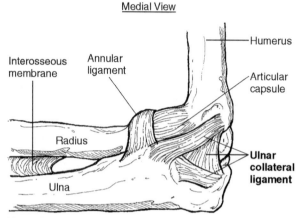

Medial View

Interosseous membrane — Annular ligament — Humerus — Articular capsule — Radius — Ulna — **Ulnar collateral ligament**

Figure 6-5

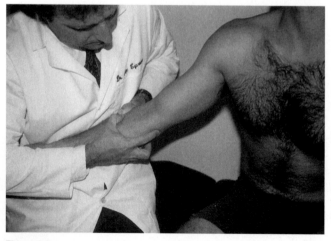

Figure 6-6

6

Lateral Aspect

Lateral Epicondyle and Wrist Extensor Tendons

DESCRIPTIVE ANATOMY

The lateral epicondyle is a relatively large protuberance at the lateral distal end of the humerus. Attached to the condyle is the common extensor tendon. From this tendon arise the carpi radialis brevis, extensor digitorum, extensor digiti minimi, and extensor carpi ulnaris. The brachioradialis and extensor carpi radialis longus and brevis are attached superior to the lateral epicondyle at the supracondylar ridge (Fig. 6-7).

PROCEDURE

With the patient's elbow flexed to 90°, palpate the lateral epicondyle and supracondylar ridge with your index and middle fingers (Fig. 6-8). Note any tenderness, inflammation, and temperature elevation at either location. These signs may indicate an inflammation of the lateral epicondyle (epicondylitis) or a strain of the extensor tendons of the wrist.

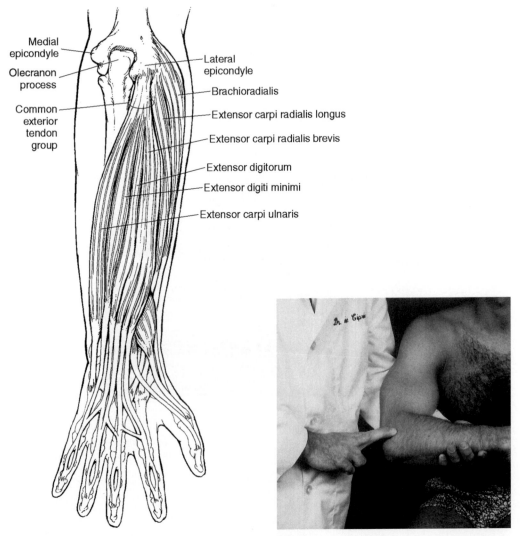

Medial epicondyle
Olecranon process
Common exterior tendon group

Lateral epicondyle
Brachioradialis
Extensor carpi radialis longus
Extensor carpi radialis brevis
Extensor digitorum
Extensor digiti minimi
Extensor carpi ulnaris

Figure 6-7

Figure 6-8

Radial Collateral Ligament and Annular Ligament

DESCRIPTIVE ANATOMY

Radial collateral ligament and annular ligaments are thick structures that extend from the lateral epicondyle of the humerus to the annular ligament and lateral aspect of the ulnar. The annular ligament encircles the radial head (Fig. 6-9). The radial collateral ligament stabilizes the humeroulnar articulation laterally.

PROCEDURE

With your index and middle fingers, palpate the area of the radial collateral ligament from the lateral epicondyle to the annular ligament (Fig. 6-10). Check for tenderness, which may indicate a sprain caused by forced varus stress.

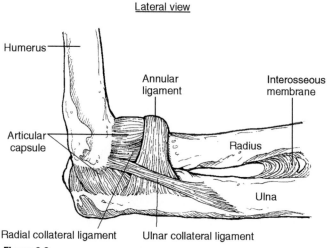

Lateral view

Humerus

Annular ligament

Interosseous membrane

Articular capsule

Radius

Ulna

Radial collateral ligament   Ulnar collateral ligament

Figure 6-9

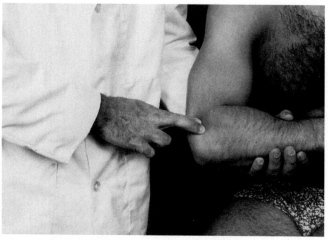

Figure 6-10

Posterior Aspect

Olecranon Process and Bursa

DESCRIPTIVE ANATOMY

The olecranon process is posterior to the elbow at the proximal end of the ulnar. It is covered by the olecranon bursa, which is not normally palpable (Fig. 6-11).

PROCEDURE

With the patient's elbow flexed to 90°, palpate the olecranon process and bursa for tenderness, inflammation, and increased temperature (Fig. 6-12). A thick, boggy feeling may indicate olecranon bursitis. Check the posterior aspect of the olecranon border for rheumatoid nodules, which indicate rheumatoid arthritis.

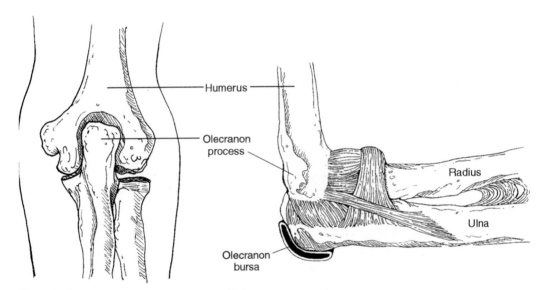

Humerus

Olecranon
process

Radius

Ulna

Olecranon
bursa

Figure 6-11

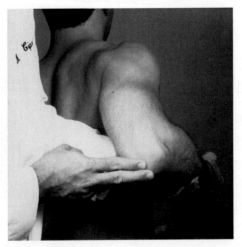

Figure 6-12

Triceps Muscle

DESCRIPTIVE ANATOMY

The triceps muscle has three heads; the long head crosses both the glenohumeral joint and the elbow joint, and it inserts into the olecranon process (Fig. 6-13).

PROCEDURE

With the patient's elbow slightly flexed, have the patient lean on a table. This will facilitate the palpation of the muscle. With your thumb and index finger, palpate the length of the muscle down to the olecranon process, looking for any tenderness or defects secondary to trauma (Fig. 6-14). This may indicate a strain or active trigger points of the triceps muscle. A hard mass may indicate myositis ossificans secondary to repeated trauma.

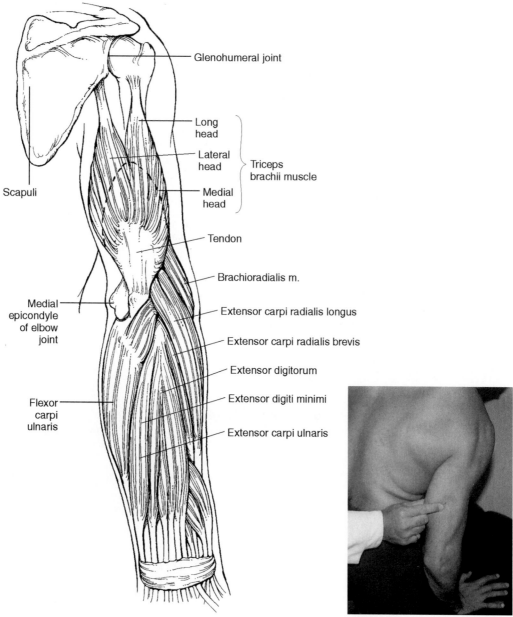

Labels in Figure 6-13:
- Glenohumeral joint
- Long head
- Lateral head
- Triceps brachii muscle
- Scapuli
- Medial head
- Tendon
- Brachioradialis m.
- Medial epicondyle of elbow joint
- Extensor carpi radialis longus
- Extensor carpi radialis brevis
- Extensor digitorum
- Flexor carpi ulnaris
- Extensor digiti minimi
- Extensor carpi ulnaris

Figure 6-13

Figure 6-14

Anterior Aspect

Cubital Fossa

LOCATION

The cubital fossa is the triangular space bordered by the brachioradialis laterally and the pronator teres medially. The base is an imaginary line between the two epicondyles. The structures that pass between the fossa are the biceps tendon, brachial artery, median nerve, and musculocutaneous nerve (Fig. 6-15).

PROCEDURE

With the patient's elbow slightly flexed and the patient resisting flexion, palpate the cubital fossa with your index finger, looking for the biceps tendon, which lies medial to the brachioradialis muscle (Fig. 6-16). Tenderness may indicate a strain in the musculotendinous junction. A ruptured tendon is not palpable in the fossa, and a bulbous gathering of muscle is evident in the upper arm.

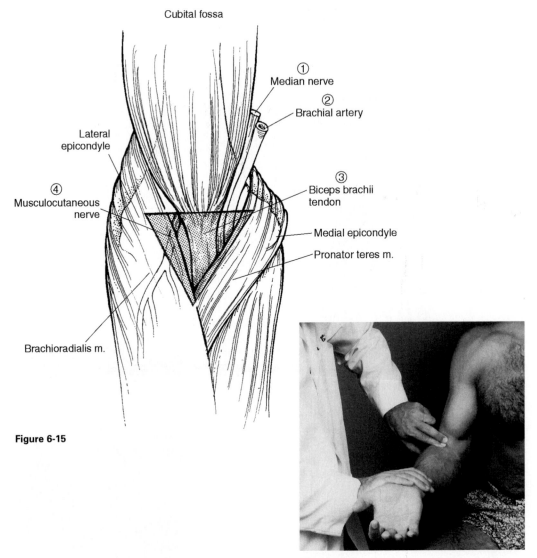

Cubital fossa

① Median nerve

② Brachial artery

Lateral epicondyle

③ Biceps brachii tendon

④ Musculocutaneous nerve

Medial epicondyle

Pronator teres m.

Brachioradialis m.

Figure 6-15

Figure 6-16

ELBOW RANGE OF MOTION

Flexion (1)

With the patient seated, elbow extended, place the goniometer in the sagittal plane with the center at the elbow joint (Fig. 6-17). This is the neutral position for the elbow joint for flexion and extension. Instruct the patient to flex the arm as far as possible while following the forearm with one arm of the goniometer (Fig. 6-18).

NORMAL RANGE

Normal range is 141° ± 4.9° or greater from the 0 or neutral position (2).

Muscles	Nerve Supply
1. Brachialis	Musculocutaneous
2. Biceps brachii	Musculocutaneous
3. Brachioradialis	Radial
4. Pronator teres	Median
5. Flexor carpi ulnaris	Ulnar

6

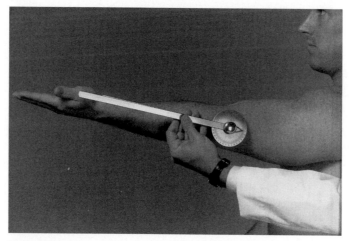

Figure 6-17

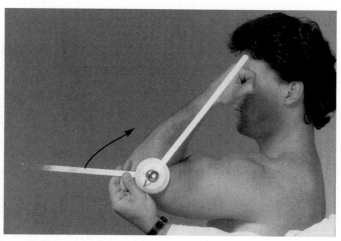

Figure 6-18

Extension (1)

With the elbow in full extension, place the goniometer in the sagittal plane with the center at the elbow joint. Instruct the patient to extend the elbow further while following the forearm with one arm of the goniometer (Fig. 6-19).

NORMAL RANGE

Normal range is 0.3° ± 2.0° from full extension (2).

Muscles	Nerve Supply
1. Triceps	Radial
2. Anconeus	Radial

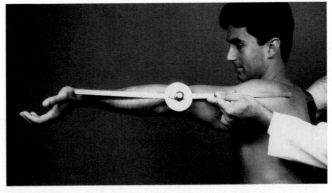

Figure 6-19

Supination (1)

With the patient's elbow in 90° of flexion and the thumb facing upward, place the goniometer in the coronal plane (Fig. 6-20). This is the neutral position for supination and pronation. Instruct the patient to rotate the thumb outward while you follow the thumb with one arm of the goniometer (Fig. 6-21).

NORMAL RANGE

Normal range is 81° ± 4° or more from the 0 or neutral position (2).

Muscles	Nerve Supply
1. Supinator	Radial
2. Biceps brachii	Musculocutaneous

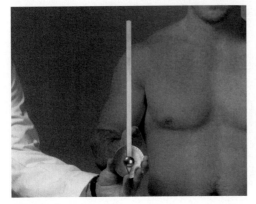
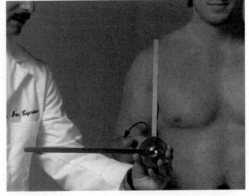

Figure 6-20   **Figure 6-21**

Pronation (1)

With the patient's elbow in 90° of flexion and the thumb facing upward, place the goniometer in the coronal plane (Fig. 6-22). Instruct the patient to rotate the thumb inward while you follow the thumb with one arm of the goniometer (Fig. 6-23).

NORMAL RANGE

Normal range is 75° ± 6.3° or greater from the 0 or neutral position (2).

Muscles	*Nerve Supply*
1. Pronator quadratus	Median
2. Pronator teres	Median
3. Flexor carpi radialis	Median

6

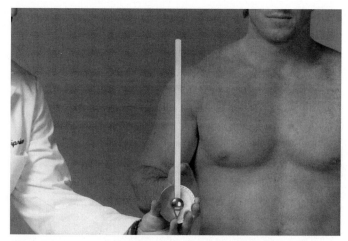

Figure 6-22

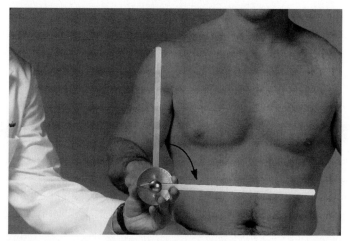

Figure 6-23

LATERAL EPICONDYLITIS (TENNIS ELBOW)

CLINICAL DESCRIPTION

Lateral epicondylitis is a repetitive injury of the common extensor tendon at the lateral epicondyle of the humerus. Repetitive actions include lifting, hammering, and tight gripping with repeated impact during sports activities. This injury causes microtearing and microavulsion at the origin of the extensor carpi radialis tendon. Secondary inflammation develops at the epicondyle after this mechanical injury. Symptoms persist because of constant traction and movement of the wrist and hand.

CLINICAL SIGNS AND SYMPTOMS
• Local lateral elbow pain
• Weakness of the forearm

Cozen's Test (3)

Sensitivity/Reliability Scale

0   1   2   3   4

PROCEDURE

With the patient seated, stabilize the patient's forearm. Instruct the patient to make a fist and extend it (Fig. 6-24). Then force the extended wrist into flexion against resistance (Fig. 6-25).

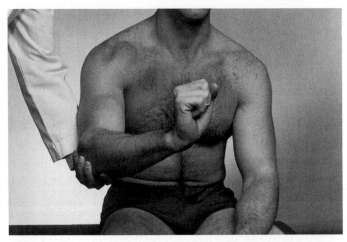

Figure 6-24

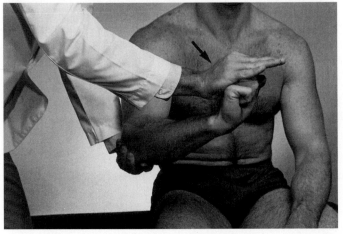

Figure 6-25

RATIONALE

The tendons that extend the wrist are attached to the lateral epicondyle (Fig. 6-26). They are the extensor carpi radialis brevis, extensor digitorum, extensor digiti minimi, and extensor carpi ulnaris. If the condyle itself or the common extensor tendons that attach to it are inflamed, then forcing the extended wrist into flexion can reproduce irritation to the lateral epicondyle and its attaching tendons. If pain is elicited at the lateral epicondyle, suspect inflammation of the lateral epicondyle (epicondylitis).

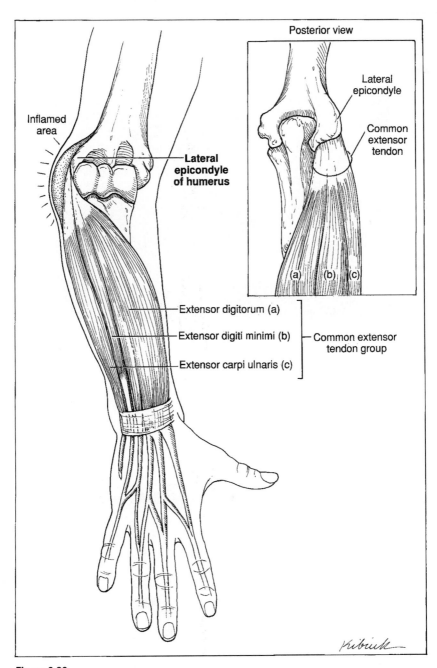

Figure 6-26

Mill's Test (4)

Sensitivity/Reliability Scale

0   1   2   3   4

PROCEDURE

With the patient seated, instruct the patient to pronate the arm and flex the wrist. Then instruct him or her to supinate the arm against resistance (Fig. 6-27).

RATIONALE

The tendon of the supinator muscle, which supinates the wrist, is attached to the lateral epicondyle. If the condyle itself or the tendon of the supinator that attaches to the condyle is inflamed, resisting supination of the wrist may reproduce irritation to the lateral epicondyle and its attaching tendons. If pain is elicited at the lateral epicondyle, suspect inflammation of the lateral epicondyle (epicondylitis).

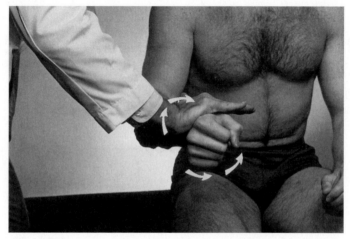

Figure 6-27

Kaplan's Sign (5)

Sensitivity/Reliability Scale
0   1   2   3   4

PROCEDURE

With the patient in the seated position and the elbow slightly flexed, instruct the patient to grip a dynamometer and record the findings (Fig. 6-28). Next, place a tennis elbow brace slightly below the patient's epicondyles (Fig. 6-29). Again, instruct the patient to grip the dynamometer and record the findings.

RATIONALE

Gripping the dynamometer unsupported increases the traction on the common extensor tendon at the lateral epicondyles, which causes pain and produces weakness of the hand and forearm. When a support is placed distal to the epicondyle, pain is reduced and strength is increased because traction to the common extensor tendon is relieved.

> **SUGGESTED DIAGNOSTIC IMAGING**
> * Plain film radiography
>   AP elbow view
>   Lateral elbow view

6

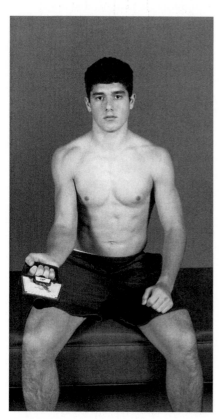

Figure 6-28

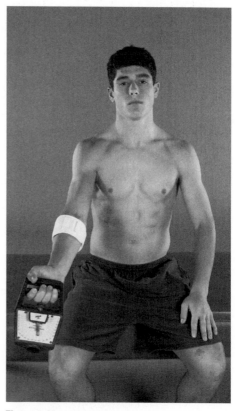

Figure 6-29

MEDIAL EPICONDYLITIS (GOLFER'S ELBOW)

CLINICAL DESCRIPTION

Medial epicondylitis is a repetitive injury of the common flexor tendon at the medial epicondyle of the humerus. Repetitive actions include lifting, hammering, and tight gripping with repetitive impact during sports activities. This injury causes microtearing and microavulsion at the origin of the flexor carpi radialis tendon. Secondary inflammation develops at the epicondyle after this mechanical injury. Symptoms persist due to constant traction and movement of the wrist and hand.

> **CLINICAL SIGNS AND SYMPTOMS**
> - Local medial elbow pain
> - Weakness of the forearm

Golfer's Elbow Test (6)

Sensitivity/Reliability Scale

0 1 2 3 4

PROCEDURE

Tell the seated patient to extend the elbow and supinate the hand. Instruct the patient to flex the wrist against resistance (Fig. 6-30).

RATIONALE

The tendons that flex the wrist, the flexor carpi radialis and flexor carpi ulnaris, are attached to the medial epicondyle (Fig. 6-31). If the condyle itself or the common flexor tendons that attach to it are inflamed, resisting wrist flexion may reproduce irritation to the medial epicondyle and its attaching tendons. If pain is elicited at the medial epicondyle, suspect inflammation of the medial epicondyle (epicondylitis).

> **SUGGESTED DIAGNOSTIC IMAGING**
> - Plain film radiography
>   AP elbow view
>   Lateral elbow view

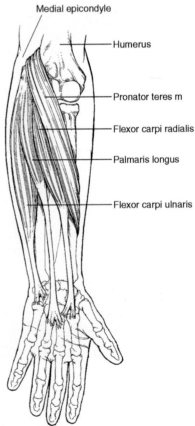

Medial epicondyle

Humerus

Pronator teres m

Flexor carpi radialis

Palmaris longus

Flexor carpi ulnaris

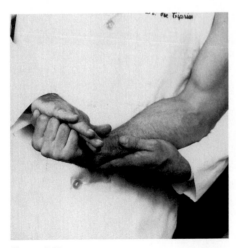

Figure 6-30

Figure 6-31

LIGAMENTOUS INSTABILITY

CLINICAL DESCRIPTION

Ligamentous instability at the elbow is relatively uncommon. The radial collateral ligament at the lateral aspect of the elbow and the ulnar collateral ligament at the medial aspect of the elbow are affected. This injury may be due to forced elbow hyperextension, forced abduction of the extended arm, or forced adduction of the extended arm. Forced adduction of the extended arm will damage the radial collateral ligament. Forced abduction of the extended arm will damage the ulnar collateral ligament. Severe instability may include an avulsion fracture or a complete dislocation of the elbow.

> **CLINICAL SIGNS AND SYMPTOMS**
> - Medial or lateral elbow pain
> - Local swelling

Adduction Stress Test (7)

Sensitivity/Reliability Scale

0   1   2   3   4

6

PROCEDURE

With the patient sitting, stabilize the medial arm and place adduction pressure on the patient's lateral forearm (Fig. 6-32).

RATIONALE

Placing adduction pressure on the lateral forearm applies stress to the radial collateral ligament (Fig. 6-33). Gapping and pain indicate radial collateral ligament instability.

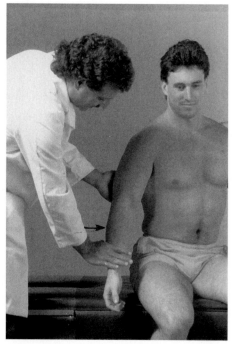

Figure 6-32

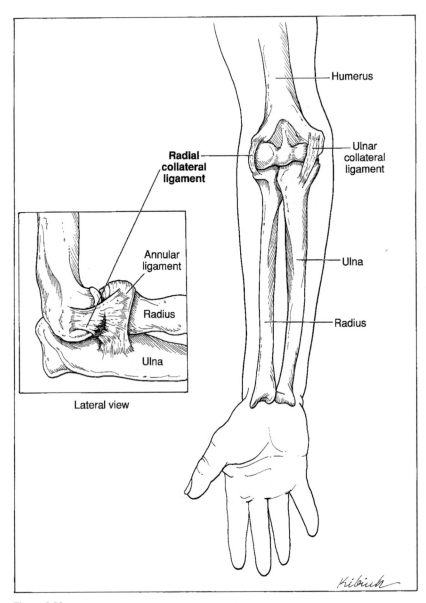

Figure 6-33

Abduction Stress Test (7)

PROCEDURE

With the patient sitting, stabilize the lateral arm and place abduction pressure on the medial forearm (Fig. 6-34).

RATIONALE

Placing an abduction pressure on the medial forearm applies stress to the ulnar collateral ligament. Gapping and pain indicate ulnar collateral ligament instability.

> **SUGGESTED DIAGNOSTIC IMAGING**
>
> - Plain film radiography
>   - AP elbow view
>   - Lateral elbow view
> - Computed tomography
> - Magnetic resonance imaging

6

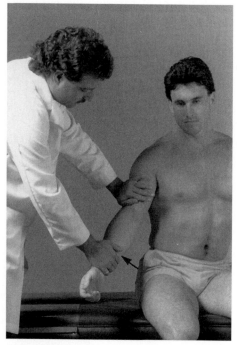

Figure 6-34

NEUROPATHY/COMPRESSION SYNDROMES

CLINCAL DESCRIPTION

Neuropathy and compression syndromes of the elbow are peripheral neurological disorders caused by trauma, overuse, arthritis, or postural considerations. These disorders may cause paresthesia and weakness to the forearm and/or hand. The nerve most affected is the ulnar nerve. The sites of compression or entrapment may include the groove between the olecranon process and medial epicondyle or the cubital tunnel (Fig. 6-35).

> **CLINICAL SIGNS AND SYMPTOMS**
> - Forearm and/or hand paresthesia
> - Forearm and/or hand weakness

Tinel's Sign (8)

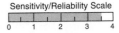

Sensitivity/Reliability Scale

0   1   2   3   4

PROCEDURE

With the patient seated, tap the ulnar nerve in the groove between the olecranon process and the medial epicondyle with a neurological reflex hammer (Fig. 6-36). The ulnar nerve passes in this groove.

RATIONALE

This test is designed to elicit pain caused by a neuritis or neuroma of the ulnar nerve. Pain indicates a positive test. The nerve can become damaged in the following ways:

1. Excessive use or repetitive injuries or trauma of the elbow
2. Arthritis of the elbow joint
3. Cubital tunnel compression, between the heads of the flexor carpi ulnaris muscle
4. Postural habits that compress the nerve, such as sleeping with elbows flexed and hands under head
5. Recurrent nerve subluxations or dislocations

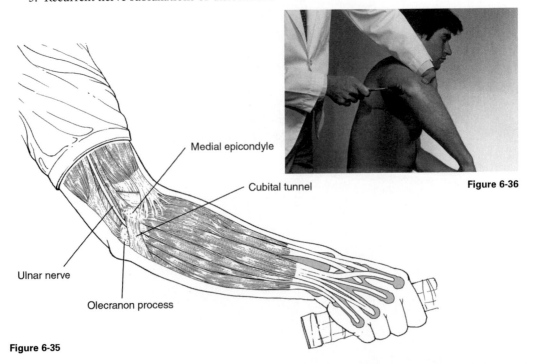

Medial epicondyle

Cubital tunnel

Figure 6-36

Ulnar nerve

Olecranon process

Figure 6-35

Wartenberg's Sign (9)

Sensitivity/Reliability Scale

0   1   2   3   4

PROCEDURE

Instruct the seated patient to place the hand on the table. Passively spread the patient's fingers (Fig. 6-37). Instruct the patient to bring the fingers together (Fig. 6-38).

RATIONALE

The ulnar nerve controls abduction of the fingers. Inability to abduct the little finger to the rest of the hand indicates ulnar nerve neuritis (Fig. 6-39).

6

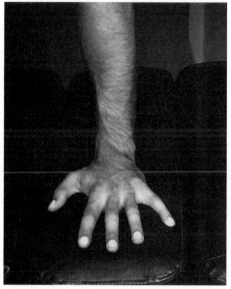

Figure 6-37

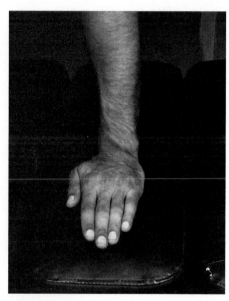

Figure 6-38

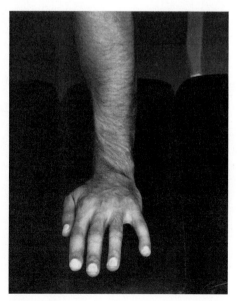

Figure 6-39

Elbow Flexion Test (10)

Sensitivity/Reliability Scale

0   1   2   3   4

PROCEDURE

Instruct the seated patient to flex the elbow completely for 5 minutes (Fig. 6-40).

RATIONALE

Flexion of the elbow may compress the ulnar nerve in the cubital tunnel. Paresthesia along the medial aspect of the forearm and hand may indicate compression of the ulnar nerve in the cubital tunnel (cubital tunnel syndrome) (Fig. 6-41). It can also be trapped between the heads of the flexor carpi ulnaris or by scar tissue in the ulnar groove.

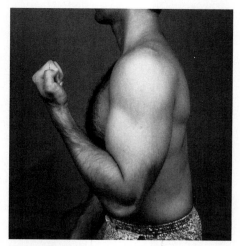

Figure 6-40

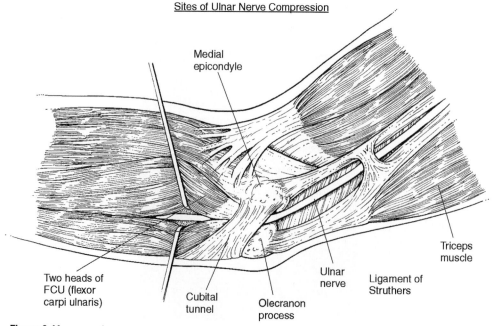

Sites of Ulnar Nerve Compression

Medial
epicondyle

Triceps
muscle

Two heads of
FCU (flexor
carpi ulnaris)

Cubital
tunnel

Olecranon
process

Ulnar
nerve

Ligament of
Struthers

Figure 6-41

Pinch Grip Test (11)

PROCEDURE

Instruct the patient to pinch the tips of the index finger and thumb together (Fig. 6-42).

RATIONALE

Normally the pinch is tip to tip. The test is positive if the pulps of the thumb and index finger touch (Fig. 6-43). This result is caused by an injury to the anterior interosseous nerve, which is a branch of the median nerve. It may also indicate an entrapment syndrome of the anterior osseous nerve between the two heads of the pronator teres muscle (Fig. 6-44).

> **SUGGESTED DIAGNOSTIC AND FUNCTIONAL TESTING**
> • Electrodiagnostic studies

6

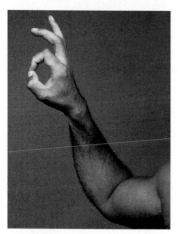

Figure 6-42

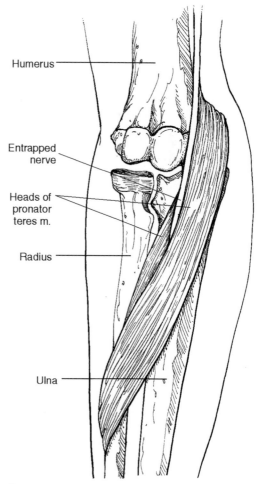

Humerus

Entrapped nerve

Heads of pronator teres m.

Radius

Ulna

Figure 6-44

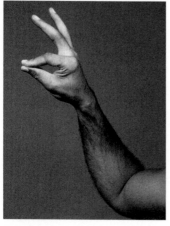

Figure 6-43

References

1. American Academy of Orthopaedic Surgeons. The Clinical Measurement of Joint Motion. Chicago: American Academy of Orthopaedic Surgeons, 1994.
2. Boone DC, Azen SP. Normal range of motion in male subjects. J Bone Joint Surg 1979;61A: 756–759.
3. Lucas GL. Examination of the Hand. Springfield, IL: Charles C. Thomas, 1972.
4. Mills GP. The treatment of tennis elbow. Br Med J 1928;1:12–13.
5. Kaplan EB. Treatment of tennis elbow by denervation. J Bone Joint Surg 1959;41A:147.
6. McRae R. Clinical Orthopedic Examination. New York: Churchill Livingstone, 1976;41.
7. Hoppenfeld S. Physical examination of the spine and extremities. New York: Appleton-Century-Crofts, 1976;127.
8. Tinel J. Nerve wounds; symptomatology of peripheral nerve lesions caused by war wounds. Joll CA, ed, Rothwell F, trans. New York: William Wood, 1918.
9. Volz RC, Morrey BF. The physical examination of the elbow. In: Morrey BF, ed. The Elbow and Its Disorder. Philadelphia: WB Saunders, 1986.
10. Magee DJ. Orthopedic Physical Assessment. 2nd ed. Philadelphia: WB Saunders, 1992.
11. Wiens E, Lane S. The anterior interosseous nerve syndrome. Can J Surg 1978;21:354.

General References

Boyd HB. Tennis elbow. J Bone Joint Surg Am 1973;55:1183–1187.

Cyriax J. Pathology and treatment of tennis elbow. J Bone Joint Surg 1936;18:921.

Cyriax J. Textbook of Orthopaedic Medicine. Vol 1. Diagnosis of soft tissue lesions. London: Bailliéré Tindall, 1982.

Kapandji IA. The physiology of the Joints. Vol 1. Upper Limb. New York: Churchill Livingstone, 1970.

McKee GK. Tennis elbow. Br Med J 1937;2:434.

Mennell JM. Joint Pain. Boston: Little, Brown, 1964.

Nagler W, Johnson E, Gardner R. The pain of tennis elbow. Current Concepts Pain Analg, 1986.

Nirschl R, Pettrone F. Tennis elbow. J Bone Joint Surg 1979;61A(6):836.

Post M. Physical examination of the musculoskeletal system. Chicago: Year Book, 1987.

Roles NC, Maudsley RH. Radial tunnel syndrome: resistant tennis elbow as a nerve entrapment. J Bone Joint Surg Br 1972;54:499.

WRIST ORTHOPAEDIC TESTS

Wrist Orthopaedic Examination

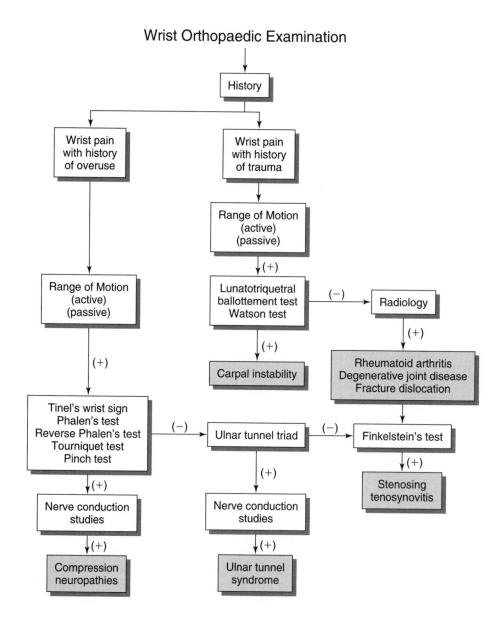

WRIST PALPATION

Anterior Aspect

Flexor Tendons

DESCRIPTIVE ANATOMY

Six wrist and digit flexor tendons cross the wrist (Fig. 7-1):
> Flexor carpi ulnaris
> Palmaris longus
> Flexor digitorum profundus
> Flexor digitorum superficialis
> Flexor pollicis longus
> Flexor carpi radialis

PROCEDURE

Palpate each tendon just proximal to the flexor retinaculum, noting any tenderness or calcific deposits (Fig. 7-2). Tenderness may indicate tenosynovitis of the suspected flexor tendon.

NOTE

Small pealike swelling may appear at the anterior or posterior aspect of the wrist. These ganglia are benign tenosynovial tumors and are usually symptom free but may become tender and painful when distended.

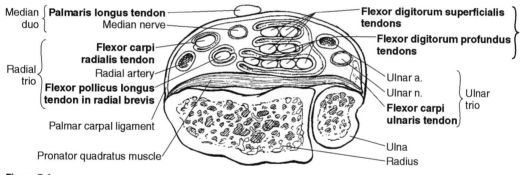

Figure 7-1

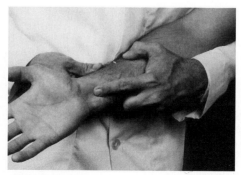

Figure 7-2

Carpal Tunnel

DESCRIPTIVE ANATOMY

The carpal tunnel is deep to the palmaris longus at the anterior surface of the wrist. It is bound by the pisiform and the hook of the hamate medially, the tubercle of the scaphoid and tubercle of the trapezium laterally, the flexor retinaculum anteriorly, and the carpal bones posteriorly (Fig. 7-3). Inside the tunnel lie the median nerve and the finger flexor tendons from the forearm to the hand. This tunnel is a common site of compression neuropathy.

PROCEDURE

The actual tunnel and structures within the tunnel are not palpable. The borders of the tunnel should be palpated for deformity and/or tenderness (Fig. 7-4). The area over the tunnel should be palpated for increase in symptoms, such as numbness, tingling, pain, and weakness in the hand. These symptoms may indicate carpal tunnel syndrome.

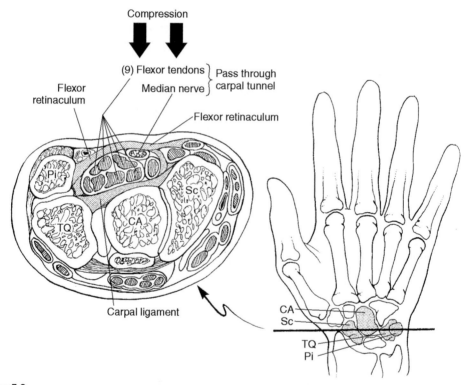

Figure 7-3

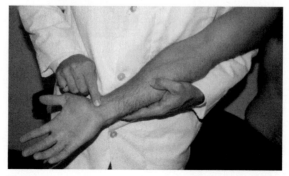

Figure 7-4

Guyon's Canal (Ulnar Tunnel)

DESCRIPTIVE ANATOMY

The tunnel, or canal, of Guyon is between the pisiform and the hook of the hamate. It contains the ulnar nerve and artery (Fig. 7-5). It is also a common site of compression neuropathy.

PROCEDURE

The ulnar artery and nerve are not palpable in the tunnel. Palpating over the tunnel may increase tenderness to the area and the symptoms to the ulnar distribution of the hand (Fig. 7-6).

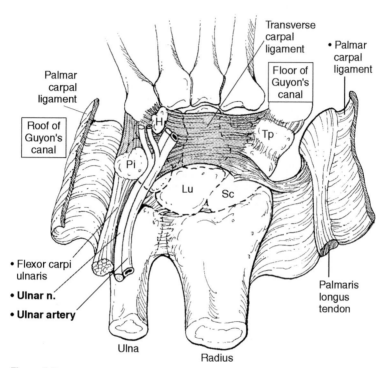

Figure 7-5

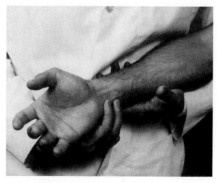

Figure 7-6

Radial and Ulnar Arteries

DESCRIPTIVE ANATOMY

The radial and ulnar arteries are the two branches of the brachial artery that supply the hand with blood flow. The radial artery lies lateral at the anterior lateral aspect of the wrist, and the ulnar artery is at the anterior medial aspect of the wrist (Fig. 7-7).

PROCEDURE

Palpate each artery individually and determine the amplitude of both pulses bilaterally (Figs. 7-8 and 7-9). A decrease in amplitude may indicate a compression of the respective artery between the elbow and the wrist if the brachial artery is palpated and not compromised. A common site of compression of the ulnar artery is the tunnel of Guyon.

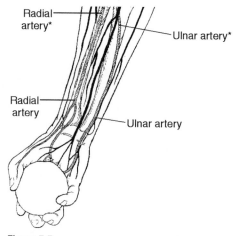

Figure 7-7

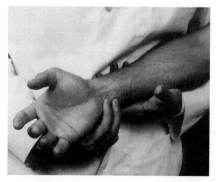

Figure 7-8

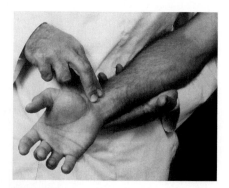

Figure 7-9

Posterior Aspect

Ulnar Styloid Process and Radial Tubercle

DESCRIPTIVE ANATOMY

The ulnar styloid process is at the posterior aspect of the wrist proximal to the fifth digit. The radial tubercle is at the posterior aspect of the wrist proximal to the thumb (Fig. 7-10).

PROCEDURE

Palpate the ulnar styloid process and radial tubercle for tenderness, pain, swelling, or deformity (Figs. 7-11 and 7-12). Pain at the radial tubercle following trauma may indicate a fracture, such as Colles', a fracture of the distal radius with dorsal angulation. Pain at the ulnar styloid may be associated with a distal ulnar fracture. Tenderness, swelling, or deformity at either site may indicate rheumatoid arthritis.

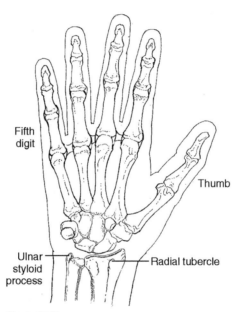

Fifth digit

Thumb

Ulnar styloid process

Radial tubercle

Figure 7-10

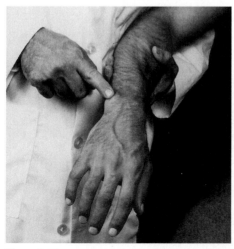

Figure 7-11

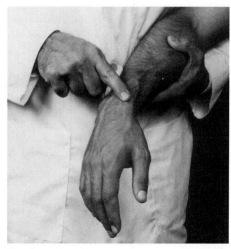

Figure 7-12

7

Extensor Tendons

DESCRIPTIVE ANATOMY

There are six fibro-osseous tunnels at the posterior aspect of the wrist. The extensor tendons to the hand pass through these tunnels, which are bound by the extensor retinaculum superficially and are lined with a synovial sheath. From the thumb laterally, these are the tunnels and their respective tendons (Fig. 7-13):

    Tunnel 1   Adductor pollicis longus, extensor pollicis brevis
    Tunnel 2   Extensor carpi radialis longus and brevis
    Tunnel 3   Extensor pollicis longus
    Tunnel 4   Extensor digitorum and extensor indexes
    Tunnel 5   Extensor digiti minimi
    Tunnel 6   Extensor carpi ulnaris

PROCEDURE

Support the patient's hand with your fingers while palpating the wrist with both your thumbs (Fig. 7-14). Note any crepitus or restriction of movement. Crepitus may indicate tenosynovitis of one of the extensor tendons.

NOTE

A small pealike swelling may appear at the anterior or posterior aspect of the wrist. These are benign tenosynovial tumors and are usually symptom free but may become tender and painful when distended.

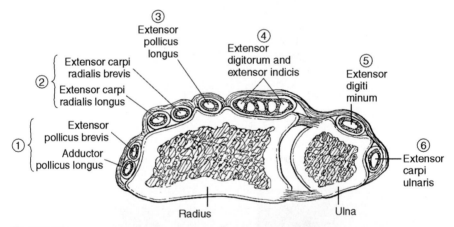

Figure 7-13

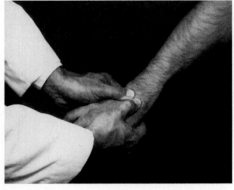

Figure 7-14

Wrist Range of Motion

Flexion (1)

With the patient's wrist in the neutral position, place the goniometer in the sagittal plane with the center at the ulnar styloid process (Fig. 7-15). Instruct the patient to flex the wrist downward, and follow the hand with one arm of the goniometer (Fig. 7-16).

NORMAL RANGE

Normal range is 75 ± 7.6° or greater from the 0 or neutral position (2).

Muscles	*Nerve Supply*
Flexor carpi radialis	Median
Flexor carpi ulnaris	Ulnar

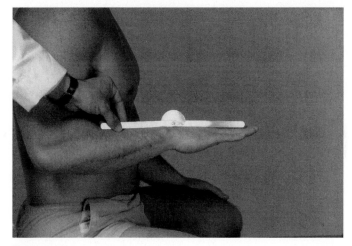

Figure 7-15

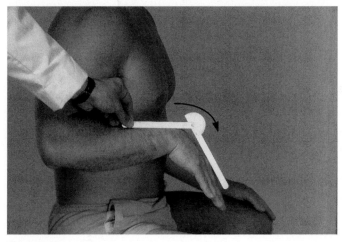

Figure 7-16

Extension (1)

With the patient's wrist in the neutral position, place the goniometer in the sagittal plane with the center at the ulnar styloid process (Fig. 7-17). Instruct the patient to extend the wrist backward while you follow the hand with one arm of the goniometer (Fig. 7-18).

NORMAL RANGE

Normal range is 74 ± 7.6° or greater from the 0 or neutral position (2).

Muscles	Nerve Supply
Extensor carpi radialis longus	Radial
Extensor carpi radialis brevis	Radial
Extensor carpi ulnaris	Radial

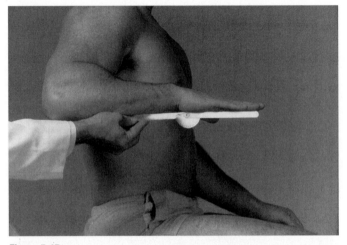

Figure 7-17

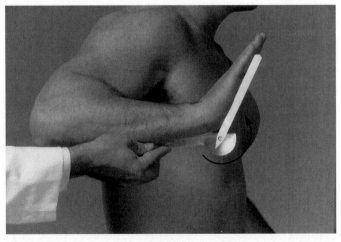

Figure 7-18

Ulnar Deviation (1)

With the patient's wrist in the neutral position and the hand supinated, place the goniometer in the coronal plane with the center at the radial–ulnar junction (Fig. 7-19). Instruct the patient to deviate the wrist medially, and follow the hand with one arm of the goniometer (Fig. 7-20).

NORMAL RANGE

Normal range is $35 \pm 3.8°$ or greater from the 0 or neutral position (2).

Muscles	*Nerve Supply*
Flexor carpi ulnaris	Ulnar
Extensor carpi ulnaris	Radial

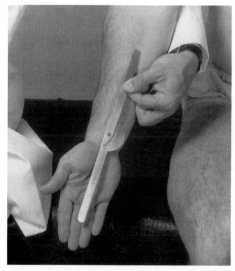

Figure 7-19

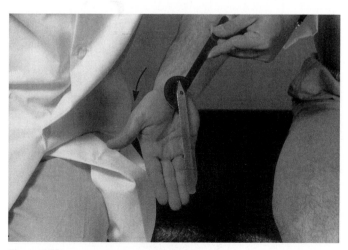

Figure 7-20

Radial Deviation (1)

With the patient's wrist in the neutral position and the hand supinated, place the goniometer in the coronal plane with the center at the radial–ulnar junction (Fig. 7-21). Instruct the patient to deviate the wrist laterally, and follow the hand with one arm of the goniometer (Fig. 7-22).

Normal Range

Normal range is 21 ± 4° or greater from the 0 or neutral position (2).

Muscles	*Nerve Supply*
Extensor carpi radialis	Median
Extensor carpi radialis longus	Radial
Abductor pollicis longus	Radial
Extensor pollicis brevis	Radial

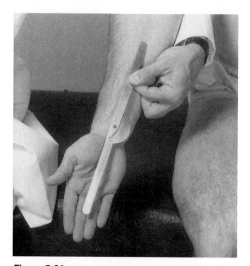

Figure 7-21

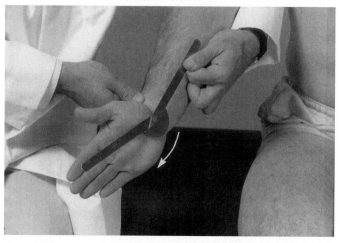

Figure 7-22

CARPAL TUNNEL SYNDROME

DESCRIPTION

Carpal tunnel syndrome is a compression neuropathy of the median nerve. Compression occurs under the flexor retinaculum at the wrist. The stage of the condition from sensory loss to motor loss with atrophy correlates directly with a degree of compression and the chronicity of the symptoms. Most cases present at an early stage with intermittent sensory symptoms only.

CLINICAL SIGNS AND SYMPTOMS
• Loss of sensation of the tips of the first three fingers • Hand and wrist pain • Weakness of grip

Tinel's Wrist Sign (3)

Sensitivity/Reliability Scale

0   1   2   3   4

PROCEDURE

With the patient's hand supinated, stabilize the wrist with one hand. With your opposite hand, tap the palmar surface of the wrist with a neurological reflex hammer (Fig. 7-23).

7

RATIONALE

Tingling in the hand along the distribution of the median nerve (thumb, index finger, middle finger, and medial half of the ring finger) indicates carpal tunnel syndrome, a compression of the median nerve by inflammation of the flexor retinaculum, anterior dislocation of the lunate bone, arthritic changes, or tenosynovitis of the flexor digitorum tendons (see Fig. 7-25).

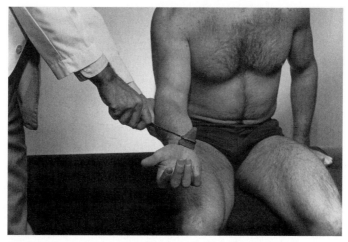

Figure 7-23

Phalen's Test (4,5)

Sensitivity/Reliability Scale

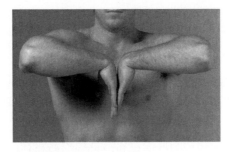

PROCEDURE

Flex both wrists and approximate them to each other. Hold for 60 seconds (Fig. 7-24).

RATIONALE

When both wrists are flexed, the flexor retinaculum provides increased compression of the medial nerve in the carpal tunnel. Tingling in the hand along the distribution of the median nerve (thumb, index finger, middle finger, and medial half of the ring finger) indicates compression of the median nerve in the carpal tunnel (Fig. 7-25) by inflammation of the flexor retinaculum, anterior dislocation of the lunate bone, arthritic changes, or tenosynovitis of the flexor digitorum tendons.

Figure 7-24

Figure 7-25

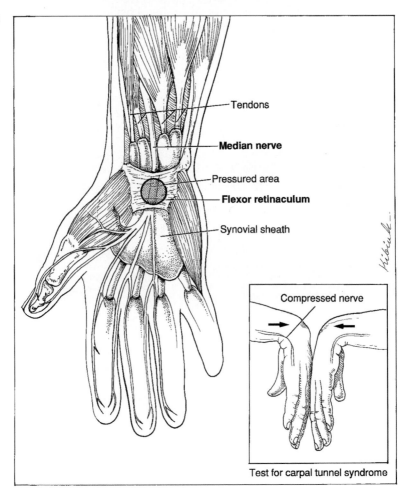

Tendons

Median nerve

Pressured area

Flexor retinaculum

Synovial sheath

Compressed nerve

Test for carpal tunnel syndrome

Reverse Phalen's Test (6)

PROCEDURE

Instruct the patient to extend the affected wrist and have the patient grip your hand. With your opposite thumb, press on the carpal tunnel (Fig. 7-26).

RATIONALE

Extending the hand and applying pressure to the carpal tunnel further constricts the tunnel. Tingling in the thumb, index finger, and lateral half of the ring finger may indicate compression of the medial nerve in the carpal tunnel by inflammation of the flexor retinaculum, anterior dislocation of the lunate bone, arthritic changes, or tenosynovitis of the flexor digitorum tendons.

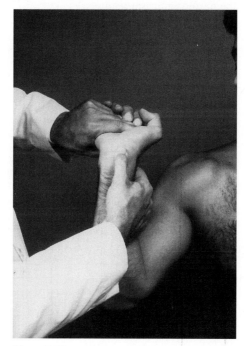

Figure 7-26

7

Carpal Compression Test (7)

Sensitivity/Reliability Scale

0   1   2   3   4

PROCEDURE

With the patient's wrist and hand extended, grasp the patient's wrist with both hands and place direct pressure with both thumbs over the median nerve in the carpal tunnel for up to 30 seconds (Fig. 7-27).

RATIONALE

Placing a mechanical pressure over the carpal tunnel increases pressure to the median nerve. Tingling in the hand along the distribution of the median nerve (thumb, index finger, middle finger, and medial half of the ring finger), indicates compression of the median nerve in the carpal tunnel by inflammation of the flexor retinaculum, anterior dislocation of the lunate bone, arthritic changes, or tenosynovitis of the flexor digitorum tendons.

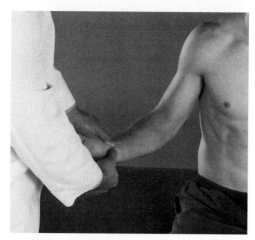

Figure 7-27

Tourniquet Test (8)

Sensitivity/Reliability Scale
0   1   2   3   4

Procedure

Wrap a sphygmomanometer cuff around the affected wrist and inflate it to just above the patient's systolic blood pressure. Hold for 1 to 2 minutes (Fig. 7-28).

Rationale

The inflated sphygmomanometer cuff induces mechanically increased pressure to the median nerve. Tingling in the hand along the distribution of the median nerve (thumb, index finger, middle finger, and medial half of the ring finger) indicates compression of the median nerve in the carpal tunnel by inflammation of the flexor retinaculum, anterior dislocation of the lunate bone, arthritic changes, or tenosynovitis of the flexor digitorum tendons.

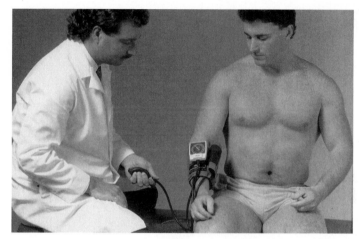

Figure 7-28

Pinch Test (9)

Sensitivity/Reliability Scale
0   1   2   3   4

Procedure

Instruct the patient to pinch a piece of paper between the thumb, index, and middle fingers while you attempt to pull it away (Fig. 7-29).

Rationale

The median nerve innervates the lumbrical muscles, which are used to pinch the piece of paper. With compression of the median nerve, the patient may have numbness and/or cramping of the fingers or mid palm region within 1 minute.

Suggested Diagnostic and Functional Testing
- Magnetic resonance imaging
- Electromyography

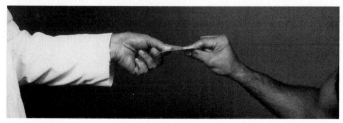

Figure 7-29

ULNAR TUNNEL SYNDROME

DESCRIPTION

The ulnar nerve travels through the tunnel of Guyon and innervates the muscles to the little and ring fingers. Ulnar tunnel syndrome is a compression neuropathy of the ulnar nerve. Compression occurs at the tunnel of Guyon at the wrist (see Fig. 7-5). The stage of the condition from sensory loss to motor loss with atrophy correlates directly with a degree of compression and the chronicity of the symptoms. Most cases present at an early stage with intermittent sensory symptoms only.

> **CLINICAL SIGNS AND SYMPTOMS**
> - Pain over the little and ring finger
> - Weakness of grip
> - Difficulty with finger spreading
> - Claw hand

Ulnar Tunnel Triad

PROCEDURE

Inspect and palpate the patient's wrist, looking for tenderness over the ulnar tunnel, clawing of the ring finger, and hypothenar wasting (Fig. 7-30).

RATIONALE

All three of these signs are indicative of ulnar nerve compression possibly in the tunnel of Guyon.

> **SUGGESTED DIAGNOSTIC AND FUNCTIONAL TESTING**
> - Magnetic resonance imaging
> - Electromyography

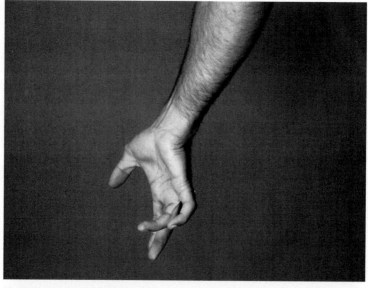

Figure 7-30

STENOSING TENOSYNOVITIS

DESCRIPTION

Stenosing tenosynovitis in the wrist affects the tendon and sheath of the abductor pollicis longus and the extensor pollicis brevis (Fig. 7-31). It is also termed de Quervain's or Hoffman's disease. Swelling of the tendons and thickening of the sheaths that the tendons pass through, is due to an overuse condition of the wrist and thumb.

CLINICAL SIGNS AND SYMPTOMS
- Painful wrist and thumb during movement
- Swelling over the radial styloid
- Tendons and sheath tender to palpation

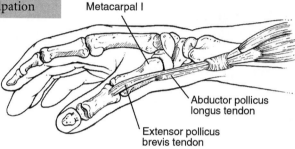

Figure 7-31

Finkelstein's Test (10)

Sensitivity/Reliability Scale
0 1 2 3 4

PROCEDURE

Instruct the patient to make a fist with the thumb across the palmar surface of the hand (Fig. 7-32) and to stress the wrist medially (Fig. 7-33).

RATIONALE

Making a fist and stressing it medially stress the abductor pollicis longus and extensor pollicis brevis tendons. Pain distal to the styloid process of the radius indicates stenosing tenosynovitis of the abductor pollicis longus and extensor pollicis brevis tendons (de Quervain's disease).

SUGGESTED DIAGNOSTIC IMAGING
- Magnetic resonance imaging
- CT arthrography

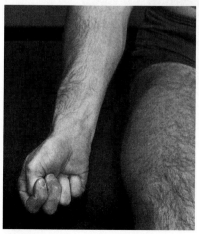

Figure 7-32

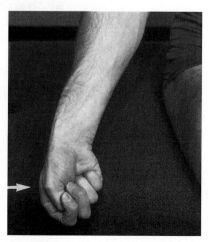

Figure 7-33

CARPAL INSTABILITY

DESCRIPTION

Carpal instability or the propensity for carpal bone dislocation or fracture is due to trauma, overuse injury, or rheumatoid arthritis. The ligaments of the wrist permit little movement of the intercarpal joints. Trauma may sprain the ligaments, which may subluxate one or more of the carpal bones. Severe trauma may cause an incomplete fracture or chondral fracture. Rheumatoid arthritis may cause weakening of the intercarpal ligaments, permitting the propensity for dislocation or subluxation of the one or more of the carpal bones.

> ### CLINICAL SIGNS AND SYMPTOMS
> - Wrist pain
> - Apprehension on movement
> - Crepitus on Movement

Lunatotriquetral Ballottement Test (11)

Sensitivity/Reliability Scale
0   1   2   3   4

PROCEDURE

With one hand, grasp the triquetrum on the affected side with your thumb and index finger. With your opposite hand, grasp the lunate, also with the thumb and index finger (Fig. 7-34). Move the lunate anteriorly and posteriorly, noting any pain, laxity, or crepitus.

RATIONALE

The lunate and triquetrum are held together by a fibrous articular capsule and by dorsal, palmar, and interosseous ligaments. The lunate is the most commonly dislocated of the carpal bones. Most of the time it dislocates anteriorly and affects the radiolunate and the ligaments between the lunate and the triquetrum. Pain, laxity, or crepitus indicates instability of the lunatotriquetral articulation, causing a propensity of the lunate to subluxate or dislocate. This instability may lead to carpal tunnel syndrome, medial nerve palsy, flexor tendon constriction, or progressive avascular necrosis of the lunate.

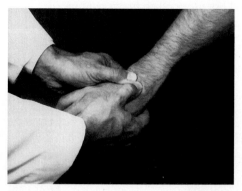

Figure 7-34

Watson's Test (11)

PROCEDURE

With one hand, stabilize the radius and the ulna. With the opposite hand, grasp the scaphoid, moving it anteriorly and posteriorly (Fig. 7-35).

RATIONALE

The scaphoid is prone to subluxate or dislocate with hyperextension trauma. Pain, laxity, or crepitus indicates an instability of the scaphoid with propensity to subluxate or dislocate.

SUGGESTED DIAGNOSTIC IMAGING
- Plain film radiography
  AP wrist view
  Lateral wrist view
  Scaphoid view
  Clenched fist view

7

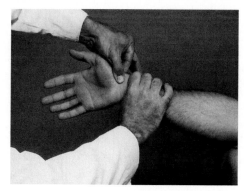

Figure 7-35

References

1. American Academy of Orthopaedic Surgeons. The Clinical Measurement of Joint Motion. Chicago: American Academy of Orthopaedic Surgeons, 1994.
2. Boone DC, Azen SP. Normal range of motion in male subjects. J Bone Joint Surg 1979;61A: 756–759.
3. Tinel J. Nerve Wounds: Symptomatology of Peripheral Nerve Lesions Caused by War Wounds. Joll CA, ed, Rothwell F, trans. New York: William Wood, 1918.
4. Phalen GS. The carpal tunnel syndrome: 17 years experience in diagnosis and treatment of 654 hands. J Bone Joint Surg 1966;48A: 211–228.
5. American Society for Surgery of the Hand. The Hand: Examination and Diagnosis. Aurora, CO, 1978.
6. Post M. Physical examination of the musculoskeletal system. Chicago: Year Book, 1987.
7. Durken JA. A new diagnostic test for carpal tunnel syndrome. J Bone Joint Surg Am1991;73: 535–538.
8. McRae R. Clinical Orthopedic Examination. New York: Churchill Livingstone, 1977.
9. Ditmars DM, Houin HP. Carpal tunnel syndrome. Hand Clin 1986;2:723–737.
10. Finkelstein H. Stenosing tenosynovitis at the radial styloid process. J Bone Joint Surg 1930;12:509.
11. Taleisnik J. Carpal instability. J Bone Joint Surg 1988;70A:1262–1268.

General References

de Quervain F. Clinical surgical diagnosis for students and practitioners. 4th ed. Snowman J, trans. New York: William Wood, 1913.

Ditmars DM, Houin HP. Carpal tunnel syndrome. Hand Clin 1986;2:525—532.

Green DP. Carpal dislocations. In: Operative Hand Surgery. New York: Churchill Livingstone, 1982.

Hoppenfeld S. Physical Examination of the Spine and Extremities. New York: Appleton-Century-Crofts, 1976;127.

Kapandji IA. The Physiology of the Joints. Vol. I. Upper Limb. New York: Churchill Livingstone, 1970.

Stevenson TM. Carpal tunnel syndrome. Proc R Soc Med 1966;59:824.

Thompson WAL, Koppell HP. Peripheral entrapment neuropathies of the upper extremities. N Engl J Med 1959;260:1261.

Wadsworth CT. Wrist and hand examination and interpretation. J Orthop Sports Phys Ther 1983; 5:108.

HAND ORTHOPAEDIC TESTS

HAND PALPATION

Anterior Aspect

Thenar Eminence

DESCRIPTIVE ANATOMY

The thenar eminence lies at the lateral aspect of the hand with the palm facing out. It comprises three muscles that move the thumb: abductor pollicis brevis, opponens pollicis, and flexor pollicis brevis. These muscles are innervated by a branch of the recurrent median nerve (Fig. 8-1). Severe, prolonged compression of the median nerve in the carpal tunnel may cause the muscles of the thenar eminence to atrophy.

PROCEDURE

Palpate the thenar eminence from the base of the thumb medial to the central aspect of the hand at the base of the carpal bones, then inferior and lateral to the base of the forefinger (Fig. 8-2). Look for hypertrophy or atrophy in comparison with the opposite hand. If atrophy or wasting is accompanied by pain and paresthesia along the medial nerve distribution, suspect compression of the medial nerve in the carpal tunnel.

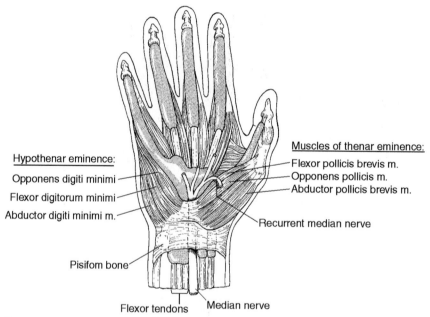

Hypothenar eminence:

Opponens digiti minimi

Flexor digitorum minimi

Abductor digiti minimi m.

Pisifom bone

Flexor tendons   Median nerve

Muscles of thenar eminence:

Flexor pollicis brevis m.
Opponens pollicis m.
Abductor pollicis brevis m.

Recurrent median nerve

Figure 8-1

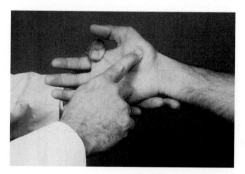

Figure 8-2

Hypothenar Eminence

DESCRIPTIVE ANATOMY

The hypothenar eminence lies at the anterior aspect of the hand from the base of the little finger to the medial aspect of the hand, ending at the pisiform (Fig. 8-1). This eminence contains the abductor digiti minimi, opponens digiti minimi, and flexor digiti minimi. These muscles are supplied by the deep branch of the ulnar nerve. Severe, prolonged compression of the nerve either in Guyon's tunnel or more proximally in the extremity may cause wasting of the hypothenar eminence.

PROCEDURE

Palpate the length of the thenar eminence from the base of the little finger to the base of the pisiform (Fig. 8-3). Look for hypertrophy or atrophy in comparison with the opposite hand. Wasting of the hypothenar eminence may indicate a compression of the ulnar nerve either in the tunnel of Guyon or more proximally in the extremity.

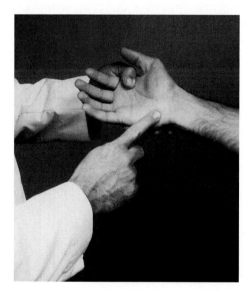

Figure 8-3

Posterior Aspect

Extensor Tendons

DESCRIPTIVE ANATOMY

The posterior aspect of the hand contains an intricate system of ligaments, fascial bands, and tendons—the extensor mechanism. This mechanism provides active extension to the fingers and contributes to the stabilization of the hand and digits. The extrinsic extensor tendons run along the entire length of the posterior aspect of the hand to each digit (Fig. 8-4). The tendons can be affected by trauma, which can strain or rupture them, and by rheumatoid arthritis, which can displace them.

PROCEDURE

With the patient's fingers and wrists extended, palpate the length of each tendon of the extensor digitorum communis from the base of the wrist to the proximal phalanx (Fig. 8-5). Note any tenderness, cysts, displacement, or loss of continuity of any of the individual tendons. Tenderness and displacement indicate rheumatoid arthritis. Loss of continuity secondary to trauma with loss of digit extension may indicate a ruptured extensor tendon. Small, easily palpable pealike cysts may develop between the second and third metacarpal bones.

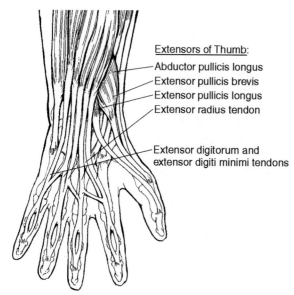

Extensors of Thumb:
- Abductor pullicis longus
- Extensor pullicis brevis
- Extensor pullicis longus
- Extensor radius tendon

- Extensor digitorum and extensor digiti minimi tendons

Figure 8-4

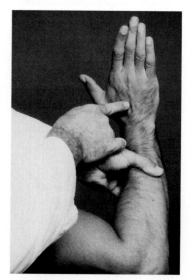

Figure 8-5

Metacarpals and Phalanges

DESCRIPTIVE ANATOMY

The metacarpal bones and phalanges are held together by a series of ligaments and joint capsules that supply stability to the joints (Fig. 8-6). The metacarpal and phalangeal bones are easily palpable from the posterior aspect of the hand. They are susceptible to traumatic fractures. The joints may become inflamed and are a common site for rheumatoid arthritis.

PROCEDURE

Palpate each individual digit and metacarpal bone (Fig. 8-7). Look for tenderness, swelling, temperature differences, and bony nodules. Tenderness and swelling following trauma may indicate a fracture. Swelling around a joint capsule may indicate an inflammatory process, such as rheumatoid arthritis. Bony nodules (Heberden's nodes) on the posterior and lateral surfaces of the distal interphalangeal joints may indicate osteoarthritis.

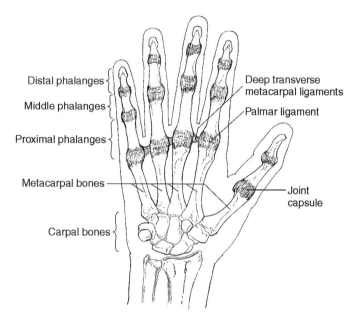

Figure 8-6

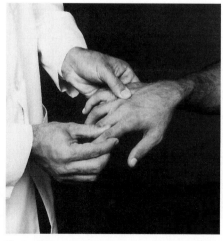

Figure 8-7

JOINT INSTABILITY

DESCRIPTION

The interphalangeal joints are the most common site of joint injuries to the hand. The injuries range from simple sprain to partial collateral ligament injury to dislocation to fracture–dislocation. Joint stability is maintained by the collateral ligaments in combination with the volar plate, which produces a three-sided box around the joints (Fig. 8-8). The most commonly affected joints are the index and little finger. Joint instability is usually due to dislocation.

> **CLINICAL SIGNS AND SYMPTOMS**
> - Joint pain
> - Joint swelling
> - Joint deformity

Varus and Valgus Stress Test (1)

Sensitivity/Reliability Scale

0   1   2   3   4

PROCEDURE

With a pinch grip, grasp the joint (either a distal or proximal interphalangeal joint) with one hand. With your opposite hand, pinch-grip the adjoining bone and apply varus (Fig. 8-9) and valgus (Fig. 8-10) stress to the joint.

RATIONALE

These procedures test the integrity of the collateral ligaments and the capsule surrounding the joints. If pain is elicited, suspect a capsule sprain, subluxation, or dislocation. Laxity may indicate a tear to the joint capsule or collateral ligaments of the joint secondary to trauma.

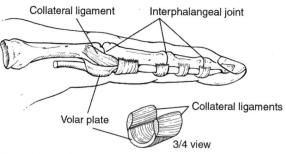

Collateral ligament   Interphalangeal joint

Collateral ligaments

Volar plate

3/4 view

Figure 8-8

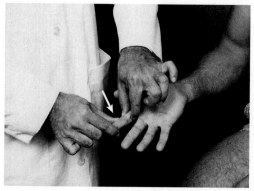

Figure 8-9

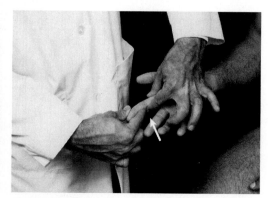

Figure 8-10

Thumb Ulnar Collateral Ligament Laxity Test (2)

Sensitivity/Reliability Scale

0   1   2   3   4

PROCEDURE

With the carpometacarpal joint in extension, stabilize the metacarpal with a pinch grip. With your opposite hand, grasp the proximal phalanx (also with a pinch grip) and push the phalanx radially (Fig. 8-11). Repeat the test with the metacarpophalangeal joint fully flexed (Fig. 8-12).

RATIONALE

When the thumb is fully extended, it normally has 6° of laxity. If laxity is greater than 6° or as much as 30°, the ulnar lateral collateral ligament and volar plate are damaged. If the joint is lax in full flexion, the ulnar collateral ligament is damaged. If there is no laxity in flexion, the ligament is intact. If there is no laxity in full flexion and more than 30° of laxity in full extension, the damage is limited to the volar plate.

SUGGESTED DIAGNOSTIC IMAGING
- Plain film radiography
    Posteroanterior hand view
    Oblique hand view
    Lateral hand view

8

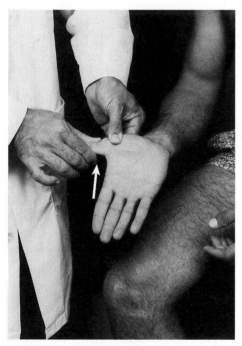

Figure 8-11

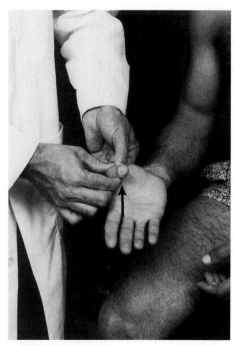

Figure 8-12

JOINT CAPSULE TESTS

Flexibility and stability of the interphalangeal joints are a function of the joint capsules. If these capsules are tight, they may have decreased joint motion; if loose, they may have increased joint motion. Decreased joint motion may also be caused by limitations in the intrinsic muscles of the hand or tight collateral ligaments. These processes may be caused by rheumatoid arthritis or osteoarthritis of the hands.

CLINICAL SIGNS AND SYMPTOMS
- Joint pain
- Joint swelling
- Joint deformity
- Limited joint motion

Bunnel-Littler Test (3)

Sensitivity/Reliability Scale

0   1   2   3   4

PROCEDURE

Instruct the patient to extend the metacarpophalangeal joint slightly. Attempt to move the proximal interphalangeal joint into flexion (Fig. 8-13). Repeat the test with the metacarpophalangeal joint in flexion (Fig. 8-14).

RATIONALE

If the proximal interphalangeal joint does not flex with the metacarpophalangeal joint in slight extension, there is a tight intrinsic muscle or a contracture of the joint capsule. If the proximal interphalangeal joint fully flexes with the metacarpophalangeal joint flexed, the intrinsic muscles are tight. A positive test indicates an inflammatory process in the fingers, such as osteoarthritis or rheumatoid arthritis.

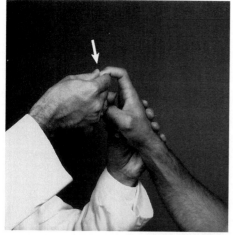

Figure 8-13

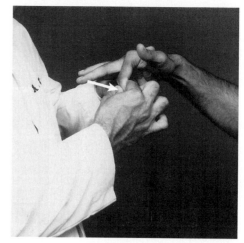

Figure 8-14

Test for Tight Retinacular Ligaments

PROCEDURE

With the proximal interphalangeal joint in the neutral position, passively attempt to flex the distal interphalangeal joint (Fig. 8-15). Repeat the test with the proximal interphalangeal joint in the flexed position (Fig. 8-16).

RATIONALE

If the distal interphalangeal joint does not flex with the proximal interphalangeal joint in the neutral position, the collateral ligaments or joint capsule is tight. If the distal interphalangeal joint flexes easily when the proximal interphalangeal joint is flexed, the collateral ligaments are tight and the capsule is normal.

SUGGESTED DIAGNOSTIC IMAGING
- Plain film radiography
  Posteroanterior hand view
  Oblique hand view
  Lateral hand view

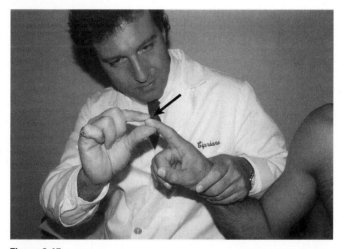

Figure 8-15

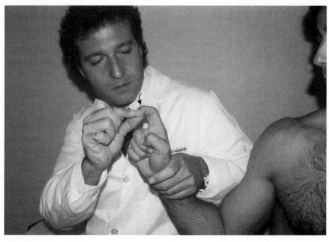

Figure 8-16

TENDON INSTABILITY

Tendon instability or rupture or may be caused by vascular impairment, tenosynovitis, overstretch, or trauma. Trauma may affect the forearm, wrist, or hand. Trauma to the forearm may injure one of more of the long tendons, such as the flexor digitorum profundus and extensor digitorum, which originates in the forearm and flexes and extends all of the joints in the fingers.

> **Clinical Signs and Symptoms**
> - Forearm, wrist, or hand pain
> - Limited or absent joint motion

Profundus Test (3)

Sensitivity/Reliability Scale

0   1   2   3   4

Procedure

Instruct the patient to flex the suspected distal phalanx while you stabilize the proximal phalanx (Fig. 8-17).

Rationale

Inability to flex the distal phalanx indicates a divided flexor digitorum profundus tendon.

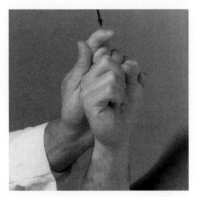

Figure 8-17

Flexor and Extensor Pollicis Longus Test (4)

Sensitivity/Reliability Scale

0   1   2   3   4

PROCEDURE

Stabilize the proximal phalanx of the thumb. Instruct the patient to flex (Fig. 8-18) and extend the distal phalanx (Fig. 8-19).

RATIONALE

Inability to flex the digit indicates an injured flexor pollicis longus tendon. Inability to extend the digit indicates an injury to the extensor pollicis longus tendon.

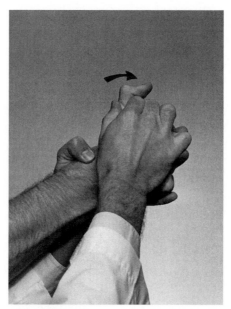

Figure 8-18

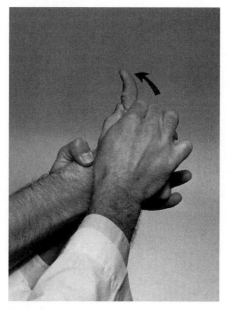

Figure 8-19

8

Extensor Digitorum Communis Test

Sensitivity/Reliability Scale

0　1　2　3　4

PROCEDURE

With the fingers flexed (Fig. 8-20), instruct the patient to extend the fingers (Fig. 8-21).

RATIONALE

Inability to extend any of the fingers indicates an injury to that particular portion of the extensor digitorum communis tendon (Fig. 8-22).

SUGGESTED DIAGNOSTIC IMAGING

- Plain film radiography
  Posteroanterior hand view
  Oblique hand view
  Lateral hand view

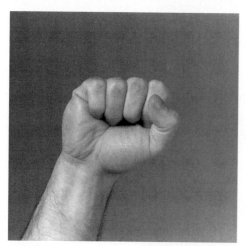

Figure 8-20

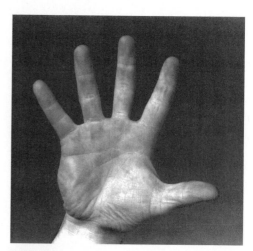

Figure 8-21

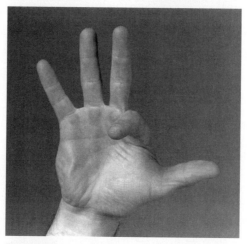

Figure 8-22

References

1. Hartley A. Practical joint assessment. St. Louis: Mosby, 1991.
2. Louis D et al. Rupture and displacement of the ulnar collateral ligament of the metacarpopha-langeal joint of the thumb. J Bone Joint Surg Am 1986;68:1320.
3. Hoppenfeld S. Physical Examination of the Spine and Extremities. New York: Appleton-Century-Croft, 1976.
4. Post M. Physical Examination of the Musculoskeletal System. Chicago: Year Book, 1988.

General References

Cailliet R. Hand Pain and Impairment. 4th ed. Philadelphia: Davis, 1994.

Eaton RG. Joint Injuries of the Hand. Springfield, IL: Charles C. Thomas, 1971.

Green DP. Operative Hand Surgery, 3rd ed. New York: Churchill Livingstone, 1993.

Jebson PJL, Kasdan ML. Hand Secrets. Philadelphia: Hanley & Belfus, 1998.

Maitland GD. The Peripheral Joints: Examination and Recording Guide. Adelaide, Australia: Virgo, 1973.

McRae R. Clinical Orthopedic Examination. New York: Churchill Livingstone, 1976.

Nicholas JS. The swollen hand. Physiotherapy 1977; 63:285.

Stern PJ. Tendinitis, overuse syndromes and tendon injuries. Hand Clin 1990;6:467–476.

Wadsworth CT. Wrist and hand examination and interpretation. J Orthop Sports Phys Ther 1983;5: 108–120.

8

THORACIC ORTHOPAEDIC TESTS

Thoracic Orthopaedic Examination

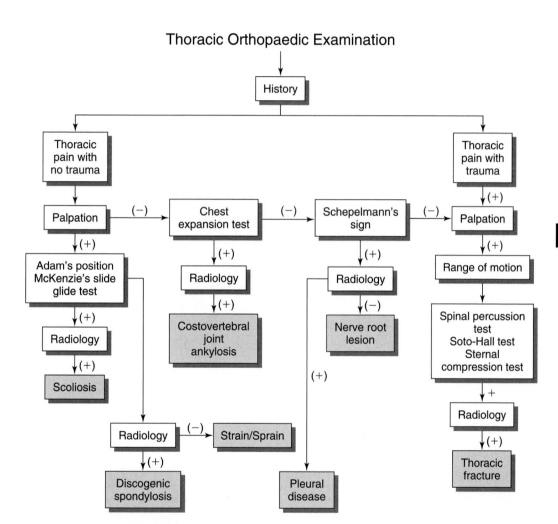

PALPATION

Anterior Aspect

Sternum

DESCRIPTIVE ANATOMY

The sternum, which lies at the anterior part of the chest wall, consists of three parts: the manubrium, body, and xiphoid process. It articulates with the costal cartilages on both sides. The manubrium also articulates with the facets of the clavicle on both sides (Fig. 9-1).

PROCEDURE

Palpate the entire length of the sternum for tenderness or abnormality (Fig. 9-2). Also palpate the costal margins and sternal clavicular articulations for tenderness, pain, and displacement (Fig. 9-3). Pain and tenderness following trauma may indicate a fractured sternum or bruised costal cartilages. Tender sternocostal or sternoclavicular articulations may indicate a sprain or subluxation of the suspect articulation.

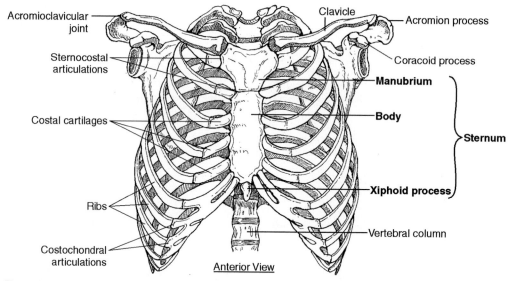

Figure 9-1

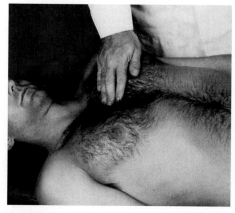

Figure 9-2

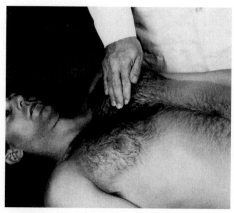

Figure 9-3

Ribs, Costal Cartilages, and Intercostal Spaces

DESCRIPTIVE ANATOMY

The ribs at the anterior aspect of the rib cage are attached to the sternum by costal cartilages, forming the costochondral articulation. They also articulate with the sternum, forming the sternocostal articulations (Fig. 9-4).

PROCEDURE

Palpate each costal cartilage with its associated rib from the lateral aspect of the sternum laterally to the axilla. Then palpate into each intercostal space (Fig. 9-5). Tender costal cartilages may indicate costochondritis (Tietze's syndrome). Tender intercostal spaces may indicate an irritated intercostal nerve or a herpes zoster viral infection. Associated with this infection may be red vesicular eruptions along the course of the intercostal nerve in the intercostal space. Tenderness that follows trauma may indicate a fractured rib.

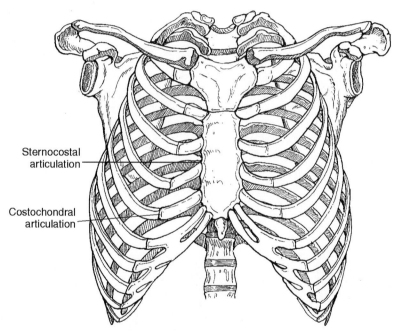

Sternocostal articulation

Costochondral articulation

Figure 9-4

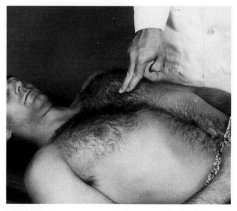

Figure 9-5

Posterior Aspect

Scapula

DESCRIPTIVE ANATOMY

At the posterior aspect of the thorax, the scapula articulates with the posterior aspect of the ribs. It also forms part of the glenoid fossa, which articulates with the head of the humerus. On the anterior aspect, the acromion articulates with the clavicle, forming the acromioclavicular joint. The scapula normally extends from T2 to T7. It has three borders: medial, lateral, and superior (Fig. 9-6).

PROCEDURE

Starting with the medial border, palpate all three borders, noting any tenderness (Figs. 9-7 to 9-9). Next, palpate the spine of the scapula, noting any tenderness or abnormality (Fig. 9-10). Finally, palpate the posterior surfaces above the spine of the scapula for the supraspinatus muscle (Fig. 9-11) and below the spine for the infraspinatus muscle (Fig. 9-12). Note any tenderness, atrophy, or spasm.

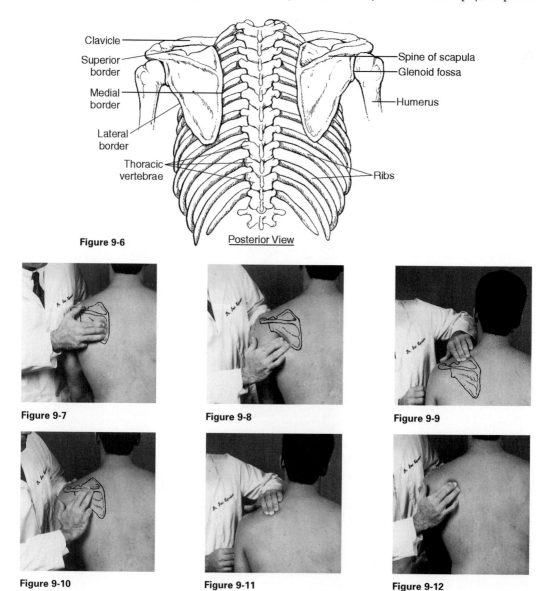

Figure 9-6

Posterior View

Figure 9-7

Figure 9-8

Figure 9-9

Figure 9-10

Figure 9-11

Figure 9-12

Parathoracic Musculature

DESCRIPTIVE ANATOMY

The thoracic spinal muscles are arranged in three layers: superficial, intermediate, and deep. The superficial layers include the trapezius, latissimus dorsi, levator scapulae, and rhomboid muscles (Fig. 9-13). The intermediate layer contains the serratus posterior, serratus superior, and serratus inferior muscles (Fig. 9-14). The deep muscles of the back are ones that maintain posture and move the spinal column. These muscles, the erector spinae group, consist of the spinalis, longissimus, and iliocostalis (Fig. 9-14).

PROCEDURE

Palpate the superficial layer by moving your fingers in a transverse fashion over the belly of the muscle, noting any abnormal tone or tenderness (Fig. 9-15). Palpate the deep layer with the fingertips directly adjacent to the spinous processes (Fig. 9-16), noting any abnormal tone or tenderness. Any abnormal tone or tenderness may indicate an inflammatory process in the muscle, such as muscle strain, myofascitis, or fibromyalgia.

9

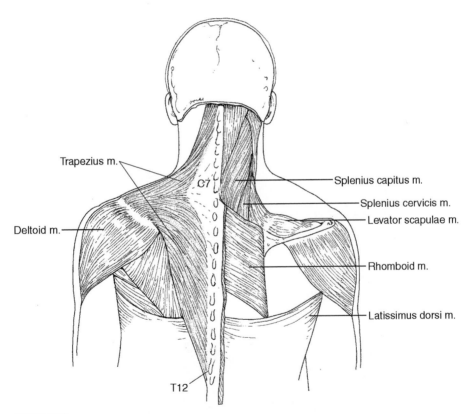

Figure 9-13

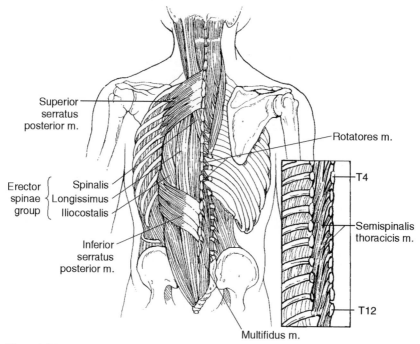

Superior serratus posterior m.

Rotatores m.

Erector spinae group { Spinalis Longissimus Iliocostalis

T4

Semispinalis thoracicis m.

Inferior serratus posterior m.

T12

Multifidus m.

Figure 9-14

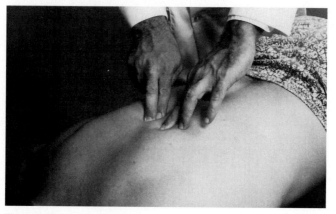

Figure 9-15

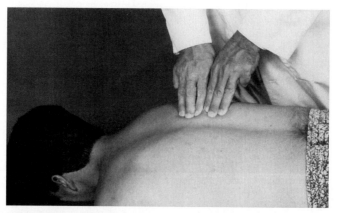

Figure 9-16

Spinous Processes

DESCRIPTIVE ANATOMY

The T1 to T12 vertebrae have relatively prominent spinous processes that are easily palpable (Fig. 9-17). The tip of each spinous process is below the transverse process of the same vertebra.

PROCEDURE

With the patient seated and thorax slightly flexed, palpate each spinous process with your index and or middle finger, noting any pain, tenderness, and abnormal alignment. Each process should be palpated individually (Fig. 9-18). Next, push each spinous process laterally, noting any rotational mobility (Fig. 9-19). Tenderness upon static spinous palpation may indicate subluxation of a thoracic vertebra. Tenderness secondary to flexion or extension injury may indicate supraspinous ligament sprain, especially in the upper thoracic vertebra. Abnormal gross alignment may indicate scoliosis.

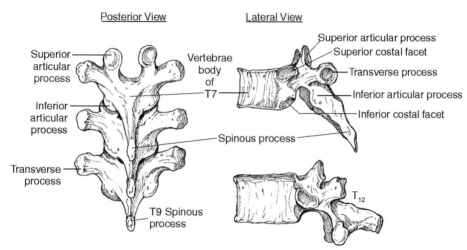

Figure 9-17

9

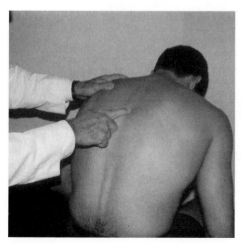

Figure 9-18

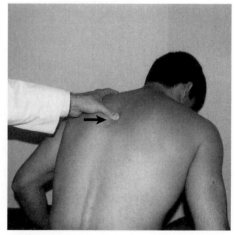

Figure 9-19

Ribs and Intercostal Spaces

DESCRIPTIVE ANATOMY

The ribs at the posterior aspect of the rib cage are attached to the vertebral body and transverse process by a capsule and a series of ligaments and muscles (Fig. 9-20). The ribs can bend slightly under stress without breaking. Between the ribs in the intercostal spaces are three layers of intercostal muscles and an intercostal nerve. This nerve can become infected with the herpes zoster virus, which invades the spinal ganglia and produces sharp burning pain in the area supplied by the affected intercostal nerve.

PROCEDURE

Palpate each individual rib from the lateral aspect of the spinal column laterally to the axilla. Then palpate each intercostal space (Fig. 9-21). Tenderness or pain following trauma may indicate a fractured rib. Tender intercostal spaces may indicate an irritated intercostal nerve or a herpes zoster viral infection. Associated with this infection may be red vesicular eruptions along the course of the intercostal nerve in the intercostal space.

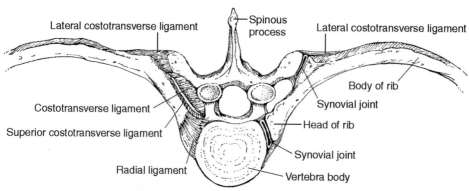

Figure 9-20

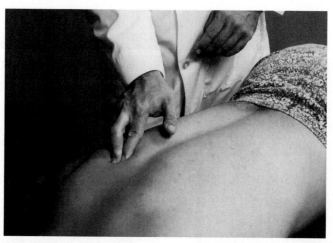

Figure 9-21

THORACIC RANGE OF MOTION

Flexion: Inclinometer Method (1)

With the patient seated, place one inclinometer in the sagittal plane at the T1 level and the other inclinometer at the T12 level, also in the sagittal plane (Fig. 9-22). Zero out both inclinometers. Instruct the patient to place hands on hips and to flex forward the thoracic spine (Fig. 9-23). Record both inclinations and subtract the T12 from the T1 inclination to arrive at the thoracic flexion angle.

NORMAL RANGE

Normal range is 50° or greater from the neutral or 0 position.

Muscles	Nerve Supply
Rectus abdominous	T6–T12
External abdominal oblique	T7–T12
Internal abdominal oblique	T7–T12, L1

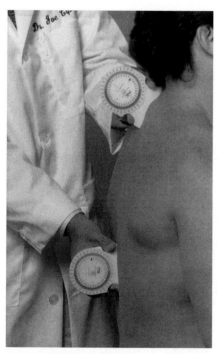

Figure 9-22

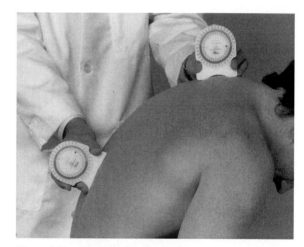

Figure 9-23

9

Lateral Flexion: Inclinometer Method (1)

With the patient standing, place one inclinometer flat against the T1 spinous process and the other flat against the L1 spinous process (Fig. 9-24). Zero out both inclinometers. Instruct the patient to flex the thoracic spine to one side and then the other (Fig. 9-25) and record your findings. Subtract the T1 inclination angle from the T12 inclination angle to arrive at your thoracic lateral flexion angle.

NORMAL RANGE

Normal range is 20° to 40° from the neutral or 0 position.

Muscles	*Nerve Supply*
Lateral Flexion to the Same Side	
Iliocostalis thoracis	T1–T12
Longissimus thoracis	T1–T12
Intertransversarii	T1–T12
Internal abdominal oblique	T1–T12, L1
External abdominal oblique	T7–T12
Quadratus lumborum	T7–T12
Lateral Flexion to the Opposite Side	
Semispinalis thoracis	T1–T12
Multifidus	T1–T12
Rotatores	T1–T12
External abdominal oblique	T7–T12
Transversus abdominis	T7–T12, L1

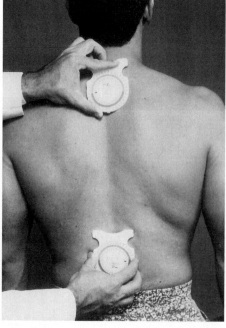

Figure 9-24

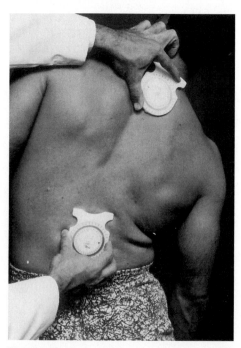

Figure 9-25

Rotation: Inclinometer Method (1)

With the patient seated, instruct the patient to flex forward as far as possible, bracing with the arms. Place one inclinometer at the T1 level and the other at the T12 level, both in the coronal plane (Fig. 9-26). Zero out both inclinometers. Instruct the patient to rotate the trunk to one side; record both T1 and T12 inclinations (Fig. 9-27). Subtract the T12 from the T1 inclination to arrive at the thoracic rotation angle. Perform this measurement with rotation to the opposite side.

NORMAL RANGE

Normal range is 30° or greater from the neutral or 0 position.

Muscles	*Nerve Supply*
Rotation to Same Side	
Iliocostalis thoracis	T1–T12
Longissimus thoracis	T1–T12
Intertransversarii	T1–T12
Internal abdominal oblique	T1–T12, L1
Rotation to Opposite Side	
1. Semispinalis thoracis	T1–T12
2. Multifidus	T1–T12
3. Rotatores	T1–T12
4. External abdominal oblique	T1–T12
5. Transversus abdominis	T1–T12, L1

9

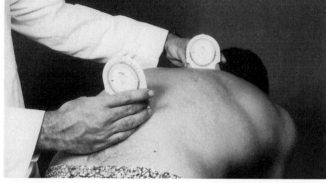

Figure 9-26

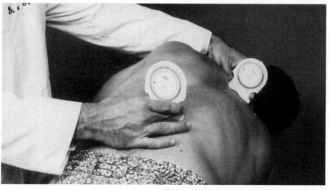

Figure 9-27

SCOLIOSIS/ KYPHOSIS SCREENING

CLINICAL DESCRIPTION

Scoliosis is an abnormal spinal deformity in the coronal plane (Fig. 9-28). It is progressive until skeletal maturity and is the most common type of spinal deformity. Hyperkyphosis is an abnormal spinal deformity in the sagittal plane that increases the posterior convex angulation (Fig. 9-29). These deformities can be congenital or acquired and are more prevalent in females than in males. Some of the problems associated with spinal deformities are pain, diminished pulmonary function, neurological compromise, and loss of self-image. Spinal deformities are best evaluated through radiography. Measurement of the scoliotic curve is accomplished using the Cobb-Lippman technique (2). A line is drawn at the superior end plate at the top of the curve, where the angle of inclination toward the concavity of the curve is most acute. Then draw a line at the inferior end plate at the bottom of the curve. Tangential lines are drawn to these end plates and the angle at their intersection is measured (Fig. 9-30).

> **CLINICAL SIGNS AND SYMPTOMS**
> - Visual deformity
> - Paraspinal pain
> - Diminished pulmonary function
> - Neurological compromise

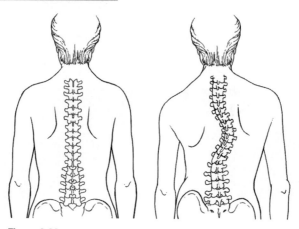

Figure 9-28

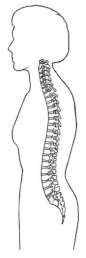
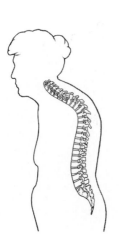

Figure 9-29

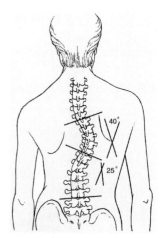

Figure 9-30

Adam's Position

Sensitivity/Reliability Scale
0   1   2   3   4

PROCEDURE

With the patient standing, stand directly behind the patient and inspect and palpate the entire length of the spine, looking for scoliosis, hyperkyphosis, or kyphoscoliosis (Fig. 9-31). Next, instruct the patient to flex forward at the hips. Again, inspect and palpate for scoliosis, kyphosis, or kyphoscoliosis (Fig. 9-32).

RATIONALE

If scoliosis, kyphosis, or kyphoscoliosis is present with the patient standing and if the angle reduces upon forward flexion, the scoliosis is a functional adaptation of the spine and surrounding soft tissue structures. It may be caused by poor posture, overdevelopment of unilateral spinal and/or upper extremity musculature, nerve root compromise, leg length deficiency, or hip contracture. This type of scoliosis is usually mild to moderate, measuring less than 25°.

If scoliosis, kyphosis, or kyphoscoliosis is present with the patient standing and if the angle does not reduce upon forward flexion, suspect a structural deformity, such as hemivertebra, compression fracture of a vertebral body, or idiopathic scoliosis.

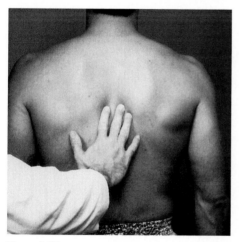

Figure 9-31

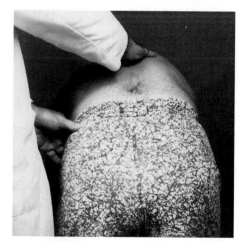

Figure 9-32

9

McKenzie's Slide Glide Test (2)

Sensitivity/Reliability Scale

| 0 | 1 | 2 | 3 | 4 |

PROCEDURE

With the patient standing, stand to one side of the patient. With your shoulder, block the thoracic spine. With both hands, grasp the patient's pelvis and pull it toward you; hold this position for 10 to 15 seconds (Fig. 9-33). Repeat this test to the opposite side. If the patient has evident scoliosis, the side toward which the spine curves should be tested first.

RATIONALE

This test is performed on patients with symptomatic scoliosis. Blocking the shoulder and moving the pelvis stress the area of the scoliosis. If the symptoms increase on the affected side, the scoliosis is contributing to the patient's symptoms.

> **SUGGESTED DIAGNOSTIC IMAGING**
> - Plain film radiography
>   Anteroposterior (AP) thoracic view
>   Lateral thoracic view with concavity toward the bucky
>   AP thoracolumbar view

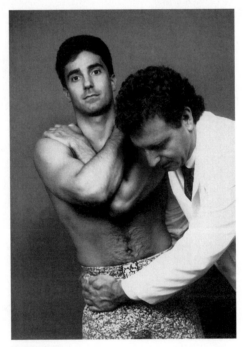

Figure 9-33

THORACIC FRACTURES

CLINICAL DESCRIPTION

Fractures of the thoracic spine are categorized as anterior or posterior. The anterior aspect of the spine is the vertebral body, and the posterior aspect consists of the posterior arch, facet joints, and spinous processes. Fractures of the thoracic spine may disrupt the spinal canal, which may lead to neurological compromise. If disruption of the spinal canal is compromised, neurological evaluation is essential. Plain radiographs in both the AP and lateral planes should be reviewed. In the AP view you may visualize fracture lines and abnormalities in alignment, angulation, or translation. In the lateral view, you may visualize fracture lines, alignment, angulation, and translation.

CLINICAL SIGNS AND SYMPTOMS

- Thoracic pain
- Anterior chest pain
- Upper extremity neurological compromise
- Lower extremity neurological compromise

Spinal Percussion Test (3,4)

Sensitivity/Reliability Scale

0   1   2   3   4

PROCEDURE

With the patient sitting and head slightly flexed, percuss the spinous process (Fig. 9-34) and associated musculature (Fig. 9-35) of each of the thoracic vertebrae with a neurological reflex hammer.

RATIONALE

Local pain may indicate a fractured vertebra without neurological compromise or ligamentous sprain. Radicular pain may indicate a fractured vertebra with neurological compromise or a disc defect with neurological compromise.

NOTE

This test is not specific; other conditions will also elicit a positive pain response. A ligamentous sprain will cause a positive sign on percussion of the spinous processes. Percussing the paraspinal musculature will elicit a positive sign for muscular strain.

9

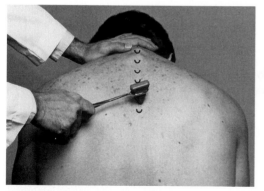

Figure 9-34

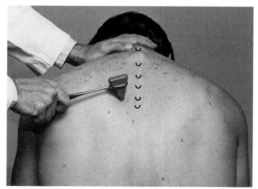

Figure 9-35

Soto-Hall Test (5)

Sensitivity/Reliability Scale
0   1   2   3   4

PROCEDURE

With the patient supine, assist him or her in flexing the chin to the chest (Fig. 9-36).

RATIONALE

Local pain indicates osseous, discal, or ligamentous pathology. This test is nonspecific. It merely isolates the cervical and thoracic spine in passive flexion. If this test is positive, perform tests for strain, sprain, fractures, and space-occupying lesions.

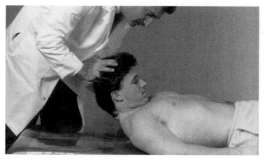

Figure 9-36

Sternal Compression Test

PROCEDURE

Sensitivity/Reliability Scale
0   1   2   3   4

With the patient supine, push down on the sternum (Fig. 9-37).

RATIONALE

Pressure to the sternum compresses the lateral borders of the ribs. If a fracture is sustained at or near the lateral border of the ribs, the pressure on the sternum will cause the fracture to become more pronounced, producing or exacerbating pain in the area of the fracture.

NOTE

Be cautious if you suspect a fractured rib, especially if it is displaced. If trauma has occurred and you suspect a fractured rib, the area should be radiographed before this test.

SUGGESTED DIAGNOSTIC IMAGING
- Plain film radiography
    - AP thoracic view (spine)
    - AP thoracic view (ribs)
    - Posteroanterior (PA) chest
    - Lateral thoracic view (spine)
    - Breathing lateral thoracic
    - Oblique thoracic (ribs)
- Computed tomography (CT)
- Bone scan

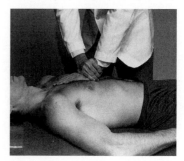

Figure 9-37

NERVE ROOT LESIONS

CLINICAL DESCRIPTION

Thoracic nerve roots lesions may be due to a thoracic trauma. There is greater mobility at the thoracolumbar junction (T11–T12) than at T1 to T10 because of the afforded stabilization of the rib cage. That is why there is a greater chance of injury between T10 and T12.

Thoracic injuries include wedge fractures, burst fractures, and fracture–dislocations. Any of these injuries may lead to a nerve root lesion in the thoracic spine. Compression by a mass or tumor in the spine may also lead to neurological compromise.

> **CLINICAL SIGNS AND SYMPTOMS**
> - Thoracic pain
> - Anterior abdominal pain
> - Loss of abdominal sensation

Passive Scapular Approximation Test (6)

Sensitivity/Reliability Scale

0 1 2 3 4

PROCEDURE

With the patient standing, grasp the patient's shoulders (Fig. 9-38). Passively approximate the scapulae by pushing the shoulders backward (Fig. 9-39).

RATIONALE

Passively approximating the scapulae places motion-induced traction on the T1 and T2 nerve roots. Pain in the scapular area indicates a T1 and/or T2 nerve root compression or irritation.

9

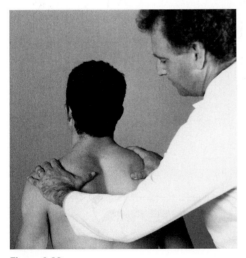

Figure 9-38

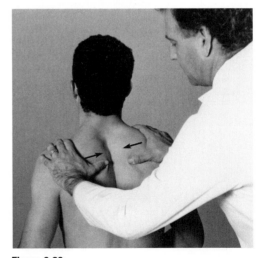

Figure 9-39

Beevor's Sign (7)

Sensitivity/Reliability Scale

0   1   2   3   4

PROCEDURE

With the patient supine, instruct the patient to hook the fingers behind the neck and raise the head toward the feet. This test should mimic a sit-up (Fig. 9-40).

RATIONALE

The umbilicus of the patient who has no thoracic root lesion will not move during this test because the abdominal muscles are equally innervated and of equal strength. If a root lesion is present, the umbilicus will move in the following manner:

If the umbilicus moves superiorly, suspect a bilateral T10 to T12 nerve root lesion. If it moves superiorly and laterally, suspect a unilateral T10 to T12 nerve root lesion on the opposite side. If the umbilicus moves inferiorly, suspect a bilateral T7 to T10 nerve root lesion. If it moves inferiorly and laterally, suspect a unilateral T7 to T10 nerve root lesion on the opposite side.

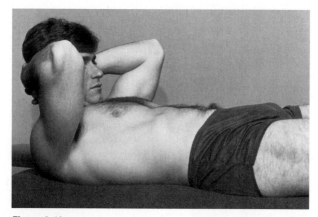

Figure 9-40

Schepelmann's Sign

Sensitivity/Reliability Scale
0   1   2   3   4

PROCEDURE

Instruct the seated patient to flex at the waist to the left and right (Fig. 9-41).

RATIONALE

Pain on the side of lateral bending indicates intercostal neuritis. Pain on the convex side indicates fibrous inflammation of the pleura or intercostal sprain. When the patient bends sideways, the intercostal nerves on the side of bending are compressed. If the intercostal nerves are irritated, pain on the side of bending will be elicited. Also, when the patient bends sideways, the pleura is stretched on the opposite side of bending. If the pleura is inflamed, pain will be elicited opposite the side of bending. Pain may also be elicited because of injury to or spasm of the thoracic or intercostal muscles.

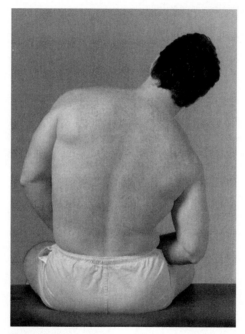

Figure 9-41

9

SUGGESTED DIAGNOSTIC IMAGING

- Plain film radiography
  - AP thoracic view
  - AP lumbar view
  - Lateral thoracic view
  - Lateral lumbar view
  - Lumbar oblique views
- Thoracolumbar MRI
- CT
- Bone scan

COSTOVERTEBRAL JOINT ANKYLOSIS

CLINICAL DESCRIPTION

Costovertebral joint ankylosis is stiffness or fixation of the costovertebral joints associated with ankylosing spondylitis. This is a chronic seronegative inflammatory disease that affects the axial skeleton. The prevalence is 1 to 3 per 1000 people; it is more common in females than in males. It affects not only the costovertebral joints but also the sacroiliac and hip joints. The disease, which usually starts in the lumbar spine and migrates cephalad to the cervical spine, is a slowly progressing one that takes decades to develop.

> **CLINICAL SIGNS AND SYMPTOMS**
> - Lumbar and thoracic pain
> - Lumbar and thoracic stiffness
> - Improved symptoms during activity
> - Loss of kyphosis
> - Chest tightness
> - Limited chest expansion

Chest Expansion Test (8)

PROCEDURE

With the patient seated, place a tape measure around the patient's chest at the level of the nipple. Instruct the patient to exhale, and record the measurement (Fig. 9-42). Next, instruct the patient to inhale maximally; record the measurement (Fig. 9-43).

RATIONALE

The normal chest expansion for a man is 2 inches or more. The normal chest expansion for a woman is 1 inch or more. A decrease in the normal chest expansion indicates an ankylosing condition, such as ankylosing spondylitis at the costotransverse or costovertebral articulation.

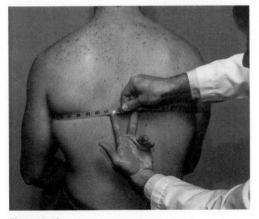

Figure 9-42   **Figure 9-43**

> **SUGGESTED DIAGNOSTIC IMAGING**
> - Plain film radiology
>   - AP lumbar view
>   - AP thoracic view
>   - Lateral lumbar view
>   - Lateral thoracic view

References

1. American Medical Association. Guides to the Evaluation of Permanent Impairment. 5th ed. Chicago: AMA, 2000.
2. McKenzie RA. The Lumbar Spine: Mechanical Diagnosis and Therapy. Waikanae, New Zealand: Spinal Publications, 1981.
3. O'Donoghue D. Treatment of injuries to athletes. 4th ed. Philadelphia: Saunders, 1984.
4. Turek SL. Orthopaedics. 5th ed. Philadelphia: Lippincott, 1977.
5. Soto-Hall R, Haldeman K. A useful diagnostic sign in vertebral injuries. Surg Gynecol Obstet: 1972; 827–831.
6. Cyriax J. Textbook of Orthopaedic Medicine. Vol 1. Diagnosis of Soft Tissue Lesions. London: Bailliere Tindall, 1982.
7. Rodnitzky RC. Van Allen's Pictorial Manual of Neurological Tests. 3rd ed. Chicago: Year Book Medical, 1989.
8. Moll JMH, Wright V. An objective clinical study of chest expansion. Ann Rheum Dis 1982;31: 1–9.

General References

Boissonault WG. Examination in Physical Therapy Practice. Screening for Medical Disease. New York: Churchill Livingstone, 1991.

Cyriax JH. Cyriax's Illustrated Manual of Orthopaedic Medicine. 2nd ed. London: Butterworth, 1993.

Goodman CC, Snyder TE. Differential Diagnosis in Physical Therapy. Philadelphia: Saunders, 1990.

Kapandji IA. The physiology of joints. Vol. 3. The Trunk and the Vertebral Column. New York: Churchill Livingstone, 1974.

Moore Kl. Clinically oriented anatomy. 3rd ed. Baltimore: Williams & Wilkins, 1992.

Post M. Physical examination of the musculoskeletal system. Chicago: Year Book Medical, 1987.

Skinner HB. Current Diagnosis & Treatment in Orthopedics. 2nd ed. New York: Lange, 2000.

White AA. Kinematics of the normal spine as related to scoliosis. J Biomech Engl 1971;4:405.

9

10

LUMBAR ORTHOPAEDIC TESTS

Lumbar Orthopaedic Examination

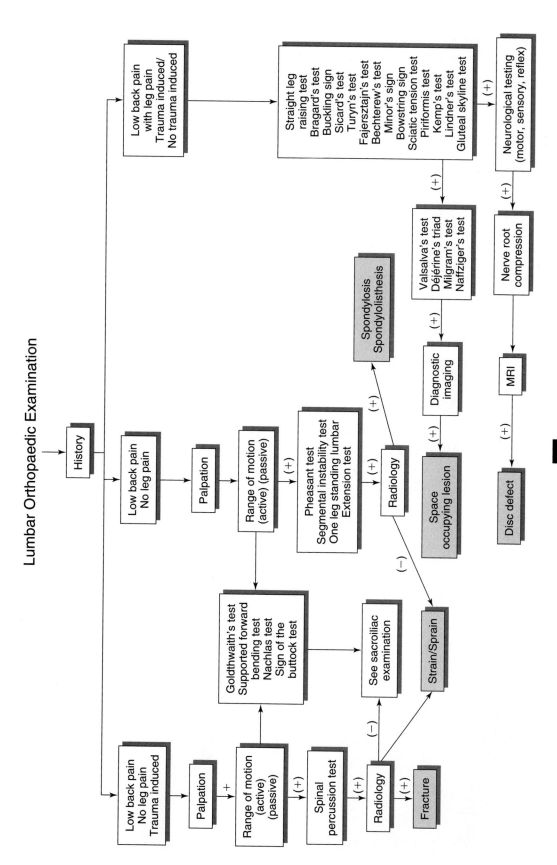

Low back pain with leg pain
Trauma induced/
No trauma induced

Straight leg raising test
Bragard's test
Buckling sign
Sicard's test
Turyn's test
Fajersztajn's test
Bechterew's test
Minor's sign
Bowstring sign
Sciatic tension test
Piriformis test
Kemp's test
Lindner's test
Gluteal skyline test

Neurological testing (motor, sensory, reflex)

(+)

Valsalva's test
Déjérine's triad
Milgram's test
Naffziger's test

(+) Nerve root compression

(+) Diagnostic imaging

(+) Spondylosis Spondylolisthesis

(+) Space occupying lesion

(+) MRI

(+) Disc defect

10

History

Low back pain
No leg pain

Palpation

Range of motion (active) (passive)

(+) Pheasant test
Segmental instability test
One leg standing lumbar Extension test

(+) Radiology

(−) Strain/Sprain

Goldthwaith's test
Supported forward bending test
Nachlas test
Sign of the buttock test

See sacroiliac examination

Low back pain
No leg pain
Trauma induced

Palpation

+ Range of motion (active) (passive)

(+) Spinal percussion test

(+) Radiology

(+) Fracture

(−) Strain/Sprain

PALPATION

Spinous Processes

DESCRIPTIVE ANATOMY

The five lumbar spinous processes are large and easily palpable with the spinal column in the flexed position (Fig. 10-1). The fifth lumbar vertebra is the lowest movable segment. In 5% of the population, the fifth lumbar vertebra is congenitally fused to the sacrum, a condition called sacralization. The person with this condition has only four palpable lumbar spinous processes. In other people, the first sacral segment is not fused to the other segments. This condition is called lumbarization, and six spinous processes may be palpable in the lumbar spine. A common abnormality in the lumbar spinous processes is spina bifida, a congenital defect found in 10% of the population. Spina bifida results from a failure of the vertebral arches to grow together and ossify. It is prevalent in the L5 or S1 segment. Another common abnormality in the L4 to L5 or L5 to S1 interval is spondylolisthesis. This is a fracture of the pars interarticularis that can cause forward movement of one vertebra on another.

PROCEDURE

With the patient seated and flexed forward, palpate each spinous process with your index finger and forefinger (Fig. 10-2). First look for any irregularities, such as spondylolisthesis, spina bifida, lumbarization, or sacralization. Next, place anterior pressure on each process with your thumb (Fig. 10-3) and note any rigidity or springing. Rigidity may indicate hypomobility and springing may indicate hypermobility.

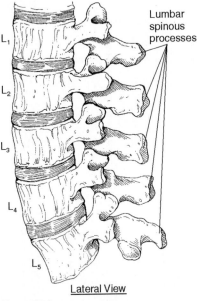

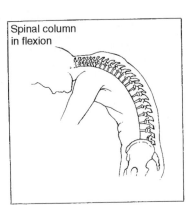

Lumbar spinous processes

Spinal column in flexion

Lateral View

Figure 10-1

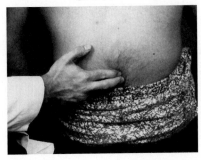

Figure 10-2

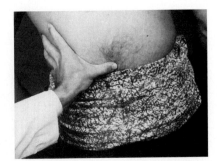

Figure 10-3

Intrinsic Spinal Muscles

DESCRIPTIVE ANATOMY

The intrinsic muscles in the lumbar spine are the erector spinae group (spinalis, longissimus, and iliocostalis). In the lower spine, these muscles come together to form the sacrospinalis group (Fig. 10-4).

PROCEDURE

With the patient prone, palpate the lumbar portions of the erector spine group diagonally from medial to lateral (Fig. 10-5). Note any tenderness, inflammation, muscle spasm, or palpable bands, which may indicate muscle strain, myofascitis, fibromyalgia, or active trigger points.

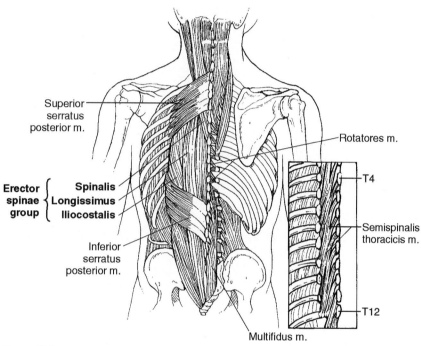

Figure 10-4

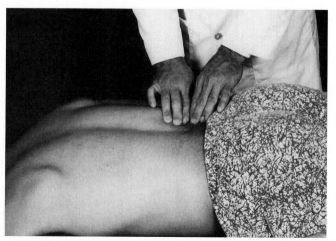

Figure 10-5

Quadratus Lumborum

DESCRIPTIVE ANATOMY

The quadratus lumborum is lateral to the thoracolumbar fascia. It is attached to the transverse processes of the lumbar vertebra, the iliac crest, and the 12th rib (Fig. 10-6). It is a common site for myofascial lower back pain.

PROCEDURE

With the patient prone, palpate the quadratus lumborum from the 12th rib to the iliac crest (Fig. 10-7). This muscle is lateral to the erector spinae group. Note any tenderness, inflammation, muscle spasm, or palpable bands, which may indicate a muscle strain, myofascitis, fibromyalgia, or active trigger points.

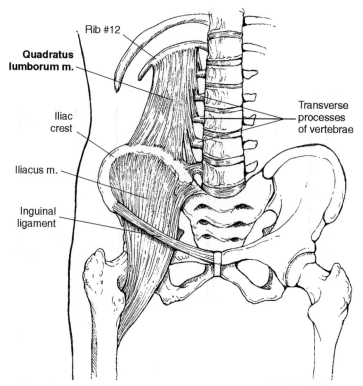

Figure 10-6

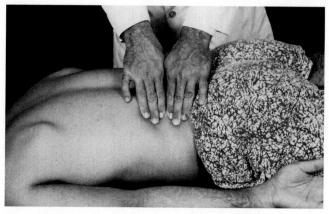

Figure 10-7

Gluteal Muscles

DESCRIPTIVE ANATOMY

The gluteal muscles consist of the gluteus maximus, gluteus medius, and gluteus minimus. These muscles extend, abduct, and rotate the thigh. They all originate from the ilium and insert into the femur (Fig. 10-8). They can be tender and spastic secondary to trauma. Pain can be referred to the gluteal muscles from a defect in an intervertebral disc, and they can lose muscle tone because of nerve root involvement. The gluteal muscles may have active myofascial trigger points that can refer pain to the posterior thigh, similar to a sciatic pain pattern from an L5–S1 disc defect with nerve root compression.

PROCEDURE

With the patient prone, palpate using strong pressure, starting just lateral to the sacrum and moving toward the greater trochanter of the femur (Fig. 10-9). Note any tenderness, spasm, loss of muscle tone, and tender trigger points. Tenderness and spasm secondary to trauma may indicate a muscle strain. A herniated intervertebral disc with nerve root compression may also cause tenderness and spasm to the area. An active myofascial trigger point may cause local tenderness with a referred component to the posterior thigh.

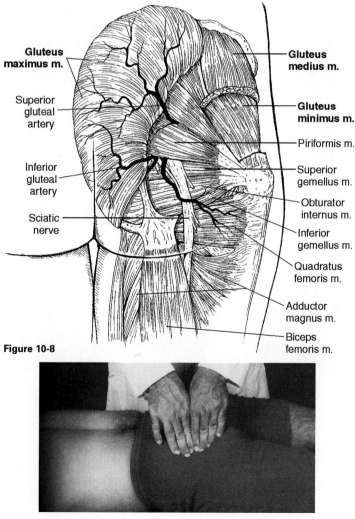

Figure 10-8

Gluteus maximus m.

Superior gluteal artery

Inferior gluteal artery

Sciatic nerve

Gluteus medius m.

Gluteus minimus m.

Piriformis m.

Superior gemellus m.

Obturator internus m.

Inferior gemellus m.

Quadratus femoris m.

Adductor magnus m.

Biceps femoris m.

10

Figure 10-9

Piriformis Muscle

DESCRIPTIVE ANATOMY

The piriformis muscle is clinically significant because of its proximity to the sciatic nerve (Fig. 10-8). It may become inflamed and spastic and compress the sciatic nerve, causing pain along the entire course of the nerve. It originates from the sacrum and inserts into the greater trochanter of the femur.

PROCEDURE

To locate the piriformis, bisect the tip of the coccyx and the posterior superior iliac spine (Fig. 10-10). This is the inferior border of the piriformis. Palpate the muscle, noting any tenderness or spasm (Fig. 10-11). If the patient has lower extremity radicular pain, note whether palpation of the piriformis increases that pain. Tenderness and spasm in the piriformis may indicate muscle strain caused by overuse. Because of the proximity of the sciatic nerve to this muscle, a radicular component to the posterior thigh may also be involved. A local tender area may indicate an active myofascial trigger point, which may also cause a radicular pain to the posterior thigh.

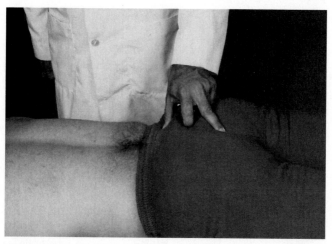

Figure 10-10

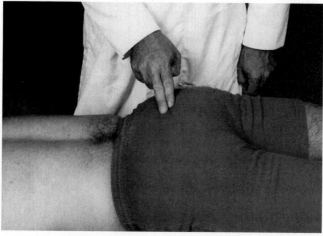

Figure 10-11

Sciatic Nerve

DESCRIPTIVE ANATOMY

The sciatic nerve is composed of the nerve roots from L4 to S3. The nerve runs through the greater sciatic foramen of the pelvis through the gluteal muscles and below the piriformis (see Fig. 10-8). Once it passes the piriformis, it runs deep to the gluteus maximus midway between the greater trochanter and the ischial tuberosity. In some cases, the sciatic nerve pierces the piriformis muscle rather than passing below it.

PROCEDURE

Starting midway between the greater trochanter and the ischial tuberosity, palpate the sciatic nerve and follow the nerve as far down the lower extremity as possible (Fig. 10-12). Note any tenderness, burning, or inflammation. If the patient has any tenderness, burning, or referred pain into the extremity, suspect an irritation of the sciatic nerve.

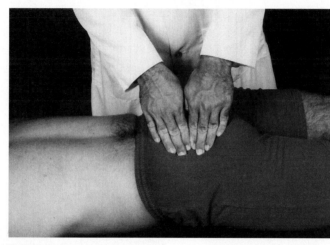

Figure 10-12

10

LUMBAR RANGE OF MOTION

Flexion: Inclinometer Method (1)

With the patient standing and the lumbar spine in the neutral position, place one inclinometer over the T12 spinous process in the sagittal plane. Place the second inclinometer at the level of the sacrum, also in the sagittal plane (Fig. 10-13). Zero out both inclinometers. Instruct the patient to flex the trunk forward. Record the inclinations of both inclinometers (Fig. 10-14). Subtract the sacral inclination from the T12 inclination to obtain the lumbar flexion angle.

NORMAL RANGE (2)

Male aged 15–30	66°		Female aged 15–30	67°
Male aged 31–60	58°		Female aged 31–60	60°
Male aged > 61	49°		Female aged > 61	44°

Muscles	Nerve Supply
Psoas major	L1–L3
Rectus abdominis	T6–T12
External abdominal oblique	T7–T12
Internal abdominal oblique	T7–T12, L1
Transversus abdominis	T7–T12, L1

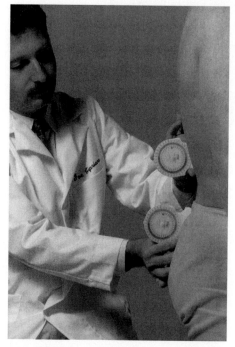

Figure 10-13

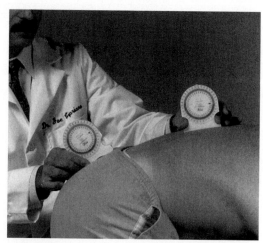

Figure 10-14

Extension: Inclinometer Method (1)

With the patient standing and the lumbar spine in the neutral position, place one inclinometer slightly lateral to the T12 spinous process in the sagittal plane. Place the second inclinometer at the sacrum, also in the sagittal plane (Fig. 10-15). Zero out both inclinometers. Instruct the patient to extend the trunk backward. Record the inclination of both inclinometers (Fig. 10-16). Subtract the sacral inclination from the T12 inclination to obtain the lumbar extension angle.

NORMAL RANGE (2)

Male aged 15–30	38°	Female aged 15–30	42°
Male aged 31–60	35°	Female aged 31–60	40°
Male aged > 61	33°	Female aged > 61	36°

Muscles	Nerve Supply
Latissimus dorsi	C6–C8
Erector spinae	L1–L3
Transversospinalis	L1–L5
Interspinalis	L1–L5
Quadratus lumborum	T12, L1–L4

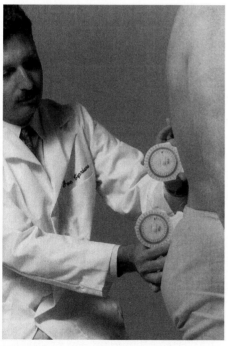

Figure 10-15

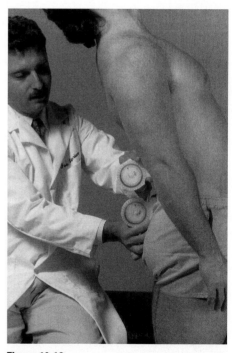

Figure 10-16

10

Lateral Flexion: Inclinometer Method (1)

With the patient standing and the lumbar spine in the neutral position, place one inclinometer flat at the T12 spinous process in the coronal plane. Place the second inclinometer at the superior aspect of the sacrum, also in the coronal plane (Fig. 10-17). Zero out both inclinometers. Instruct the patient to flex the trunk to one side. Record the inclination of both inclinometers (Fig. 10-18). Subtract the sacral inclination from the T12 inclination to obtain the lumbar lateral flexion angle. Perform measurements for both right and left lateral flexion.

NORMAL RANGE (3,4)

Male aged 20–29	38° ±5.8	Female aged 15–30	35° ±6.4
Male aged 31–60	29° ±6.5	Female aged 31–60	30° ±5.8
Male aged > 61	19° ±4.8	Female aged > 61	23° ±5.4

Muscles	*Nerve Supply*
Latissimus dorsi	C6–C8
Erector spinae	L1–L3
Transversospinalis	L1–L5
Intertransversarii	L1–L5
Quadratus lumborum	T12, L1–L4
Psoas major	L1–L3
External abdominal oblique	T7–T12

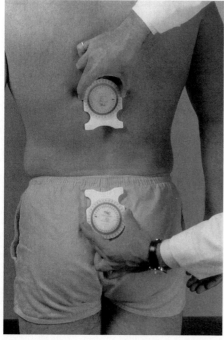

Figure 10-17

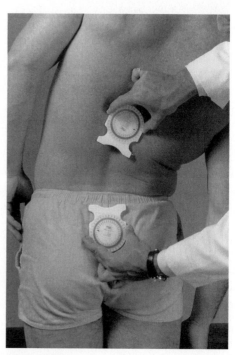

Figure 10-18

JOINT DYSFUNCTION TESTS

CLINICAL DESCRIPTION

Joint dysfunction may involve the forward displacement of one vertebra on another. These defects may be congenital or traumatic. A defect with no forward movement of one vertebra on another is a spondylolysis (Fig. 10-19). A defect with forward movement is a spondylolisthesis (Fig. 10-20). A spondylolisthesis is graded according to the amount of forward movement of one vertebra on another (Box 10-1). Spondylolisthesis is more common in males than in females and occurs 85% to 90% of the time at the L5–S1 level. There are five recognizable clinical groups of spondylolisthesis (Box 10-2). The most common is the type II lesion, called isthmic. This defect of the pars interarticularis allows for forward migration of one vertebra on another.

> **CLINICAL SIGNS AND SYMPTOMS**
> - Asymptomatic
> - Lower back pain (mild to acute disabling)
> - Rigid lumbar spine
> - Functional scoliosis
> - Lower extremity radicular pain (rare)

10

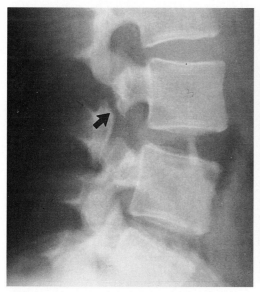 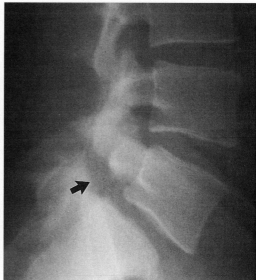

Figure 10-19.   Reprinted with permission from Yochum TR, Rowe LJ. Essentials of Skeletal Radiology. Vol 1. ed 2. Baltimore: Williams & Wilkins, 1996;244.

Figure 10-20.   Reprinted with permission from Yochum TR, Rowe LJ. Essentials of Skeletal Radiology. Vol 1. ed 2. Baltimore: Williams & Wilkins, 1996;244.

Box 10-1	Spondylolisthesis Grades
Grade 1	0–25% forward movement
Grade 2	25–50 % forward movement
Grade 3	50–75% forward movement
Grade 4	75–100% forward movement

Reprinted with permission from Myerding H. Spondylolisthesis: Surgical treatment and results. Surg Gynecol Obstet 1932;54:371–377

Box 10-2	Clinical Groups of Spondylolisthesis	
Type	**Description**	
I.	Dysplastic	Congenital malformations of primarily the superior sacral facets or the arch of L5 vertebra, which allows spondylolisthesis.
II.	Isthmic	Common in both children and adults, this lesion or defect in the pars interarticularis allows anterior vertebral migration, typically of L5. Three types are described:
	1.	Lytic: resulting from a fatigue of the pars interarticularis
	2.	Elongated pars interarticularis: The pars interarticularis is intact
	3.	Fracture
III.	Degenerative	Secondary to longstanding segmental instability with joint degeneration. Occurs most frequently at L4–L5.
IV.	Traumatic	Secondary to fractures not involving the pars interarticularis.
V.	Pathological	Local or general structural weakness secondary to bone disease.

Modified with permission from Wiltse LL, Newman PH, MacNab I. Classification of spondylolysis and spondylolisthesis. Clin Orthop Rel Res 1976;117–123.

Segmental Instability Test (5)

PROCEDURE

Place the patient prone with the legs over the examination table and the feet resting on the floor. Press down on the lumbar spine (Fig. 10-21). Next, instruct the patient to lift the legs off the floor, and again press down on the lumbar spine (Fig. 10-22).

RATIONALE

When the patient lifts the legs off the floor, the lumbar paravertebral muscle tightens, causing muscle guarding in the lumbar spine. The test is positive if pain is elicited when pressure is applied to the lumbar spine with the feet on the floor and the pain disappears when the feet are off the floor and the paravertebral muscles are tightened. Raising the feet off the floor allows the mechanical muscle guarding to protect the underlying lumbar instability, such as a spondylolisthesis.

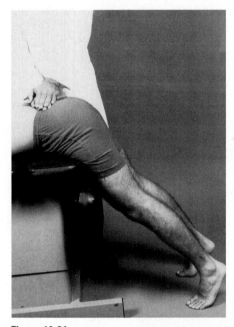

Figure 10-21

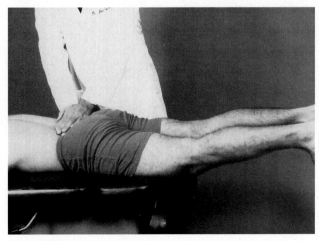

Figure 10-22

10

One Leg Standing Lumbar Extension Test (6–8)

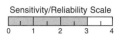
Sensitivity/Reliability Scale
0   1   2   3   4

PROCEDURE

Instruct the patient to stand on one leg (Fig. 10-23)and extend the lumbar spine. Be close to the patient to provide support if the patient loses balance (Fig. 10-24). Repeat the test with the opposite leg.

RATIONALE

Standing on one leg with lumbar extension increases the pressure to the pars interarticularis. If the pars interarticularis is fractured, lumbar pain will be produced or increased. This indicates spondylolysis or spondylolisthesis.

> **SUGGESTED DIAGNOSTIC IMAGING**
> - Plain film radiography
>   - AP lumbar view
>   - Lateral lumbar view
>   - Lumbar oblique views
>   - Sacral base view
> - Computed tomography (CT)
> - Single proton emission computed tomography (SPECT)

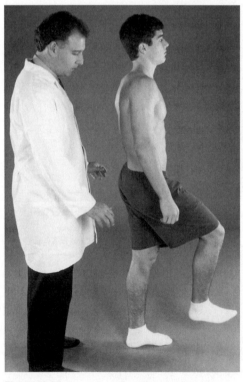

Figure 10-23

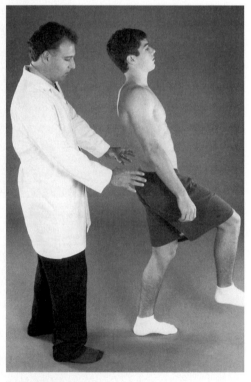

Figure 10-24

LUMBAR FRACTURES

CLINICAL DESCRIPTION

Fractures of the lumbar spine can be caused by trauma or deterioration of osteoporotic bone. The two most common types of fracture in the lumbar spine are the compression, or burst, fracture and the fracture–dislocation. The compression fracture, which can be traumatic or osteoporotic, may be stable or unstable. The stable fracture involves only the vertebral bodies; the posterior elements are intact. An unstable compression fracture involves both the vertebral bodies and the posterior elements of the vertebra. The degree of neurological damage depends on the size of the bone fragment and degree of displacement of the spinal canal.

Fracture–dislocations are a result of severe forces in flexion and rotation and are associated with multiple other traumatic injuries, such as severe abdominal or spinal trauma, in which the posterior elements are affected. This usually causes a high percentage of severe neurological compromise.

> ### CLINICAL SIGNS AND SYMPTOMS
> - Lower back pain
> - Lower extremity neurological compromise

Spinal Percussion Test (9,10)

Sensitivity/Reliability Scale
0   1   2   3   4

PROCEDURE

With the patient seated and slightly bent forward, tap the spinous process (Fig. 10-25) and associated musculature (Fig. 10-26) of each of the lumbar vertebrae with a neurological reflex hammer.

RATIONALE

Local pain may indicate a fractured vertebra with no neurological compromise. Radicular pain may indicate a fractured vertebra with neurological compromise or possibly a disc defect with neurological compromise.

10

NOTE

This test is not specific, so other conditions also elicit a positive pain response. A ligamentous sprain will cause a positive sign on percussion of the spinous processes. Percussion on the paraspinal musculature will elicit a positive sign for muscular strain.

> ### SUGGESTED DIAGNOSTIC IMAGING
> - Plain film radiography
>   AP lumbar view
>   Lateral lumbar view
> - CT
> - Bone scan

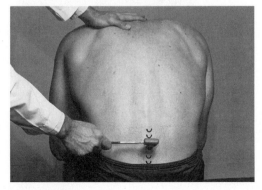

Figure 10-25

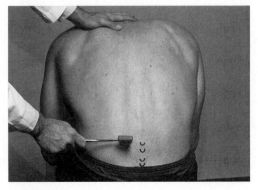

Figure 10-26

LUMBAR NERVE ROOT AND SCIATIC NERVE IRRITATION/COMPRESSION TESTS

CLINICAL DESCRIPTION

Lower extremity pain may be referred from lumbopelvic tissues or viscera or radicular pain from the nerve root complex of the spine. One of the features distinguishing between referred pain and radicular pain is that in referred pain patterns, the spinal pain is more aggravating than the lower extremity pain. In radicular pain patterns the leg pain is more aggravating than the spinal pain. Also, referred pain is poorly localized and dull, but radicular pain is sharp and well localized. One of the most important functions the clinician must perform is determination of the cause of lower extremity pain. Is the pain referred or radicular? This section will deal only with neurogenic radicular pain patterns.

Neurogenic radicular lower extremity pain may be caused by any of several factors. The most common is tension, irritation, or compression of a lumbar nerve root or roots. The irritation or compression may occur within or outside of the spinal canal. Intraspinal canal compressions may be caused by disc lesions, spinal stenosis, degenerative disc disease, hypertrophic changes, or spinal malignancy. Extraspinal canal compression may be caused by muscle dysfunction or extradural defects or masses.

CLINICAL SIGNS AND SYMPTOMS
- Lower back pain
- Lower extremity radicular pain
- Loss of lower extremity reflexes
- Loss of lower extremity muscle strength
- Loss of lower extremity sensation

Straight Leg Raising Test (11–14)

Sensitivity/Reliability Scale

0   1   2   3   4

PROCEDURE

With the patient supine, place and zero out an inclinometer at the tibial tuberosity and raise the patient's leg to the point of pain or 90°, whichever comes first (Fig. 10-27).

RATIONALE

This test primarily stretches the sciatic nerve and spinal nerve roots at the L5, S1, and S2 levels. Between 70° and 90° of hip flexion, these nerve roots are fully stretched. If pain is elicited or exacerbated after 70° of hip flexion, suspect lumbar joint pain. At 35° to 70° of hip flexion, the sciatic nerve roots tense over the intervertebral disc. If radicular pain begins or exacerbates at this level, suspect sciatic nerve root irritation by intervertebral disc pathology or an intradural lesion. At 0 to 35° of hip flexion, there is no dural movement, and the sciatic nerve is relatively slack. If pain begins or exacerbates at this level, suspect extradural sciatic involvement, that is, spastic piriformis muscle or sacroiliac joint lesions (Fig. 10-28). If dull posterior thigh pain is elicited, suspect tight hamstring muscles. If you suspect intervertebral disc pathology, continue with Bragard's and Lasègue's tests and evaluate the suspected neurological level (see Chapter 11).

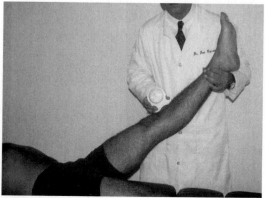

Figure 10-27

Figure 10-28

Lasègue's Test (15,16)

Sensitivity/Reliability Scale

0   1   2   3   4

PROCEDURE

With the patient supine, flex the patient's hip with the leg flexed (Fig. 10-29). Keeping the hip flexed, extend the leg (Fig. 10-30).

RATIONALE

This test is positive for sciatic radiculopathy when (*a*) no pain is elicited when the hip is flexed and the leg is flexed or (*b*) pain is present when the hip is flexed and the leg is extended. When both the hip and the leg are flexed, there is no tension on the sciatic nerve. When the hip is flexed and the leg is extended, the sciatic nerve is stretched and, if irritated, will cause pain or will exacerbate existing leg pain.

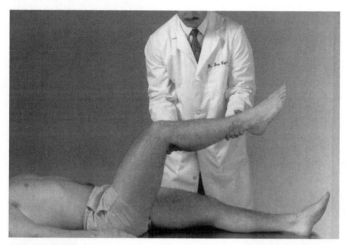

Figure 10-29

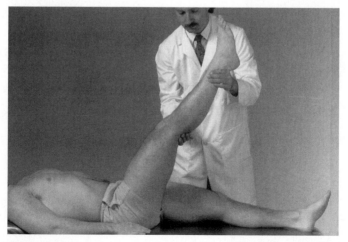

Figure 10-30

10

Slump Test (17)

Sensitivity/Reliability Scale

0   1   2   3   4

PROCEDURE

Instruct the patient to sit on the examination table with hands behind the back (Fig. 10-31). Instruct the patient to slump forward while you hold the chin level to prevent cervical flexion (Fig. 10-32). Apply overpressure with one hand to the shoulder to maintain flexion and instruct the patient to flex the cervical spine forward (Fig. 10-33). Next, apply overpressure to the cervical spine so that the cervical, thoracic, and lumbar spines are flexed (Fig. 10-34). Instruct the patient to extend one leg (Fig. 10-35); dorsiflex the foot of the extended knee with the patient holding the slumped position (Fig. 10-36). Instruct the patient to extend the cervical spine (Fig. 10-37). Repeat the test on the opposite side and with both knees extended.

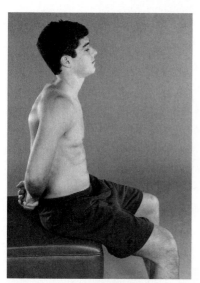

Figure 10-31

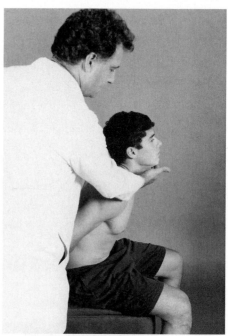

Figure 10-32

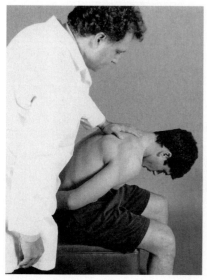

Figure 10-33

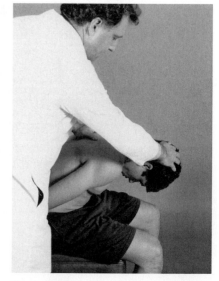

Figure 10-34

RATIONALE

Each phase of this test places on the spinal meningeal tract a motion-induced traction that increases during each phase of the test. Pain at any phase may indicate meningeal tract irritation usually caused by a disc defect. If the patient cannot extend the knee or extends the knee with pain or if the pain increases with foot dorsiflexion, the test is positive, indicating increased tension in the neuromeningeal tract. The test is also positive if the knee cannot extend fully but increases with cervical extension. If symptoms are produced in any phase of the test, stop the test to prevent any undue discomfort to the patient.

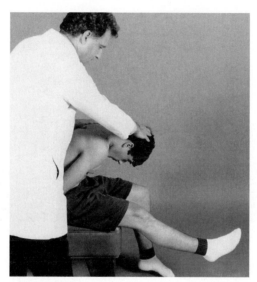

Figure 10-35

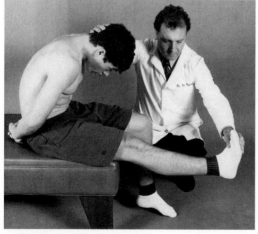

Figure 10-36

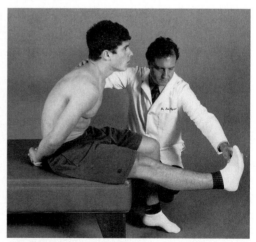

Figure 10-37

Buckling Sign

Sensitivity/Reliability Scale

0   1   2   3   4

PROCEDURE

With the patient supine, perform a straight leg raising test (Fig. 10-38).

RATIONALE

This test exerts traction pressure on the sciatic nerve. The patient with severe sciatic radiculopathy will flex the leg at the knee to reduce the traction (Fig. 10-39).

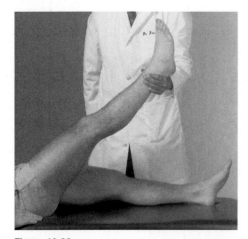

Figure 10-38

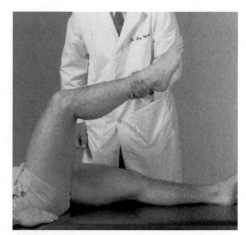

Figure 10-39

Femoral Nerve Traction Test (18)

Sensitivity/Reliability Scale

0   1   2   3   4

PROCEDURE

With the patient side-lying with the affected side up, instruct the patient to flex the unaffected extremity slightly at the hip and knee. Then grasp the affected leg and extend the hip 15° with the knee extended (Fig. 10-40). Next, flex the knee to stretch the femoral nerve further (Fig. 10-41).

RATIONALE

Extension of the hip and flexion of the knee place traction pressure on the femoral nerve and nerve roots of L2 to L4. Pain that radiates to the anterior medial thigh indicates an L3 nerve root problem. Pain extending to the mid tibia indicates a L4 nerve root problem. This test may also cause contralateral pain, indicating a nerve root compression or irritation on the opposite side.

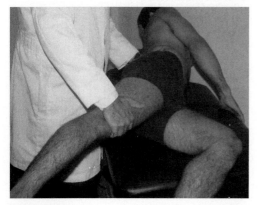

Figure 10-40

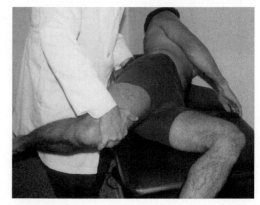

Figure 10-41

Bragard's Test (12)

Sensitivity/Reliability Scale

0   1   2   3   4

PROCEDURE

With the patient supine, raise the leg to the point of leg pain. Lower the leg 5° and dorsiflex the foot (Fig. 10-42).

RATIONALE

The raising of the leg and dorsiflexion of the foot places traction pressure on the sciatic nerve. If the dorsiflexion produces pain in the 0° to 35° range, suspect extradural sciatic nerve irritation. If pain occurs with dorsiflexion of the foot at 35° to 70°, suspect irritation of the sciatic nerve roots from a intradural problem, usually from an intervertebral disc lesion (see Straight Leg Raising Test). Dull posterior thigh pain indicates tight hamstring muscles. If you suspect intervertebral disc pathology, evaluate which neurological level is affected (see Chapter 11).

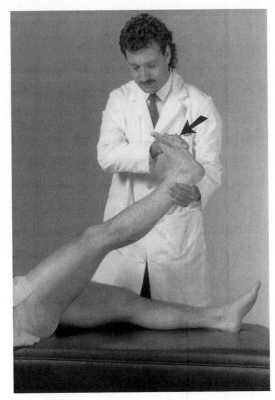

Figure 10-42

Sicard's Test

Sensitivity/Reliability Scale

0   1   2   3   4

PROCEDURE

Raise the supine patient's leg to the point of pain. Lower the leg 5° and dorsiflex the big toe (Fig. 10-43).

RATIONALE

Raising the leg and dorsiflexion of the big toe, place traction pressure on the sciatic nerve. If the dorsiflexion produces pain in the 0° to 35° range, suspect extradural sciatic nerve irritation. If pain occurs with dorsiflexion of the foot at 35° to 70°, suspect irritation of the sciatic nerve roots from an intradural problem, usually from an intervertebral disc lesion (see Straight Leg Raising Test). Dull posterior thigh pain indicates tight hamstring muscles. If you suspect intervertebral disc pathology, evaluate which neurological level is affected (see Chapter 11).

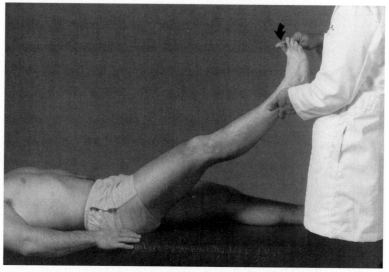

Figure 10-43

Fajersztajn's Test (19,20)

Sensitivity/Reliability Scale

0   1   2   3   4

PROCEDURE

With the patient supine, raise the unaffected leg to 75° or to the point of leg pain, and dorsiflex the foot (Fig. 10-44).

RATIONALE

This test causes ipsilateral and contralateral stretching of the nerve roots (Fig. 10-45), pulling laterally on the dural sac. A positive sign is elicited if an increase in leg pain or pain is reproduced on the affected leg side. This pain indicates a disc protrusion usually medial to the nerve root.

When the unaffected leg is raised, the nerve root on that side is stretched, causing the nerve root on the opposite side to slide down and toward the midline (Fig. 10-46). If a medial disc protrusion is present, this movement will increase tension on the nerve root opposite the side of hip flexion, increasing the pain on the affected side. If pain decreases on the affected side when the unaffected leg is raised, suspect a lateral disc protrusion, because the nerve root is being pulled away from the disc (Fig. 10-47). If this test is positive, evaluate the neurological level affected (see Chapter 11).

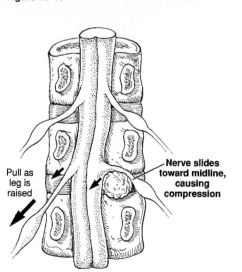

Figure 10-44

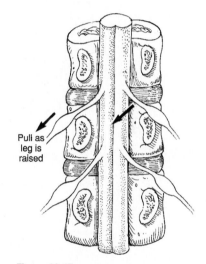

Pull as leg is raised

Figure 10-45

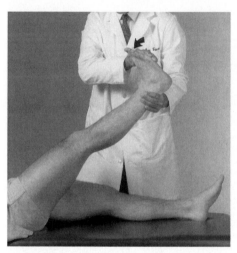

Pull as leg is raised

Nerve slides toward midline, causing compression

Figure 10-46

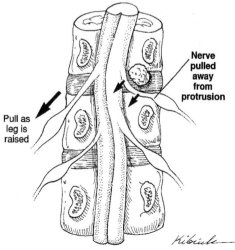

Nerve pulled away from protrusion

Pull as leg is raised

Figure 10-47

Bechterew's Test

Sensitivity/Reliability Scale

0   1   2   3   4

PROCEDURE

Seat the patient with legs hanging over the examination table. Instruct the patient to extend one knee at a time alternately (Fig. 10-48). If no positive response is elicited, instruct the patient to raise both legs together (Fig. 10-49).

RATIONALE

With the patient seated and the leg flexed, the sciatic nerve is relatively slack. Extending the leg places traction pressure on the sciatic nerve. If the patient cannot perform this test because of radicular pain or performs the test but leans back, compression to the sciatic nerve or lumbar nerve roots, either intradurally or extradurally, is indicated. This test is usually positive in disc protrusion cases.

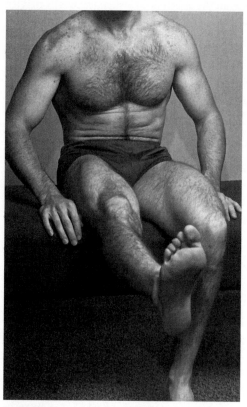

Figure 10-48

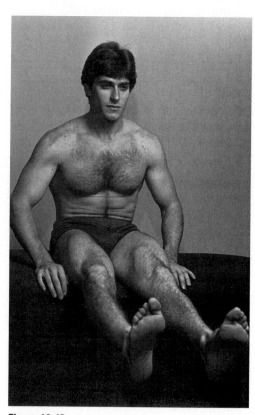

Figure 10-49

Minor's Sign

Sensitivity/Reliability Scale

0   1   2   3   4

PROCEDURE

Instruct the seated patient to stand (Fig. 10-50).

RATIONALE

The patient with sciatic radiculopathy will stand on the healthy side and keep the affected leg flexed to decrease the tension on the sciatic nerve, hence relieve pain. The patient in Figure 10-50 is demonstrating sciatic radiculopathy down the left lower extremity.

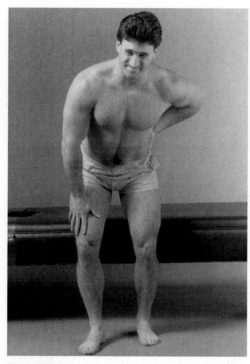

Figure 10-50

10

Knee Flexion Test (21)

Sensitivity/Reliability Scale

0   1   2   3   4

PROCEDURE

Instruct the standing patient to bend forward (Fig. 10-51).

RATIONALE

The patient with sciatic radiculopathy will flex the affected leg while bending forward. Flexion of the leg reduces the traction on the sciatic nerve, hence reduces the pain. The patient in Figure 10-52 is demonstrating sciatic radiculopathy down the right leg.

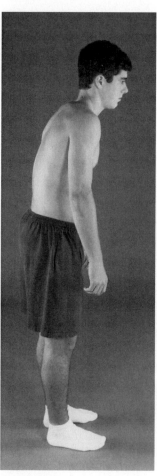

Figure 10-51

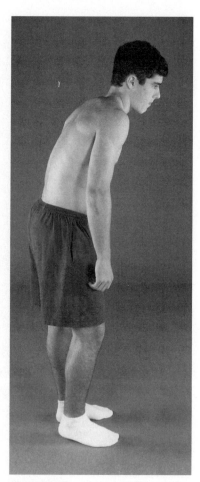

Figure 10-52

Antalgic Lean Sign (13)

Sensitivity/Reliability Scale

0   1   2   3   4

PROCEDURE

Either instruct the patient to stand or observe the patient standing (Fig. 10-53).

RATIONALE

Patients with disc protrusions that place pressure on a nerve root will lean in a direction that reduces the mechanical pressure on the disc. If the disc protrusion is lateral to the nerve root, the patient will lean away from the side pain (Fig. 10-54). Pain is relieved because when the patient leans away from the lateral disc defect, the nerve root moves medially and away from the defect, reducing pressure on the nerve root (Fig. 10-55). If the disc protrusion is medial to the nerve root, the patient will lean toward

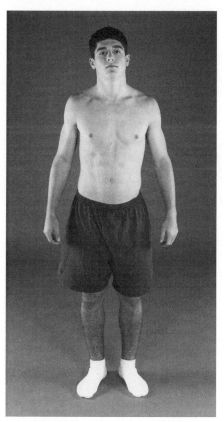

Figure 10-53

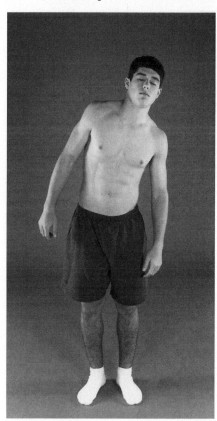

Figure 10-54

10

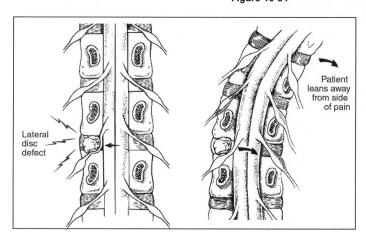

Lateral disc defect

Patient leans away from side of pain

Figure 10-55

the side of pain (Fig. 10-56). Pain of medial disc protrusion is relieved because when the patient leans toward the side of pain, the nerve root moves laterally and away from the defect, reducing pressure on the nerve root (Fig. 10-57). If the disc protrusion is central to the nerve root, the patient may assume a flexed posture (Fig. 10-58). This is because the posterior aspect of the disc is under traction, which may reduce the surface area of the disc defect that comes in contact with the nerve root (Fig. 10-59).

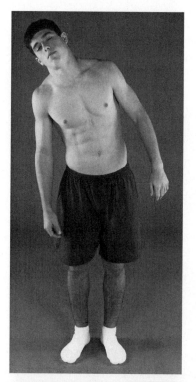

Figure 10-56

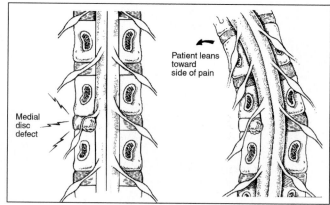

Figure 10-57

Figure 10-58

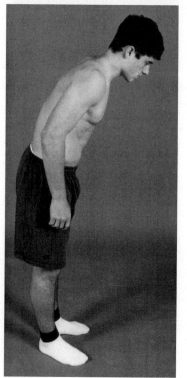

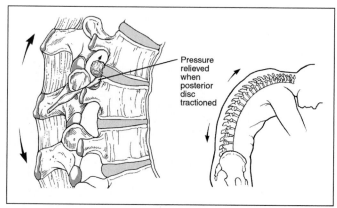

Figure 10-59

Bowstring Sign (22)

Sensitivity/Reliability Scale

0 1 2 3 4

PROCEDURE

With the patient supine, place the patient's leg atop your shoulder. At this point, firm pressure should be exerted on the hamstring muscles (Fig. 10-60). If pain is not elicited, apply pressure to the popliteal fossa (Fig. 10-61).

RATIONALE

Pain in the lumbar region or radiculopathy is a positive sign of sciatic nerve compression, either intradurally or extradurally. Applying pressure to the hamstring muscles or popliteal fossa increases tension on the sciatic nerve, thus eliciting or exacerbating the patient's pain.

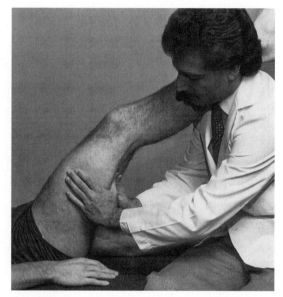

Figure 10-60

10

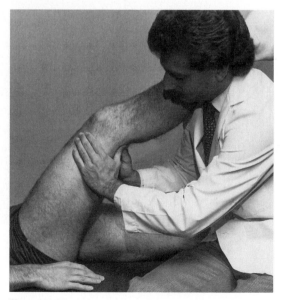

Figure 10-61

Sciatic Tension Test (23)

Sensitivity/Reliability Scale

0   1   2   3   4

PROCEDURE

With the patient seated, passively extend the affected limb to the point of pain (Fig. 10-62). Lower the limb below the point of pain and grasp the leg between your knees. With both hands, place posterior to anterior pressure in the popliteal space (Fig. 10-63).

RATIONALE

Flexing the leg places traction pressure on the sciatic nerve. Lowering the leg reduces the traction; if the sciatic nerve is irritated, the pain will ease. Placing additional pressure in the popliteal space with your fingers increases the traction pressure on the sciatic nerve, causing radicular pain if the sciatic nerve is irritated. An increase in pain indicates an irritation to the sciatic nerve, either intradurally or extradurally.

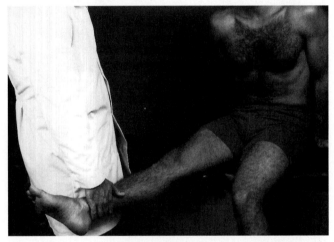

Figure 10-62

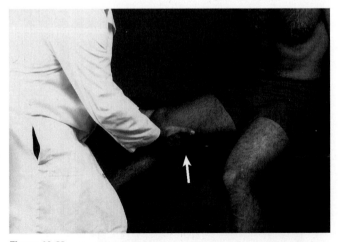

Figure 10-63

Piriformis Test (24)

PROCEDURE

Instruct the patient to lie on his or her side close to the edge of the examination table. Have the patient flex the hip and knee to 90°. Place your hand on the patient's pelvis for stabilization, and with your opposite hand press down on the patient's knee (Fig. 10-64).

RATIONALE

This test stresses the external rotators and piriformis muscle. If the sciatic nerve passes through the piriformis or if the piriformis is in spasm, it may impinge on the sciatic nerve and reproduce the pain in the buttock or radicular pain in the extremity.

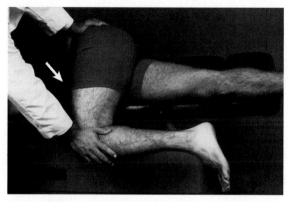

Figure 10-64

Gluteal Skyline Test (25)

10

PROCEDURE

Instruct the patient to lie prone on the examination table, head straight and arms by the sides or hanging down. Stand at the patient's feet and observe the height of the buttock. Instruct the patient to contract each gluteal muscle (Fig. 10-65).

RATIONALE

The L5, S1, S2, and inferior gluteal nerves innervate the gluteal muscles. If the affected gluteal muscle is flat and shows less contraction than the unaffected side, suspect damage to the L5, S1, S2, and inferior gluteal nerve.

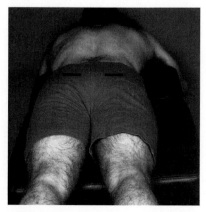

Figure 10-65

Kemp's Test

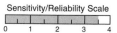

Sensitivity/Reliability Scale

0   1   2   3   4

PROCEDURE

With the patient either sitting or standing, stabilize the posterior superior iliac spine with one hand. With your other hand, reach around to the front of the patient and grasp the shoulder. Passively bend the dorsolumbar spine obliquely backward (Fig. 10-66).

RATIONALE

When the patient bends obliquely backward, the dural sac on the side of bending moves laterally. If a lateral disc lesion is present, this movement will increase the nerve root tension over that disc lesion, producing pain in the lower back, usually with a radicular component on the side of oblique bending (Fig. 10-67, *left*). On the side opposite the oblique bending, the dural sac moves medially. If a medial disc lesion is present, this movement will increase the tension over that disc lesion, producing pain in the lower back, usually with a radicular component on the side opposite the oblique bending (Fig. 10-67, *right*). If the test is positive, evaluate the affected neurological level (see Chapter 11). If the patient has local lower back pain with no radicular component, suspect lumbar muscle spasm or facet capsulitis.

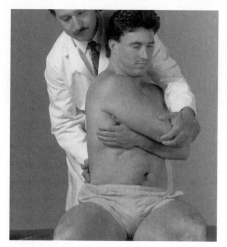

Figure 10-66

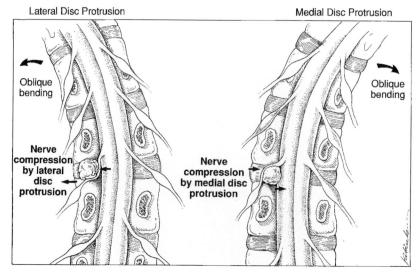

Figure 10-67   Left, lateral disk; right, medial disk.

Lindner's Sign

Sensitivity/Reliability Scale

0   1   2   3   4

PROCEDURE

With the patient supine, passively flex the patient's head (Fig. 10-68).

RATIONALE

Passive flexion of the patient's head stretches the dural sac. Reproduction of the patient's pain indicates a disc lesion at the level of pain. Sharp, diffuse pain or involuntary hip flexion may indicate meningeal irritation (see Brudzinski's Test). If you suspect disc pathology, evaluate the affected level (see Chapter 11).

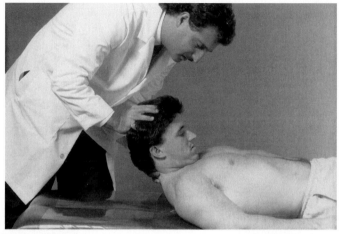

Figure 10-68

10

Heel–Toe Walk Test (13)

Sensitivity/Reliability Scale

0   1   2   3   4

PROCEDURE

Instruct the patient to walk on the toes (Fig. 10-69), then on the heels (Fig. 10-70). Observe the patient and see whether the patient can support the entire body weight on each set of toes and each heel.

RATIONALE

If an L5–S1 disc defect is creating pressure on the S1 nerve root, the patient may not be able to sustain body weight while walking on the toes. This is due to weakness of the calf muscles, which are supplied by the tibial nerve.

If an L4–L5 disc defect is creating pressure on the L5 nerve root, the patient may not be able to sustain the body weight while walking on the heels. This is due to the weakness of the anterior leg muscles, which are supplied by the common peroneal nerve.

SUGGESTED DIAGNOSTIC IMAGING

- Plain film radiology
  AP lumbar view
  Lateral lumbar view
  Oblique lumbar view
- Lumbar CT
- Lumbar MRI
- Electromyography

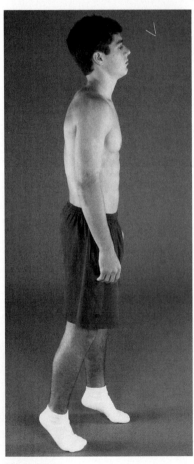

Figure 10-69

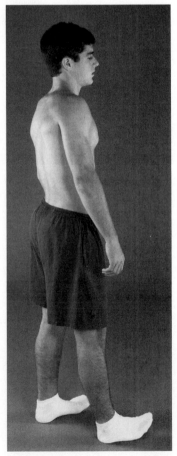

Figure 10-70

SPACE-OCCUPYING LESIONS

CLINICAL DESCRIPTION

Space-occupying lesions of the spine may lead to spinal stenosis. Spinal stenosis is narrowing of the tubular structures of the spine, which include the central canal, lateral recess, and intervertebral foramen. The condition may be congenital, developmental, acquired, traumatic, or postsurgical. It may be a disc defect, hypertrophic or degenerative change, synovial cyst, fracture, tumor, or a combination. Space-occupying lesions can affect the neurological structures of the spine, such as the spinal cord, cauda equina, or nerve roots.

CLINICAL SIGNS AND SYMPTOMS
- Lower back pain
- Lower extremity radicular pain
- Lower extremity weakness
- Loss of lower extremity reflexes
- Loss of lower extremity sensation

Valsalva's Maneuver (26)

Sensitivity/Reliability Scale

0 1 2 3 4

PROCEDURE

Instruct the seated patient to bear down as if straining at stool but concentrating the bulk of the stress at the lumbar region (Fig. 10-71). If the patient feels any increased pain, ask him or her to point to it. This test is subjective and requires an accurate response from the patient.

RATIONALE

This test increases intrathecal pressure. Local pain secondary to the increased pressure may indicate a space-occupying lesion (e.g., disk defect, mass, osteophyte) in the lumbar canal or foramen.

10

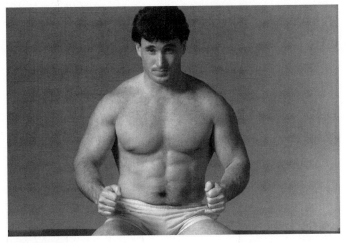

Figure 10-71

Déjérine's Triad

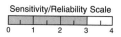
Procedure

With the patient seated, instruct him to cough, sneeze, and bear down as if straining at stool (Valsalva's maneuver).

Rationale

Pain local to the lumbar region after any of the previous actions indicates increased intrathecal pressure, most likely induced by a space-occupying lesion (e.g., disc defect, mass, osteophyte). If the patient cannot sneeze, administer a dash of pepper (Lewin's snuff test).

Milgram's Test (27)

Procedure

Instruct the supine patient to raise the legs 2 or 3 inches above the table (Fig. 10-72).

Rationale

The patient should be able to perform this test for at least 30 seconds without low back pain. If pain is present, suspect a space-occupying lesion inside or out of the spinal canal. Disc protrusion usually produces a positive test. Patients with weak abdominal muscles may not be able to perform this test.

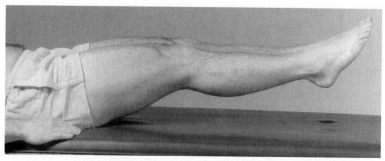

Figure 10-72

Naffziger's Test (28)

PROCEDURE

With the patient seated, compress the jugular veins, which lie approximately 1 inch lateral to the tracheal cartilage (Fig. 10-73). Hold the compression for 1 minute.

RATIONALE

Compressing the jugular veins raises the intrathecal pressure. Local pain in the lumbar region indicates a space-occupying lesion, usually a disc protrusion or prolapse. Radicular pain may indicate nerve root involvement. The theca is the covering of the spinal cord, which consists of the pia mater, arachnoid mater, and dura mater.

SUGGESTED DIAGNOSTIC IMAGING

- Plain film radiology
    AP lumbar view
    Lateral lumbar view
    Oblique lumbar view
- Lumbar CT
- Lumbar MRI
- Electromyography

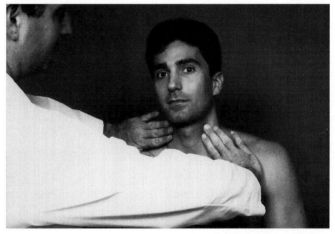

Figure 10-73

DIFFERENTIAL DIAGNOSIS: LUMBAR VERSUS SACROILIAC INVOLVEMENT

CLINICAL DESCRIPTION

Lumbar and/or radicular pain in a leg may be caused by a lumbar condition or by a pathological condition affecting the sacroiliac joint, such as sacroiliac joint syndrome, trauma, infection, inflammation, degeneration, tumor, or tumorlike condition. The most common sacroiliac joint pathology is sacroiliac joint syndrome. It can cause local lower back pain with or without a lower extremity radicular component and may be sharp or dull. The symptoms are usually unilateral and have a right-sided predominance. Weakness, paresthesia, and dysesthesia are rare. The following tests help to determine whether the patient's lower back pain is lumbar or sacroiliac related.

> **CLINICAL SIGNS AND SYMPTOMS**
> * Lower back pain
> * Sacroiliac joint pain
>   Aggravated by sitting
>   Alleviated by standing or walking
> * Lower extremity radicular pain

Goldthwaith's Test

Sensitivity/Reliability Scale

0   1   2   3   4

PROCEDURE

With the patient supine, place one hand under the lumbar spine with each finger under an interspinous space. With the other hand, perform a straight leg raising test. Note whether pain is elicited before, during, or after the spinous processes fan out (Fig. 10-74).

RATIONALE

Radicular pain before fanning out of the lumbar vertebrae indicates an extradural lesion, such as a sacroiliac joint disorder (0° to 35°). Radicular pain during lumbar fanning indicates an intradural lesion, such as an intrathecal space-occupying lesion (e.g., disc defect, osteophyte, mass) (35° to 70°). Local pain after lumbar fanning indicates a posterior lumbar joint disorder (after 70°) (see Straight Leg Raising Test).

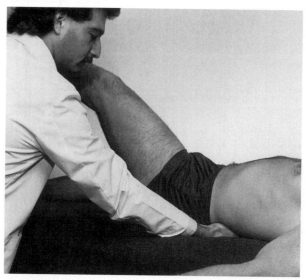

Figure 10-74

Supported Forward Bending Test

PROCEDURE

With the patient standing, instruct the patient to bend forward, keeping the knees straight (Fig. 10-75). Repeat the test, but support the ilia with your hands while bracing the patient's sacrum with your hip (Fig. 10-76).

RATIONALE

Stabilizing the ilia immobilizes the sacroiliac joints; thus, when the person bends, a lumbar lesion will elicit pain in both instances because the lumbar vertebrae are not immobilized either time. If a sacroiliac joint lesion is present, pain will be elicited only when the ilia are not immobilized.

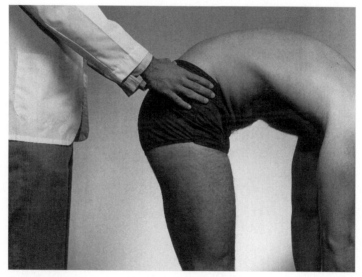

Figure 10-75

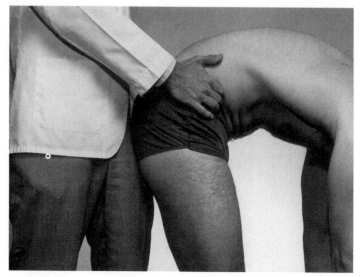

Figure 10-76

10

Nachlas Test (29)

Sensitivity/Reliability Scale

0   1   2   3   4

PROCEDURE

With the patient prone, approximate the patient's heel to the buttock on the same side (Fig. 10-77).

RATIONALE

Flexing the leg to the buttock stretches the quadriceps muscles and the femoral nerve, which is the largest branch of the lumbar plexus (L2–L4). Radicular pain into the anterior thigh may indicate compression or irritation of the L2 to L4 nerve roots by an intradural lesion (e.g., disc defect, spur, mass), a lumbar plexus, or femoral nerve compression or irritation by an extradural lesion (piriformis muscle hypertrophy). Stretching the quadriceps muscles causes the sacroiliac joint and the lumbosacral joints to move inferiorly. Pain in the buttock may indicate a sacroiliac joint lesion. Pain in the lumbosacral joint may indicate a lumbosacral lesion.

NOTE

Local pain at the anterior thigh and inability to touch the heel to the buttock may indicate a quadriceps muscle contracture.

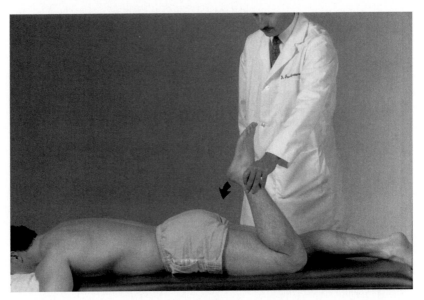

Figure 10-77

Sign of the Buttock Test (24)

PROCEDURE

With the patient supine, perform a passive straight leg raising test (Fig. 10-78). If you find restriction, flex the patient's knee and see if hip flexion increases (Fig. 10-79).

RATIONALE

If hip flexion increases and the patient's pain is exacerbated, the problem is in the lumbar spine, because there is full movement in the sacroiliac joint when the knee is flexed. This result indicates a negative sign. If hip flexion does not increase when the knee is flexed, the sacroiliac joint is dysfunctional. This dysfunction indicates pathology of the sacroiliac joint or buttocks, such as an inflammatory process, bursitis, mass, or abscess. This result is a positive sign.

> **SUGGESTED DIAGNOSTIC IMAGING**
> • Plain film radiology
>   AP lumbar view
>   Lateral lumbar view
>   AP pelvis view
>   Sacral base view
>   S-I joint views

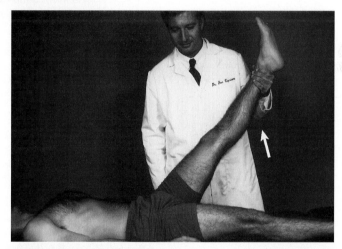

Figure 10-78

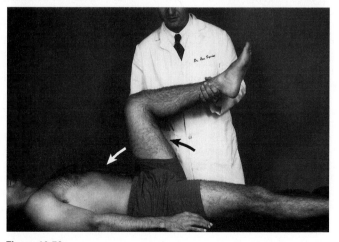

Figure 10-79

References

1. American Academy of Orthopaedic Surgeons. The Clinical Measurement of Joint Motion. Chicago: American Academy of Orthopaedic Surgeons, 1994.
2. Loebl WY. Measurement of spinal posture and range of spinal movements. Ann Phys Med 1967;9:103–110.
3. Fitzgerald GK, Wynveen KJ, Rheault W, et al. Objective assessment with establishment of normal values for lumbar spinal range of motion. Phys Ther 1983;63:1776–1781.
4. Einkauf DK, Gohdes ML, Jensen GM, et al. Objective assessment with establishment of normal values for lumbar spinal range of motion. Phys Ther 1987;67:370–375.
5. Wadsworth CT. Manual Examination and Treatment of the Spine and Extremities. Baltimore: Williams & Wilkins, 1988.
6. Gariick JG, Webb DR. Sports Injuries: Diagnosis and Management. Philadelphia: Saunders, 1990.
7. Jackson DW, Ciullo JV. Injuries of the spine in the immature athlete. In Nicholas JA, Hershmann EB, eds. The Lower Extremity and Spine in Sports Medicine. Vol 2. St. Louis: Mosby, 1986.
8. Jackson DW, Wiltse LL, Dingeman RD, Hayes M. Stress reactions involving the pars interarticularis in young athletes. Am J Sports Med 1981;9:304–312.
9. O'Donoghue D. Treatment of Injuries to Athletes. 4th ed. Philadelphia: Saunders, 1984.
10. Turek SL. Orthopaedics. 3rd ed. Philadelphia: JB Lippincott, 1977.
11. Breig A, Troup JDG. Biomechanical considerations in straight-leg-raising test: cadaveric and clinical studies of the effects of medial hip rotation. Spine 1979;4:242.
12. Fahrni WH. Observations on straight-leg-raising with special reference to nerve root adhesions. Can J Surg 1966;9:44.
13. Hoppenfeld S. Physical examination of the spine and extremities. New York: Appleton-Century-Crofts, 1976:127.
14. Urban LM. The straight-leg-raising test: a review. J Orthop Sports Phys Ther 1981;2:117.
15. Lasègue C. Considérations sur la sciatique. Arch Gen Meil 1864;24:558.
16. Wilkins RH, Brody IA. Lasègue's sign. Arch Neurol 1969;21:2110.
17. Maitland D. The slump test: examination and treatment. Aust J Physiother 1985;31:215–219.
18. Dyck P. The femoral nerve traction test with lumbar disc protrusion. Surg Neurol 1976;6:163.
19. Hudgins WR. The crossed-straight-leg-raising test. N Engl J Med 1977;297:1127.
20. Woodhall R, Hayes GJ. The well-leg-raising test of Fajersztajn in the diagnosis of ruptured lumbar intervertebral disc. J Bone Joint Surg 1950; 32A:786.
21. Rask M. Knee flexion test and sciatica. Clin Orthop 1978;134:221.
22. Cram RH. Sign of sciatic nerve root pressure. J Bone Joint Surg 1953;358:192.
23. Magee JM. Orthopaedic physical assessment. 3rd ed. Philadelphia: Saunders, 1997.
24. Hartley A. Practical joint assessment. St. Louis: Mosby, 1991.
25. Katznelson A, Nerubay J, Level A. Gluteal skyline: a search for an objective sign in the diagnosis of disc lesions of the lower lumbar spine. Spine 1982;7:74.
26. DeGowin EL, DeGowin RL. Bedside Diagnostic Examination. 2nd ed. London: Macmillan, 1960.
27. Scham SM, Taylor TKF. Tension signs in lumbar disc prolapse. Clin Orthop Relat Res 1971; 75:195.
28. Arid RB, Naffziger HC. Prolonged jugular compression: a new diagnostic test of neurologic value. Trans Am Neural Assoc 1941;66:45–48.
29. Cyriax J. Textbook of orthopaedic medicine. Vol I. 4th ed. London: Bailliéré Tindall, 1975.

General References

American Medical Association. Guides to the evaluation of permanent impairment. 3rd ed. Chicago: AMA, 1988.

Bogduk N, Twomey LT. Clinical anatomy of the lumbar spine. New York: Churchill Livingstone, 1987.

Chadwick PR. Examination, assessment and treatment of the lumbar spine. Physiotherapy 1984;70:2.

Charnley J. Orthopaedic signs in the diagnosis of disc protrusion with special reference to the straight-leg-raising test. Lancet 1951;1:156.

Cyriax J. Textbook of orthopaedic medicine. Vol 1. Diagnosis of soft tissue lesions. London: Bailliéré Tindall, 1982.

D'Ambrosia RD. Musculoskeletal Disorders: Regional Examination and Differential Diagnosis. 2nd ed. Philadelphia: JB Lippincott, 1986.

Derosa C, Portefielf J. Review for Advanced Orthopaedic Competencies: The Low Back and Sacroiliac Joint and Hip. Chicago: 1980.

Edgar MA, Park WM. Induced pain patterns on passive straight-leg-raising in lower lumbar disc protrusion. J Bone Joint Surg 1974;56B:658.

Farfan HF. Mechanical disorders of the low back. Philadelphia: Lea & Febiger, 1973.

Farfan HF, Cossette JW, Robertson GW, et al. Effects of torsion on lumbar intervertebral joints: the role of torsion in the production of disc degeneration. J Bone Joint Surg 1970; 52A:468.

Finneson BE. Low Back Pain. 2nd ed. Philadelphia: JB Lippincott, 1981.

Fisk JW. The Painful Neck and Back. Chicago: Charles C. Thomas, 1977.

Goddard BS, Reid JD. Movements induced by straight-leg-raising in the lumbo-sacral roots, nerves, and plexus and in the intrapelvic section of the sciatic nerve. J Neurol Neurosurg Psychiatry 1965;28:12.

Gracovetsky S, Farfan HF, Lamy C. The mechanism of the lumbar spine. Spine 1981;6:249–262.

Grieve GP. Common Vertebral Joint Problems. 2nd ed. New York: Churchill Livingstone, 1988.

Helfet AJ, Lee DM. Disorders of the lumbar spine. Philadelphia: JB Lippincott, 1978.

Kapandji IA. The physiology of joints. Vol 3. The Trunk and the Vertebral Column. New York: Churchill Livingstone, 1974.

Loeser JD. Pain due to nerve injury. Spine 1985;10:232.

Macnab I. Backache. Baltimore: Williams & Wilkins, 1977.

Mayer TG, Tencer AF, Kristoferson S, et al. Use of non-invasive techniques for quantification of spinal range-of-motion in normal subjects and chronic low back dysfunction patients. Spine 1984;9:588–595.

McKenzie RA. The Lumbar Spine: Mechanical Diagnosis and Therapy. Waikanae, New Zealand: Spinal Publications, 1981.

McRae R. Clinical Orthopaedic Examination. New York: Churchill Livingstone, 1976.

Nachemson A. Towards a better understanding of low back pain: a review of the mechanics of the lumbar disc. Rheumatol Rehabil 1975; 14:1210.

Panjabi M, Krag M, Chung T. Effects of disc injury on mechanical behavior of the human spine. Spine 1984;9:707.

Post M. Physical Examination of the Musculoskeletal System. Chicago: Year Book, 1987.

Ruge D, Wiltse LL. Spinal disorder diagnosis and treatment. Philadelphia: Lea & Febiger, 1977.

Travell JG, Simmons DG. Myofascial Pain and Dysfunction: The Trigger Point Manual. Vol 2. The Lower Extremities. Baltimore: Williams & Wilkins, 1992.

White AA, Panjabi MM. Clinical biomechanics of the spine. Toronto: JB Lippincott, 1978.

Wooden MJ. Preseason screening of the lumbar spine. J Orthop Sports Phys Ther 1981;3:6.

10

11

LUMBAR NERVE ROOT LESIONS

T12, L1, L2, L3

CLINICAL DESCRIPTION

Nerve roots in the lumbar spine exit the spinal column through laterally placed intervertebral foramina. The nerve roots in the lower thoracic and lumbar spine gradually exit their intervertebral foramen at its upper aspect. This causes the nerve root in these areas to be affected by the intervertebral disc above the exiting nerve root (Fig. 11-1). The lower thoracic area and upper lumbar area (T12–L2) are transitions to this anatomic consideration and in this area may be affected either by

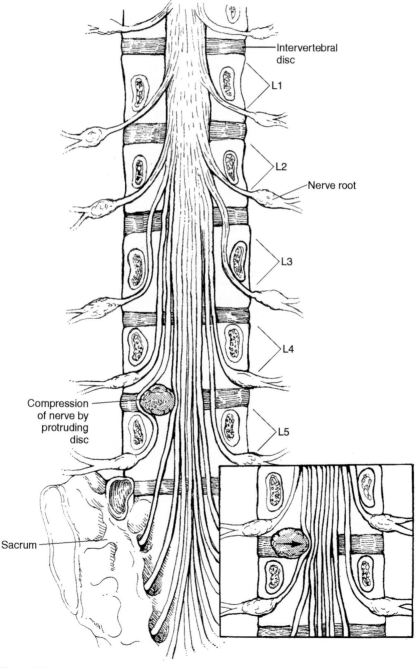

Figure 11-1

the intervertebral disc at the same interval or the disc at the level above the exiting nerve root. This situation may depend on the laterality of the disc defect. The L3 to L5 nerve roots exit the intervertebral foramen at the upper end of the foramen 80% of the time, and they are usually affected by the intervertebral disc above the exiting nerve root. Because of its anatomic position, the S1 nerve root is usually affected by the L5–S1 intervertebral disc. If a lumbar nerve root lesion is suspected, you must evaluate three clinical aspects of the neurological examination: sensory dysfunction, motor dysfunction, and reflex dysfunction.

The sensory deficit evaluation addresses the segmental cutaneous innervation of the skin. It is tested with a sterile or disposable Neurotip or pinwheel in specific dermatomal patterns. Two dermatomal maps are provided here. Figure 11-2 indicates the body areas of intact sensation when roots above and below an isolated root are interrupted, sensation loss when one or more continuous roots are interrupted, or the pattern of herpetic rash and hypersensitivity in isolated root involvement. Figure 11-3 presents the hyposensitivity to pin scratch in various root lesions and is consistent with electrical skin resistance studies showing axial dermatomes extending to the distal extremities. This pattern is useful in evaluating paresthesias and hyperesthesias secondary to root irritation. This is the pattern that will be delineated to evaluate sensory root dysfunction. Since a fair amount of segmental overlap exists, a single unilateral lesion may affect more than one dermatomal level. Motor function is tested by evaluating the muscle strength of specific muscles innervated by a particular nerve root or roots using the muscle grading chart adopted by the American Academy of Orthopaedic Surgeons (Box 11-1). The reflex arc is tested by evaluating the superficial stretch reflex associated with the particular nerve root. These reflexes are graded by the Wexler scale (Box 11-2).

Box 11-1	Muscle Grading Chart
5	Complete range of motion against gravity with full resistance
4	Complete range of motion against gravity with some resistance
3	Complete range of motion against gravity
2	Complete range of motion with gravity eliminated
1	Evidence of slight contractility; no joint motion
0	No evidence of contractility

Box 11-2	Wexler Scale
0	No response
+1	Hyporeflexia
+2	Normal
+3	Hyperreflexia
+4	Hyperreflexia with transient clonus
+5	Hyperreflexia with sustained clonus

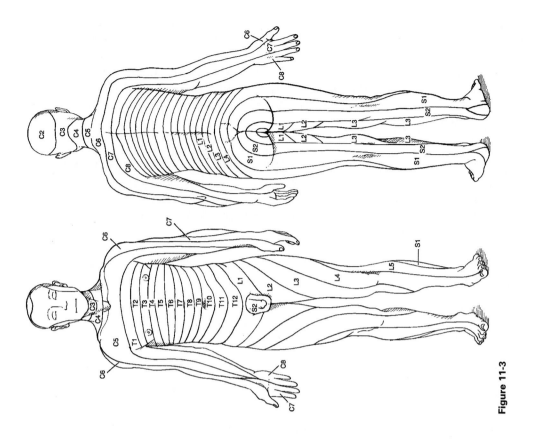

Figure 11-3

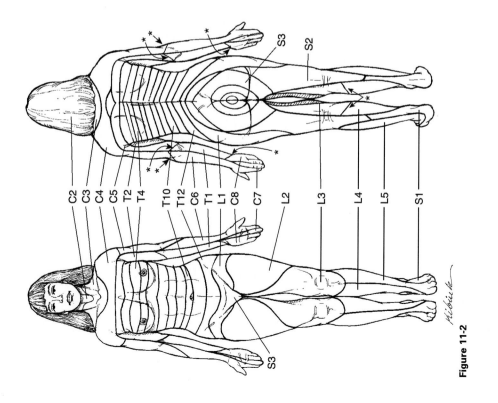

Figure 11-2

The clinical presentation of nerve root lesions depends on two important factors: the **location** and the **severity** of the injury or pathology. These two factors determine the lesion's clinical presentation. The possibilities range from no clinical signs or slight clinical manifestation, such as slight loss of sensation and pain, to total denervation with complete loss of function (motor, sensory, and reflex) in the structures innervated by the involved nerve root. Each nerve root has its own sensory distribution, muscle test or tests, and a stretch reflex, which will be grouped to facilitate identification of the suspected level.

The clinical evaluation is not made solely on one aspect of the neurological package but is determined by the combination of history, inspection, palpation, the three individual tests (motor, reflex, and sensory), and appropriate diagnostic imaging and/or functional neurological testing, such as electromyography. Furthermore, the injury or pathology may not necessarily affect a nerve root; it may affect the lumbar plexus, a trunk of that plexus, or a named nerve. Depending on the severity and location of the injury or pathology, various combinations of neurological dysfunction may be revealed.

T12, L1, L2, L3

The T12, L1, L2, and L3 nerve roots exit the spinal canal at their respective levels. The T12 and L1 nerve roots can be affected by the intervertebral disc at their respective levels or levels above them, depending on the size and laterality of the disc defect (Fig. 11-4).

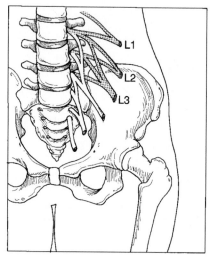

Figure 11-4

Motor

Iliopsoas: T12, L1, L2, L3 Nerve Root Innervation

PROCEDURE

With the patient sitting at the edge of the examination table, instruct the patient to raise the thigh off the table. Place your hand on the patient's knee and instruct the patient to continue to raise the thigh against your resistance (Fig. 11-5). Perform the test on the opposite thigh. Grade according to the muscle grading chart and evaluate bilaterally.

RATIONALE

A grade 0 to 4 unilaterally may indicate a neurological deficit of the T12, L1, L2, or L3 nerve root. Suspect a weak or strained iliopsoas muscle if the sensory portion of the T12, L1, L2, or L3 neurological package is intact.

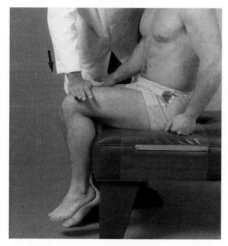

Figure 11-5

Reflex

There is no reflex test.

Sensory

PROCEDURE

With a pin, stroke the dermatomal area corresponding to each nerve root (Fig. 11-6) and evaluate bilaterally.

RATIONALE

Unilateral hypoesthesia may indicate a neurological deficit of the corresponding T12, L1, L2, or L3 nerve root or the femoral nerve.

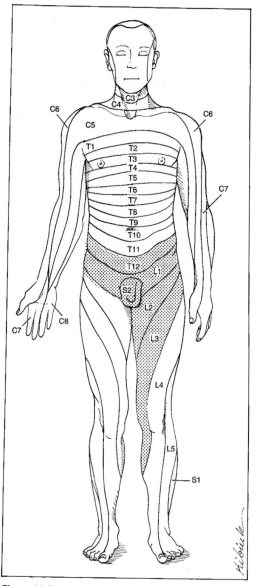

Figure 11-6

L2, L3, L4

The L2, L3, and L4 nerve roots can be affected by the intervertebral disc at their respective levels or levels above them, depending on the size and laterality of the disc defect (Fig. 11-7).

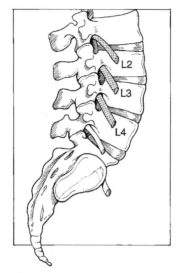

Figure 11-7

Motor

Quadriceps Muscle: L3, L4 Femoral Nerve Innervation

PROCEDURE

With the patient sitting at the edge of the examination table, instruct the patient to extend the knee. Place one hand on the patient's thigh for stabilization and place the other hand on his or her leg. Exert pressure on the leg while instructing the patient to resist flexion (Fig. 11-8). Grade according to the muscle grading chart and evaluate bilaterally.

RATIONALE

A grade 0 to 4 unilaterally may indicate a neurological deficit of the L2, L3, or L4 nerve root or femoral nerve. Suspect a weak or strained quadriceps muscle if the sensory portion of the L2, L3, or L4 neurological package is intact.

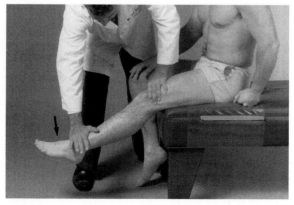

Figure 11-8

Reflex

Patella Reflex

The patella reflex is primarily an L4 reflex and is tested with the L4 neurological level.

Sensory

PROCEDURE

With a pin, stroke the dermatomal area corresponding to each nerve root (Fig. 11-9) and evaluate bilaterally.

RATIONALE

Unilateral hypoesthesia may indicate a neurological deficit of the corresponding L2, L3, or L4 nerve roots or the femoral nerve.

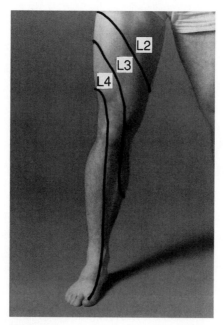

Figure 11-9

L4

The L4 nerve root exits the spinal canal between the L4 and L5 vertebrae and is usually affected by the L3-L4 intervertebral disc (Fig. 11-10).

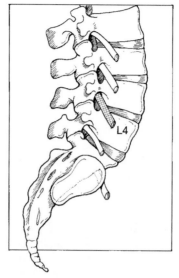

Figure 11-10

Motor

Tibialis Anterior: L4, L5 Deep Fibular Nerve Innervation

PROCEDURE

With the patient seated at the edge of the examination table, instruct the patient to dorsiflex and invert the foot. Grasp the patient's ankle with one hand and foot with your other hand, and attempt to force the foot into plantar flexion and eversion against resistance by the patient (Fig. 11-11). Grade according to the muscle grading chart and evaluate bilaterally.

RATIONALE

A grade 0 to 4 unilaterally may indicate a neurological deficit of the L4 nerve root or the deep fibular nerve. A weak or strained tibialis anterior muscle may be suspected if the sensory and reflex portions of the L4 neurological package are intact.

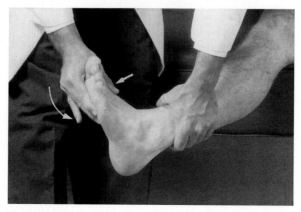

Figure 11-11

Reflex

Patella Reflex

PROCEDURE

With the patient seated at the edge of the examination table, tap the infrapatellar tendon with the neurological reflex hammer (Fig. 11-12).

RATIONALE

Unilateral hyporeflexia may indicate a nerve root deficit. Loss of reflex unilaterally may indicate an interruption of the reflex arc (lower motor neuron lesion). Unilateral hyperreflexia may indicate an upper motor neuron lesion.

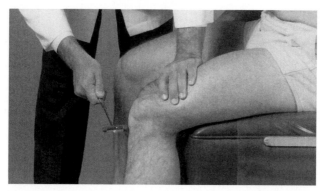

Figure 11-12

Sensory

PROCEDURE

With a pin, stroke the medial aspect of the leg and foot (Fig. 11-13) and evaluate bilaterally.

RATIONALE

Unilateral hypoesthesia may indicate a neurological deficit of the L4 nerve root.

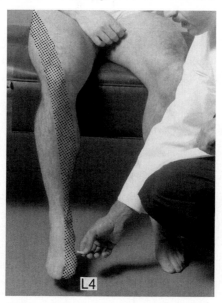

L4

Figure 11-13

L5

The L5 nerve root exits the spinal canal between the L5 vertebra and the first sacral segment and is usually affected by the L4–L5 intervertebral disc (Fig. 11-14).

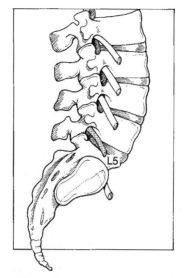

Figure 11-14

Motor

Extensor Hallucis Longus: L5, S1 Deep Fibular Nerve Innervation

PROCEDURE

With the patient seated at the edge of the examination table, grasp the patient's calcaneus with one hand for stabilization. With your opposite hand, pinch the great toe and instruct the patient to dorsiflex it against your resistance (Fig. 11-15). Grade according to the muscle grading chart and compare bilaterally.

RATIONALE

A grade 0 to 4 unilaterally may indicate a neurological deficit of the L5 nerve root or the deep fibular nerve. A weak or strained extensor hallucis longus muscle may be suspected if the sensory and reflex portions of the L5 neurological package are intact.

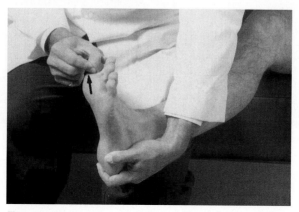

Figure 11-15

Gluteus Medius: L5, S1 Superior Gluteal Nerve Innervation

PROCEDURE

With the patient side-lying on the examination table, instruct the patient to abduct the superior leg (Fig. 11-16). Place your hand on the lateral aspect of the patient's knee and attempt to push the knee into adduction against patient resistance (Fig. 11-17). Grade according to the muscle grading chart and evaluate bilaterally.

RATIONALE

A grade 0 to 4 unilaterally may indicate a neurological deficit of the L5 nerve root or the superior gluteal nerve. A weak or strained gluteus medius muscle may be suspected if the sensory and reflex portions of the L5 neurological package are intact.

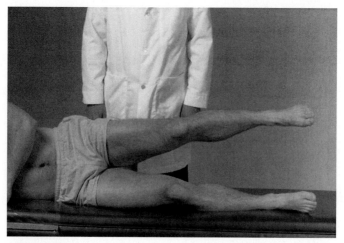

Figure 11-16

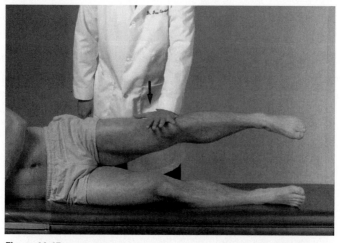

Figure 11-17

Extensor Digitorum Longus and Brevis: L5, S1 Superficial Fibular Nerve Innervation

PROCEDURE

With the patient sitting at the edge of the examination table, grasp the calcaneus to stabilize the foot. With your opposite hand, grasp the patient's second through fifth toes and instruct the patient to dorsiflex the toes against your resistance (Fig. 11-18).

RATIONALE

A grade 0 to 4 unilaterally may indicate a neurological deficit of the L5 nerve root or the superficial fibular nerve. A weak or strained extensor digitorum longus and/or brevis muscle may be suspected if the sensory and reflex portions of the L5 neurological package are intact.

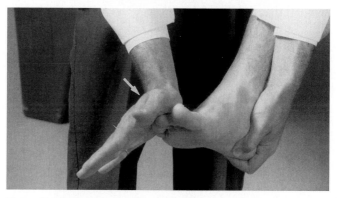

Figure 11-18

Reflex

Medial Hamstring Reflex

PROCEDURE

With the patient prone, slightly flex the patient's knee and place your thumb on the medial hamstring tendon. With a neurological reflex hammer, tap the medial hamstring tendon (Fig. 11-19). The patient should slightly flex the knee.

RATIONALE

Unilateral hyporeflexia may indicate a nerve root deficit. Loss of reflex unilaterally may indicate an interruption of the reflex arc (lower motor neuron lesion). Unilateral hyperreflexia may indicate an upper motor neuron lesion.

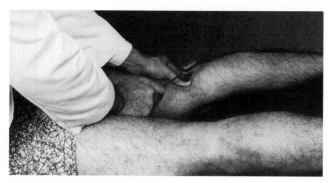

Figure 11-19

Sensory

PROCEDURE

With a pin, stroke the lateral leg and dorsum of the foot (Fig. 11-20). Evaluate bilaterally.

RATIONALE

Unilateral hypoesthesia may indicate a neurological deficit of the L5 nerve root.

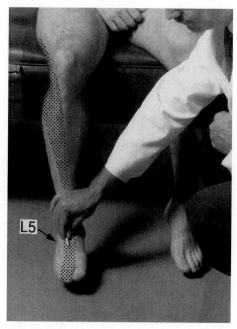

Figure 11-20

S1

The S1 nerve root exits the spinal canal through the first sacral foramen and is usually affected by the L5–S1 intervertebral disc (Fig. 11-21).

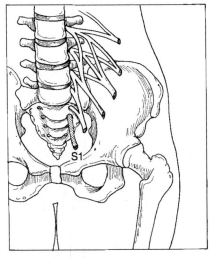

Figure 11-21

Motor

Peroneus Longus and Brevis: L5, S1 Superficial Fibular Nerve Innervation

PROCEDURE

With the patient sitting at the edge of the examination table, stabilize the calcaneus with one hand and grasp the lateral aspect of the foot with your opposite hand. Instruct the patient to plantarflex and evert the foot against your resistance (Fig. 11-22). Grade according to the muscle grading chart and evaluate bilaterally.

RATIONALE

A grade 0 to 4 unilaterally may indicate a neurological deficit of the S1 nerve root or the superficial fibular nerve. A weak or strained peroneus longus and/or brevis muscle may be suspected if the sensory and reflex portions of the S1 neurological package are intact.

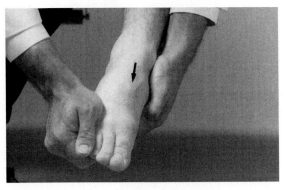

Figure 11-22

11

Reflex

Achilles Reflex

Procedure

With the patient seated at the edge of the examination table, place slight dorsiflexion on the foot. With a neurological reflex hammer, tap the Achilles tendon (Fig. 11-23). The patient should exhibit a slight plantar flexion of the foot.

Rationale

Unilateral hyporeflexia may indicate a nerve root deficit. Loss of reflex unilaterally may indicate an interruption of the reflex arc (lower motor neuron lesion). Unilateral hyperreflexia may indicate an upper motor neuron lesion.

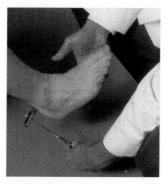

Figure 11-23

Sensory

Procedure

With a pin, stroke the lateral aspect of the foot (Fig. 11-24).

Rationale

Unilateral hypoesthesia may indicate a neurological deficit of the S1 nerve root.

Suggested Diagnostic Imaging and Functional Testing
• Lumbar magnetic resonance imaging
• Electromyography
• Somatosensory evoked potential

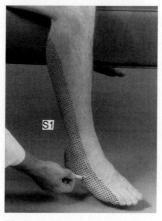

Figure 11-24

General References

Barrows HS. Guide to Neurological Assessment. Philadelphia: JB Lippincott, 1980.

Braziz PW, Masdeu JC, Biller J. Localization in Clinical Neurology. 3rd ed. New York: Little, Brown.

Bronisch FW. The Clinically Important Reflexes. New York: Grune & Stratton, 1952.

Chusid JG. Correlative Neuroanatomy and Functional Neurology. 16th ed. Los Altos, CA: Lange Medical, 1976.

DeJong RN. The Neurologic Examination. 4th ed. Hagerstown, MD: Harper & Row, 1979.

Devinsky O, Feldmann E. Examination of the Cranial and Peripheral Nerves. New York: Churchill Livingstone, 1988.

Geenberg DA, Aminoff MJ, Simon RP. Clinical neurology. 2nd ed. East Norwalk, CT: Appleton & Lange, 1993.

Hoppenfeld S. Physical examination of the spine and extremities. New York: Appleton-Century-Croft, 1976;127.

Kendall FP, McCreary EK, Provance PG. Muscles: Testing and Function. 4th ed. Baltimore: Williams & Wilkins, 1993.

Mancall E. Essentials of the neurologic examination. 2nd ed. Philadelphia: FA Davis, 1981.

Moore KL, Dailey AF. Clinically Oriented Anatomy. 4th ed. Baltimore: Lippincott Williams & Wilkins, 1999.

Parsons N. Color Atlas of Clinical Neurology. Chicago: Year Book Medical, 1989.

VanAllen MW, Rodnitzky RL. Pictorial Manual of Neurologic Tests. 2nd ed. Chicago: Year Book Medical, 1981.

11

SACROILIAC ORTHOPAEDIC TESTS

Sacroiliac Orthopaedic Examination

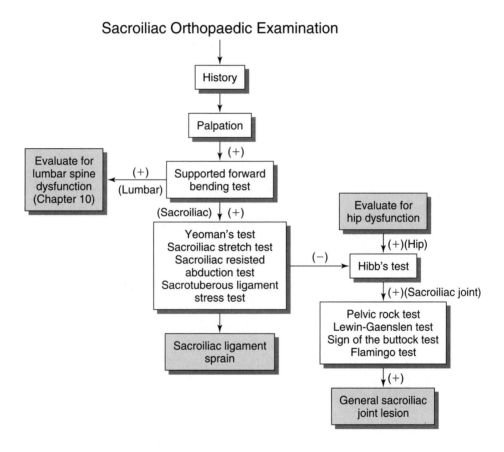

PALPATION

Posterior Superior Iliac Spine and Iliac Crest

DESCRIPTIVE ANATOMY

The iliac crest and posterior superior iliac spine are important bony landmarks used to assess postural deviations and leg length deficiencies. The iliac crest extends through the inferior margin of the flank and is easily palpable. The posterior superior iliac spine is inferior to the iliac crest and lateral to the S2 sacral segment (Fig. 12-1).

PROCEDURE

With the patient standing, palpate the iliac crest for tenderness (Fig. 12-2). Tenderness may be caused by contusions, periosteitis, or avulsion fractures. Next, place your forefingers on each iliac crest and your thumbs on the posterior superior iliac spines of each ilium (Fig. 12-3). Note any difference in longitudinal position, which may indicate a leg length discrepancy, scoliosis, sacroiliac joint subluxation, or hip joint dislocation.

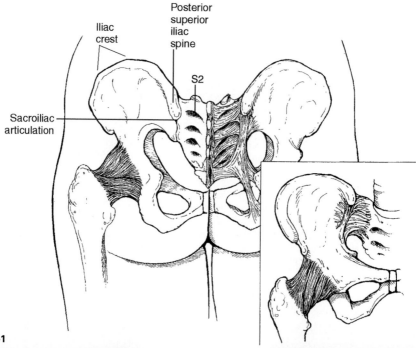

Figure 12-1

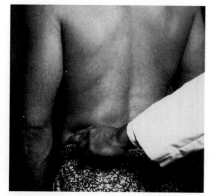

Figure 12-2

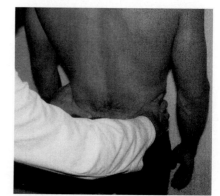

Figure 12-3

Sacroiliac Articulations

DESCRIPTIVE ANATOMY

The sacroiliac articulations are inferior and medial to the posterior superior iliac spine (Fig. 12-1). The articulations are synovial and are held together by interosseous ligaments and ventral and dorsal sacroiliac ligaments. The movement of the sacroiliac joints is limited to slight gliding and rotation. These joints are primarily weight bearing; they transfer the weight of the trunk to the hip joints.

PROCEDURE

With the patient prone, flex the patient's knee to 90° and externally rotate the hip. With your opposite hand, palpate the sacroiliac joint from just below the posterior superior iliac spine to the sacral notch (Fig. 12-4). Note any pain or tenderness that may indicate an inflammatory process in the sacroiliac joint.

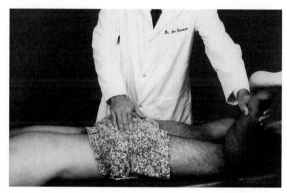

Figure 12-4

Ischial Tuberosity

DESCRIPTIVE ANATOMY

The ischial tuberosity is just below the gluteal fold (Fig. 12-1) and can be palpated easily with the hip flexed. The hamstring muscles originate from the tuberosity. The tuberosity may be injured by direct trauma or by trauma to the hamstring muscles.

12

PROCEDURE

Have the patient lie on one side and flex the hip by bringing the knee to the chest. Palpate the ischial tuberosity, noting any pain or tenderness (Fig. 12-5). Pain may indicate a contusion secondary to trauma, an avulsion fracture caused by severe hamstring pull, or ischial tuberosity bursitis.

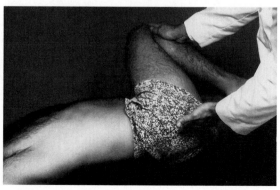

Figure 12-5

SACROILIAC SPRAIN

CLINICAL DESCRIPTION

The sacroiliac joint is a very strong cartilaginous joint that produces little movement. The sacrum is suspended between the two iliac bones and held in place by very strong interosseous dorsal sacroiliac ligaments. The joint is under great stress that predisposes it to sprains. The joint movement is limited by the tension of the sacrotuberous, sacrospinous, and sacroiliac ligaments (Fig. 12-6). These ligaments may be stretched, causing ligamentous sprain by some of the following movements:

1. Sudden contracture of the hamstrings or abdominal muscles, which exerts a rotating force on the ilium
2. Sudden unexpected twisting motions of the trunk, which may occur in sports such as football and basketball
3. Vigorous pulling while bending forward
4. A fall on one or both buttocks

The patient may have acute lower back pain and difficulty in bending. In unilateral cases it may cause the patient to elevate the hip when standing on the painful side to avoid weight bearing over the sacroiliac joint. Local tenderness is a common finding.

CLINICAL SIGNS AND SYMPTOMS
- Sacroiliac joint pain
- Abnormal gait
- Tender sacroiliac joint on palpation
- Pain on forward flexion

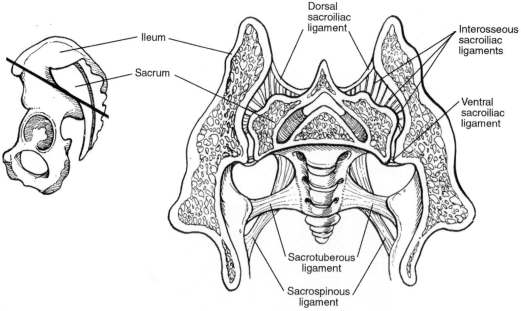

Figure 12-6

Gaenslen's Test (4)

PROCEDURE

With the patient supine and the affected side near the edge of the table, instruct the patient to approximate the knee to the chest on the unaffected side (Fig. 12-7). Then place downward pressure on the affected thigh until it is lower than the edge of the table (Fig. 12-8).

RATIONALE

Extension of the leg stresses the sacroiliac joint and anterior sacroiliac joint ligaments on the side of leg extension. Pain on that side indicates a general sacroiliac lesion, that is, anterior sacroiliac ligament sprain (iliofemoral, ischiofemoral) or inflammatory process in the sacroiliac joint.

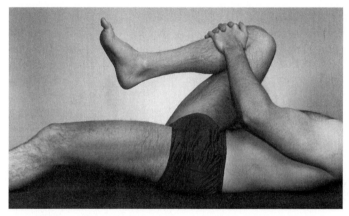

Figure 12-7

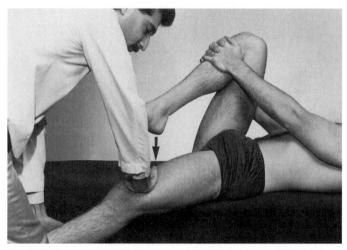

Figure 12-8

12

Lewin-Gaenslen Test

Sensitivity/Reliability Scale

0   1   2   3   4

PROCEDURE

Instruct the patient to lie on the unaffected side and flex the inferior leg (Fig. 12-9). Take the superior leg and extend it while you stabilize the lumbosacral joint (Fig. 12-10).

RATIONALE

Extension of the leg stresses the sacroiliac joint and anterior sacroiliac joint ligaments on the side of leg extension. Pain on that side indicates a general sacroiliac joint lesion, that is, anterior sacroiliac ligament sprain (iliofemoral, ischiofemoral ligaments) or inflammatory process in the sacroiliac joint.

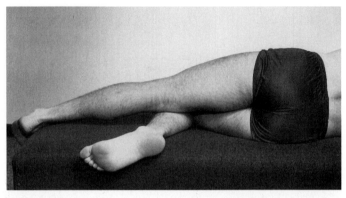

Figure 12-9

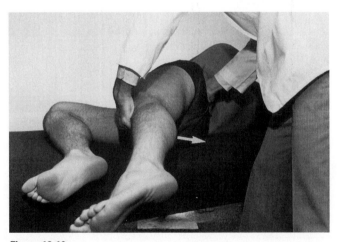

Figure 12-10

Yeoman's Test (2)

Sensitivity/Reliability Scale
0   1   2   3   4

PROCEDURE

With the patient prone, grasp the patient's lower leg and passively flex the knee, then extend the hip (Fig. 12-11).

RATIONALE

Extension of the thigh stresses the sacroiliac joint and anterior sacroiliac joint ligaments on the side of thigh extension. If pain is elicited on the ipsilateral side, suspect a sprain of the anterior sacroiliac joint ligaments, that is, the iliofemoral or ischiofemoral ligament (Fig. 12-12). Pain or an increase in pain may also indicate an inflammatory process or abscess in the sacroiliac joint.

NOTE

This test also stresses the lower lumbar vertebra by slightly extending the lumbar spine. Lumbar pain, either local or radiating, may indicate lumbar involvement. See Chapter 10 for evaluation.

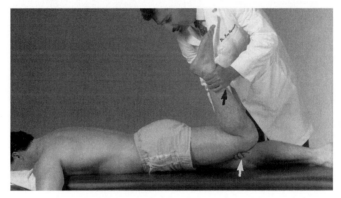

Figure 12-11

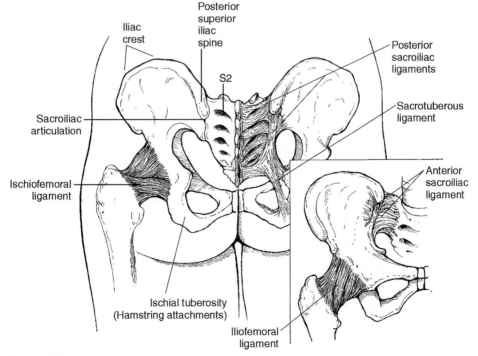

Figure 12-12

Sacroiliac Stretch Test

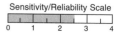

Sensitivity/Reliability Scale

0   1   2   3   4

PROCEDURE

With the patient supine, cross the patient's arms and apply posterior and lateral pressure to the anterior superior iliac spine of each ilium (Fig. 12-13).

RATIONALE

Pressure on both anterior and superior iliac spines simultaneously compresses both sacroiliac joint surfaces and stretches the anterior sacroiliac ligaments. If pain is elicited or increased in one or both joints, suspect a strain of the anterior sacroiliac ligaments, that is, iliofemoral or ischiofemoral ligament (see Fig. 12-6). Pain in the joint may also indicate an inflammatory process in the affected joint.

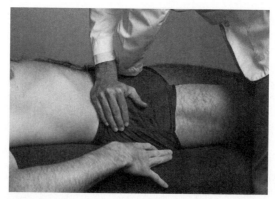

Figure 12-13

Sacroiliac Resisted Abduction Test

Sensitivity/Reliability Scale

0   1   2   3   4

PROCEDURE

Instruct the patient to lie on one side with the inferior hip and knee slightly flexed. The superior leg should be straight and abducted. Place pressure on the abducted limb against patient resistance (Fig. 12-14).

RATIONALE

Resisting abduction of the hip stresses the sacroiliac joint and abductor muscles of the hip. Increased pain in the sacroiliac joint indicates a sprain of the sacroiliac ligaments on the ipsilateral side. Pain in the affected buttock or lateral thigh indicates a strain of the abductor muscles of the thigh (tensor fasciae latae and gluteus group).

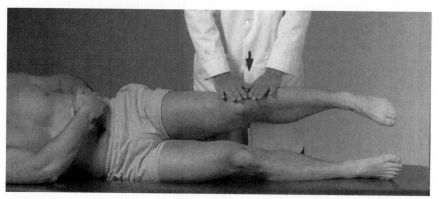

Figure 12-14

Sacrotuberous Ligament Stress Test (3)

Sensitivity/Reliability Scale

0 1 2 3 4

PROCEDURE

Place the patient supine. Fully flex the patient's knee and hip and adduct and internally rotate the hip. With your opposite hand, palpate the sacrotuberous ligament, which runs from the posterior aspect of the sacrum to the ischial tuberosity (Fig. 12-15).

RATIONALE

The sacrotuberous ligament anchors the sacrum to the ischial tuberosity. The action of hip adduction and medial hip rotation stresses the sacrotuberous ligament. Increased pain in the area of the sacrotuberous ligament may indicate a sacrotuberous ligament sprain.

SUGGESTED DIAGNOSTIC IMAGING
- Plain film radiography
  AP pelvis view

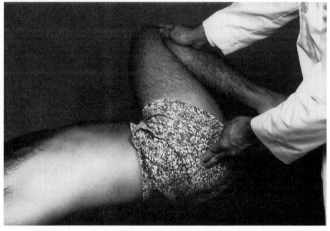

Figure 12-15

12

GENERAL SACROILIAC JOINT LESIONS

CLINICAL DESCRIPTION

The sacroiliac joint is a strong weight-bearing synovial joint with little movement. The surfaces are irregular to provide some interlocking of the sacrum to the ilium. This articulation is subject to inflammation due to trauma, overuse, or degenerative arthritis. Diffuse idiopathic skeletal hyperostosis, which produces osteophytes along the inferior aspect of the sacroiliac joint, may result in a painful joint. Ankylosing spondylitis, which is usually bilateral, may cause restriction and pain. The following tests attempt to increase the pressure in the sacroiliac joint or distract the joint to initiate or exacerbate sacroiliac joint pain.

CLINICAL SIGNS AND SYMPTOMS

- Sacroiliac joint pain
- Abnormal gait
- Tender sacroiliac joint on palpation
- Pain on forward flexion
- Pain on sitting

Hibb's Test

PROCEDURE

Sensitivity/Reliability Scale

0   1   2   3   4

With the patient prone, flex the patient's leg to the buttock and move the leg outward, internally rotating the hip (Fig. 12-16).

RATIONALE

This procedure causes a stressed internal rotation of the femoral head into the acetabular cavity and causes slight distraction on the sacroiliac joint. This test is mainly a hip joint test, but because of the sacroiliac joint distraction, it may help you evaluate sacroiliac joint lesions. Pain in the sacroiliac joint indicates a sacroiliac joint lesion, such as an inflammatory process or abscess in the sacroiliac joint or a sprain of the sacroiliac ligaments. Pain in the hip joint indicates a hip joint lesion (see Hibb's test in Chapter 13).

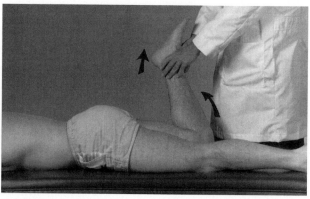

Figure 12-16

Pelvic Rock (Iliac Compression) Test (4)

Sensitivity/Reliability Scale

0   1   2   3   4

PROCEDURE

With the patient side-lying, exert a strong downward pressure on the ilium. Perform this test bilaterally (Fig. 12-17).

RATIONALE

Downward pressure on the ilium transfers a compression pressure to the joint surfaces of the sacroiliac joints. Pain in either sacroiliac joint indicates a sacroiliac joint lesion, such as an inflammatory process in the joint surfaces on the affected side.

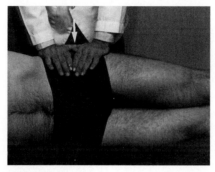

Figure 12-17

Sign of the Buttock Test (5)

Sensitivity/Reliability Scale

0   1   2   3   4

PROCEDURE

With the patient supine, perform a passive straight leg raising test (Fig. 12-18). If restriction is found, flex the patient's knee and see if hip flexion increases (Fig. 12-19).

RATIONALE

If hip flexion increases and the patient's pain is exacerbated, the problem is in the lumbar spine, because there is full movement in the sacroiliac joint when the knee is flexed. This is indicative of a negative sign. If hip flexion does not increase when the knee is flexed, the sacroiliac joint is dysfunctional. This indicates pathology of the sacroiliac joint or buttocks, such as an inflammatory process, bursitis, mass, or abscess. This is indicative of a positive sign.

12

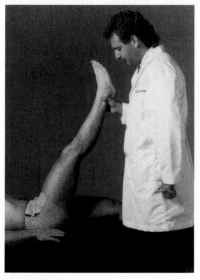

Figure 12-18

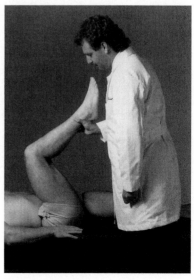

Figure 12-19

Flamingo Test (6)

Sensitivity/Reliability Scale

0   1   2   3   4

Procedure

Instruct the patient to stand on one leg at a time (Fig. 12-20). Instruct the patient to hop, which increases stress on the joint (Fig. 12-21).

Rationale

This test increases the pressure in the hip, sacroiliac articulation, and symphysis pubis articulation. Increased pain in any of these joints may indicate an inflammatory process on the standing leg side. Pain following trauma may indicate a fracture in the suspected joint. Pain in the hip joint may also indicate trochanteric bursitis.

> **Suggested Diagnostic Imaging**
> - Plain film radiography
>   AP pelvis view

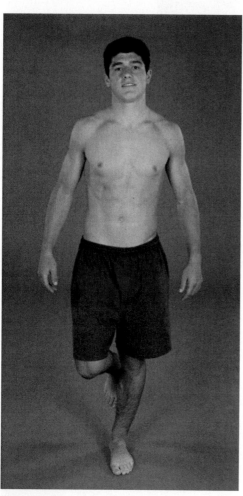

Figure 12-20

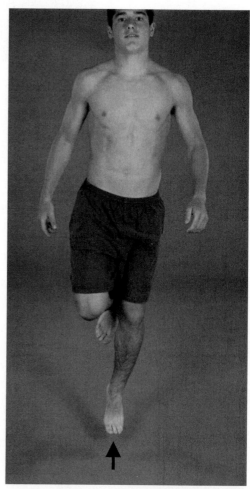

Figure 12-21

References

1. Gaenslen FJ. Sacroiliac arthrodesis. JAMA 1927;89:2031–2035.
2. Yeoman W. The relation of arthritis of the sacroiliac joint to sciatica. Lancet 1928;2:1219–1222.
3. Lee D. The Pelvic Girdle. Edinburgh: Churchill Livingstone, 1989.
4. Hoppenfeld S. Physical Examination of the Spine and Extremities. New York: Appleton-Century-Crofts, 1976:127.
5. Cyriax J. Textbook of Orthopaedic Medicine. 4th ed. Vol. I. London: Bailliéré Tindall, 1975:541.
6. Magee DJ. Orthopedic Physical Assessment. 3rd ed. Philadelphia: Saunders, 1997.

General References

Alderink GJ. The sacroiliac joint: review of anatomy, mechanics, and function. J Orthop Sports Phys Ther 1991;13:71.

DeGowin EL, DeGowin RL. Bedside Diagnostic Examination. 3rd ed. New York: Macmillan, 1976.

Gray H. Sacroiliac joint pain: the finer anatomy. New Intern Clin 1938;2:54.

Hartley A. Practical Joint Assessment. St. Louis: Mosby, 1991.

McRae R. Clinical Orthopedic Examination. New York: Churchill Livingstone, 1976

Meschan I. Roentgen Signs in Diagnostic Imaging. 2nd ed. Vol 3. Sydney: Saunders, 1985.

Norkin C, Levangie P. Joint Structure and Function: A Comprehensive Analysis. Philadelphia: FA Davis, 1987.

Post M. Physical Examination of the Musculoskeletal System. Chicago: Year Book Medical, 1987.

Wells PE. The examination of the pelvic joints. In: Grieve GP, ed. Modern Manual Therapy of the Vertebral Column. Edinburgh: Churchill Livingstone, 1986.

12

HIP JOINT ORTHOPAEDIC TESTS

Hip Joint Orthopaedic Examination

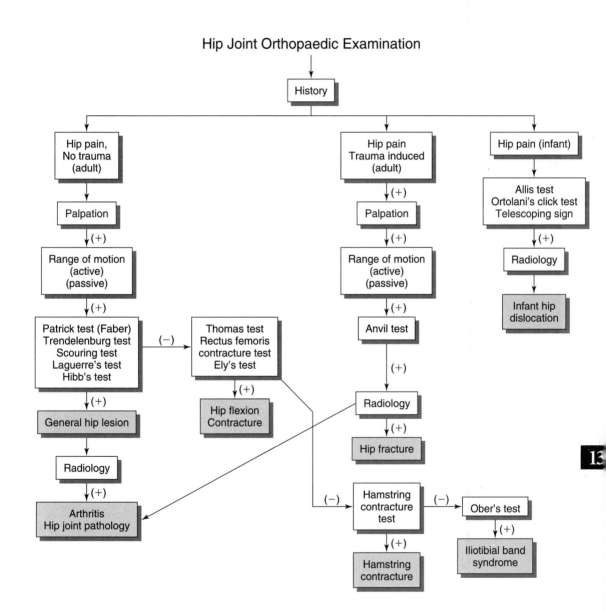

History

Hip pain, No trauma (adult)

Palpation

(+)

Range of motion (active) (passive)

(+)

Patrick test (Faber)
Trendelenburg test
Scouring test
Laguerre's test
Hibb's test

(−) →

Thomas test
Rectus femoris contracture test
Ely's test

(+)

Range of motion (active) (passive)

(+)

Hip flexion
Contracture

General hip lesion

Radiology

(+)

Arthritis
Hip joint pathology

Hip pain Trauma induced (adult)

(+)

Palpation

(+)

Range of motion (active) (passive)

(+)

Anvil test

(+)

Radiology

(+)

Hip fracture

(−) →

Hamstring contracture test

(−) →

Ober's test

(+)

Hamstring contracture

Iliotibial band syndrome

Hip pain (infant)

Allis test
Ortolani's click test
Telescoping sign

(+)

Radiology

Infant hip dislocation

13

PALPATION

Iliac Crest and Anterior, Superior, and Inferior Iliac Spine

DESCRIPTIVE ANATOMY

The iliac crest is at the inferior margin of the flank from the anterior; from the posterior, its highest point is at the level of the L4 spinous process (Fig. 13-1). The iliacus, external oblique, and tensor fasciae latae muscles originate from the iliac crest. At the anterior terminal end of the iliac crest lies the anterior superior iliac spine (Fig. 13-1). It is the attachment of the sartorius muscle and is easily palpable. The anterior inferior iliac spine is just below the anterior superior iliac spine. The rectus femoris muscle and iliofemoral ligament are attached to it (Fig. 13-1).

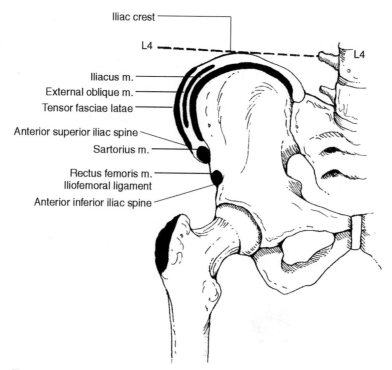

Figure 13-1

PROCEDURE

With the patient supine, palpate the iliac crests for point tenderness and swelling (Fig. 13-2). This may indicate periostitis or strain or avulsion of the iliacus, external oblique, or tensor fasciae latae muscles. Contusion to the iliac crest secondary to trauma is common in the athlete. Palpate the iliac crests with the patient standing as well, checking for unevenness of the crests (Fig. 13-3). Unevenness may be a sign of scoliosis, anatomical short leg, or contracture deformity. The anterior superior iliac spine should be palpated next (Fig. 13-4). Look for point tenderness and swelling, which may indicate a sartorius muscle strain or avulsion fracture. Just below the anterior superior iliac spine is the anterior inferior iliac spine (Fig. 13-5). With your thumb or forefinger, palpate this area and note any point tenderness or swelling. It may indicate a sprained or avulsed rectus femoris muscle or strained iliofemoral ligament.

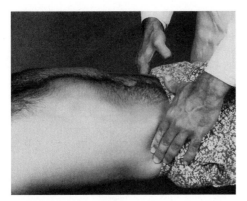

Figure 13-2

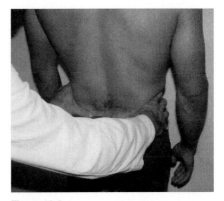

Figure 13-3

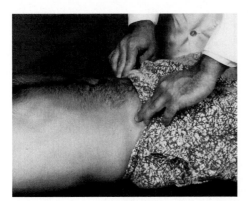

Figure 13-4

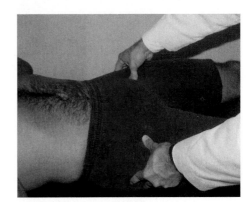

Figure 13-5

13

Greater Trochanter

DESCRIPTIVE ANATOMY

The greater trochanter is approximately 10 cm inferior and lateral to the anterior superior iliac spine (Fig. 13-6). The greater trochanter is the attachment of the gluteus medius, gluteus minimus, and vastus lateralis muscles. The trochanteric bursa also lies under these muscles.

PROCEDURE

With the patient supine, slightly abduct the thigh and palpate the greater trochanter (Fig. 13-7). Note any point tenderness or swelling. This may indicate a strain of the gluteus medius, gluteus minimus, or vastus lateralis muscles. An increase in the temperature differential associated with tenderness and swelling is an indication of trochanteric bursitis.

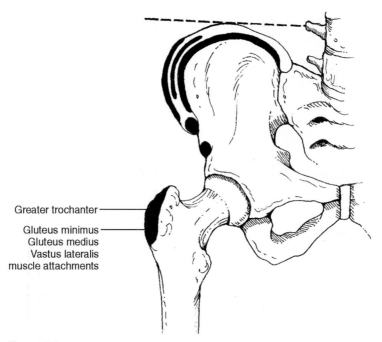

Greater trochanter
Gluteus minimus
Gluteus medius
Vastus lateralis
muscle attachments

Figure 13-6

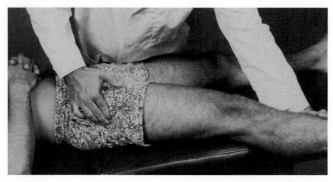

Figure 13-7

Hip Joint

DESCRIPTIVE ANATOMY

The hip joint is a ball and socket synovial joint, and the femur head is held in place by the iliofemoral, pubofemoral, and ischiofemoral ligaments (Fig. 13-8). The iliofemoral ligament is the largest and strongest of these ligaments that hold the femur into the acetabular cavity.

The hip joint at best is difficult to palpate because it lies deep in the body. Unless the joint is traumatized to the point of fracture or dislocation, palpation of the actual joint will reveal little clinical information. Palpation of the surrounding tissue may be a better indicator of hip joint pathology.

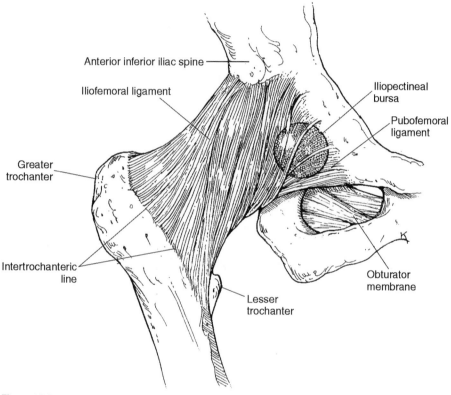

Figure 13-8

13

Tensor Fasciae Latae Muscle

DESCRIPTIVE ANATOMY

The tensor fasciae latae muscle is on the anterior lateral side of the thigh. It originates from the anterior outer lip of the iliac crest and inserts into the iliotibial band, which attaches to the lateral epicondyle of the tibia (Fig. 13-9).

PROCEDURE

With the patient laying on the unaffected side, palpate the tensor fasciae latae muscle from just below the anterior superior iliac spine down over the greater trochanter to the lateral aspect of the knee (Fig. 13-10). Note any tenderness, spasm, increase in skin temperature, or inflammation. These may indicate a strain of the muscle. If point tenderness is present, suspect an active trigger point that may refer pain to the upper half of the medial thigh. If the muscle becomes strained through microtrauma as it moves over the greater trochanter of the femur, it can cause greater trochanteric bursitis.

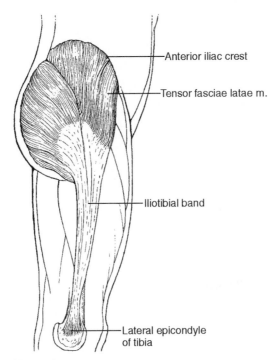

Anterior iliac crest

Tensor fasciae latae m.

Iliotibial band

Lateral epicondyle of tibia

Figure 13-9

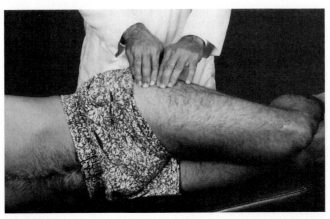

Figure 13-10

Femoral Triangle

DESCRIPTIVE ANATOMY

The femoral triangle is a clinically important region. It is bound superiorly by the inguinal ligament, medially by the adductor longus muscle, and laterally by the sartorius muscle (Fig. 13-11). The triangle contains lymph nodes and the femoral artery, vein, and nerve.

PROCEDURE

With the patient supine, palpate the inguinal ligament, which extends from the anterior superior iliac spine to the pubic tubercle. Note any tenderness, which may indicate a sprain. Next, palpate the adductor longus and sartorius muscle, again noting any tenderness or inflammation. This may indicate a strain or active trigger points in the affected muscle. Once the borders are palpated, palpate the interior of the triangle for inflamed lymph nodes, which may indicate a lower extremity or systemic infection (Fig. 13-12). Palpate the femoral artery for amplitude. A decrease in the amplitude indicates a compromise to the vascular supply to the lower extremity.

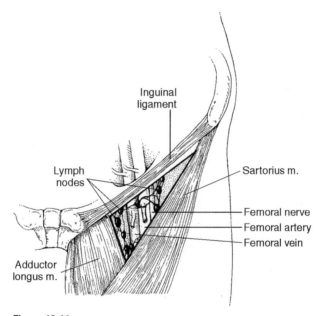

Figure 13-11

13

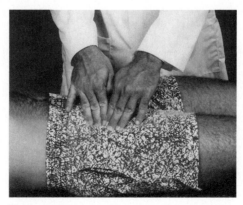

Figure 13-12

HIP RANGE OF MOTION

Flexion (1)

With the patient supine, place the goniometer in the sagittal plane at the level of the hip (Fig. 13-13). Instruct the patient to flex the hip, and follow the thigh with one arm of the goniometer (Fig. 13-14).

NORMAL RANGE (2)

Normal range is $131° \pm 6.4°$ or greater from the 0 or neutral position.

Muscles	Nerve Supply
Psoas	L1–L3
Iliacus	Femoral
Rectus femoris	Femoral
Sartorius	Femoral
Pectineus	Femoral
Adductor longus and brevis	Obturator
Gracilis	Obturator

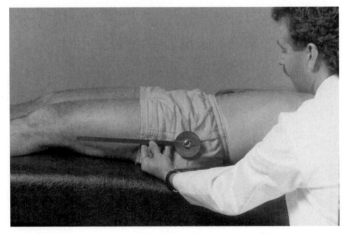

Figure 13-13

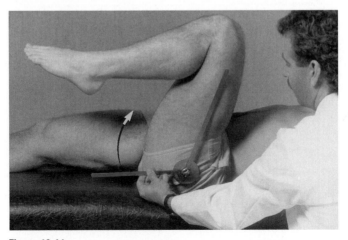

Figure 13-14

Extension (1)

With the patient prone, place the goniometer in the sagittal plane at the level of the hip joint (Fig. 13-15). Instruct the patient to raise the thigh off the table as far as possible, and follow the thigh with one arm of the goniometer (Fig. 13-16).

NORMAL RANGE (2)

Normal range is 13° ± 5.4° or greater from the 0 or neutral position.

Muscles	Nerve Supply
Biceps femoris	Sciatic
Semimembranosus	Sciatic
Semitendinosus	Sciatic
Gluteus maximus	Inferior gluteal
Gluteus medius	Superior gluteal
Adductor magnus	Sciatic

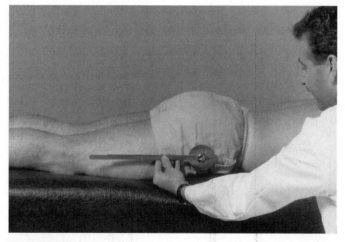

Figure 13-15

13

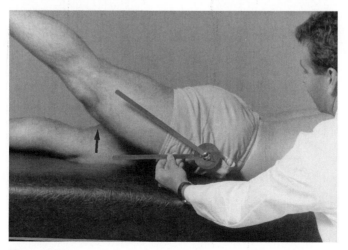

Figure 13-16

Abduction (1)

With the patient supine, place the goniometer in the coronal plane with the center at the level of the hip (Fig. 13-17). Instruct the patient to move the thigh laterally while following the thigh with one arm of the goniometer (Fig. 13-18).

NORMAL RANGE (2)

Normal range is 41° ± 6° or greater from the 0 or neutral position.

Muscles	*Nerve Supply*
Tensor fasciae latae	Superior Gluteal
Gluteus minimus	Superior Gluteal
Gluteus medius	Superior Gluteal
Gluteus maximus	Inferior Gluteal
Sartorius	Femoral

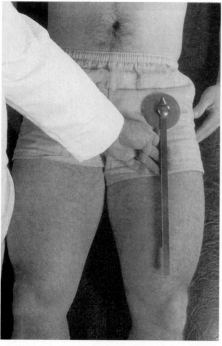

Figure 13-17

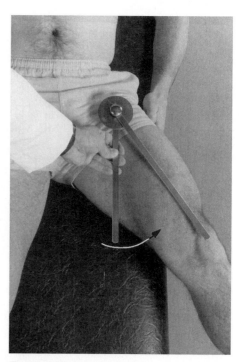

Figure 13-18

Adduction (1)

With the patient supine and the opposite hip flexed, place the goniometer in the coronal plane with the center at the level of the hip (Fig. 13-19). Instruct the patient to move the thigh medially while following the thigh with one arm of the goniometer (Fig. 13-20).

NORMAL RANGE (2)

Normal range is 27° ± 3.6° or greater from the 0 or neutral position.

Muscles	Nerve Supply
Adductor longus	Obturator
Adductor brevis	Obturator
Adductor magnus	Obturator
Gracilis	Obturator
Pectineus	Femoral

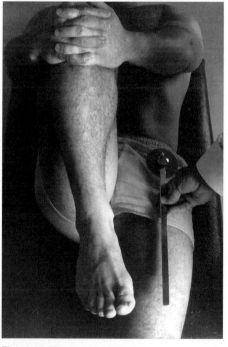

Figure 13-19

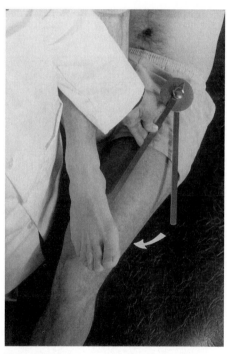

Figure 13-20

13

Internal Rotation (1)

With the patient seated, place the goniometer in front of the patella (Fig. 13-21). Instruct the patient to rotate the leg outward while following the leg with one arm of the goniometer (Fig. 13-22). This movement internally rotates the hip.

NORMAL RANGE (2)

Normal range is 44° ± 4.3° or greater from the 0 or neutral position.

Muscles	*Nerve Supply*
Adductor longus	Obturator
Adductor brevis	Obturator
Adductor magnus	Obturator
Gluteus minimus	Superior gluteal
Gluteus medius	Superior gluteal
Tensor fasciae latae	Superior gluteal
Pectineus	Femoral
Gracilis	Obturator

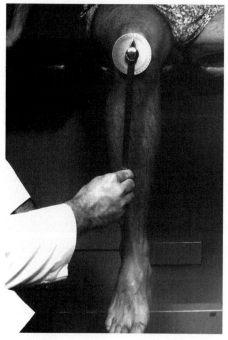

Figure 13-21

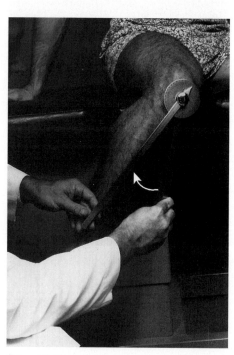

Figure 13-22

External Rotation (1)

With the patient seated, place the goniometer in front of the patella (Fig. 13-23). Instruct the patient to rotate the thigh medially while following the leg with one arm of the goniometer (Fig. 13-24).

NORMAL RANGE (2):

Normal range is 44° ± 4.8° or greater from the 0 or neutral position.

Muscles	Nerve Supply
Gluteus maximus	Inferior gluteal
Obturator internus, externus	Obturator
Quadratus femoris	N. to quadratus femoris
Piriformis	L5, S1, S2
Gemellus superior, inferior	N. to obturator internus
Sartorius	Femoral
Gluteus medius	Superior gluteal

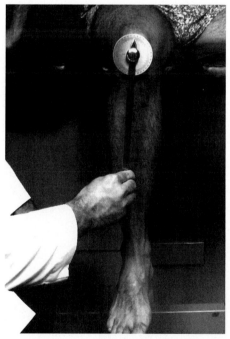

Figure 13-23

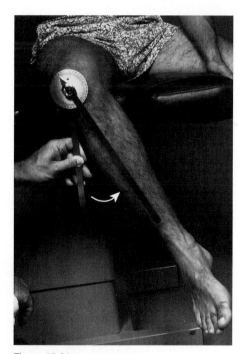

Figure 13-24

13

CONGENITAL HIP DYSPLASIA

CLINICAL DESCRIPTION

Congenital dysplasia of the hip is a condition in which the femoral head is displaced out of the acetabular cavity. The condition is often bilateral, and girls are affected more often than boys. As the name indicates, the origin is usually congenital. As a rule the acetabular cavity is shallow or more vertical than normal. The femur is often anteverted and the hip joint capsule may be lax. As the child ages, the hip becomes less flexible, and the ability to reduce the dislocation is lessened. If the hip is dislocated, there is limited abduction and a shortening of the extremity. If weight bearing has begun, the Trendelenburg test will be positive. Normally the contraction of the abductor muscle elevates the opposite side of the pelvis. If the hip is dislocated, these muscles no longer work effectively, and when the child stands on the affected leg, the opposite side on the pelvis moves down.

> **CLINICAL SIGNS AND SYMPTOMS**
> - Decreased hip flexibility
> - Limited abduction
> - Painless limp
> - Hip pain
> - Shortened extremity

Allis Test (3)

Sensitivity/Reliability Scale

0   1   2   3   4

PROCEDURE

With the infant supine, flex the knees. The patient's feet should approximate each other on the table (Fig. 13-25).

RATIONALE

A difference in the height of the knees indicates a positive test. A short knee on the affected side indicates posterior displacement of the femoral head or decreased tibial length. A long knee on the affected side indicates anterior displacement of the femoral head or an increase in tibial length.

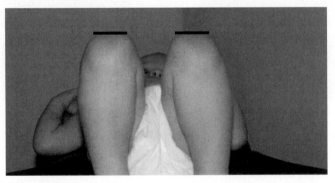

Figure 13-25

Ortolani's Click Test (4)

PROCEDURE

With the infant supine, grasp both thighs with your thumbs on the lesser trochanters. Then flex and abduct the thighs bilaterally (Fig. 13-26).

RATIONALE

A palpable and/or audible click are the signs of a positive test. The click signifies a displacement of the femoral head in or out of the acetabular cavity.

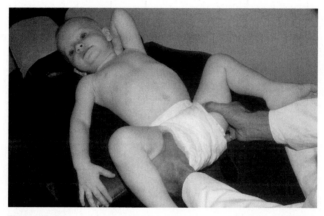

Figure 13-26

13

Telescoping Sign (5)

Sensitivity/Reliability Scale

0   1   2   3   4

PROCEDURE

With the child supine, flex the suspected hip and knee to 90°. Next, grasp the thigh and push it posterior toward the table (Fig. 13-27), then pull it anterior away from the table (Fig. 13-28).

RATIONALE

If the child has a dislocated hip or a hip that has potential to dislocate, excessive movement or a click will occur with this procedure. Normally, little motion occurs when this action is performed. This excessive movement is called telescoping.

> **SUGGESTED DIAGNOSTIC IMAGING**
>
> - Ultrasonography
> - Plain film radiography
>   Anteroposterior (AP) hip view
>   AP frog leg view
>   AP pelvis view

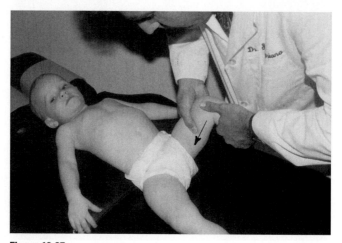

Figure 13-27

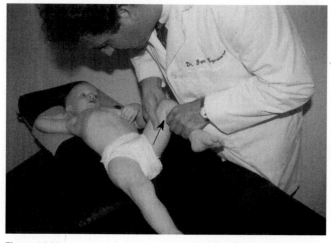

Figure 13-28

HIP FRACTURES

CLINICAL DESCRIPTION

Hip fractures occur most frequently in elderly patients, usually the result of a fall. The most common types of hip fractures are intertrochanteric and intracapsular. Intertrochanteric fractures and femoral neck fractures for the most part do not disrupt the blood supply to the femoral head. Intracapsular fractures disrupt the blood supply to the femoral head, which may lead to nonunion or avascular necrosis. In femoral neck fractures the extremity may be slightly shortened and externally rotated. Osteoporosis and osteoarthritis usually play a significant role in the region. Occasionally the fracture may be occult, with no trauma, and may show up only with a bone scan or magnetic resonance imaging (MRI).

CLINICAL SIGNS AND SYMPTOMS
- Hip pain
- Shortened extremity
- Externally rotated extremity
- Referred pain to medial thigh

Anvil Test

Sensitivity/Reliability Scale

0   1   2   3   4

PROCEDURE

With the patient supine, tap the inferior calcaneus with your fist (Fig. 13-29).

RATIONALE

Tapping the inferior calcaneus transfers quick, sharp compression-type blows to the hip joint. Local pain in the hip joint following trauma may indicate a femoral head fracture or joint pathology.

NOTE

Local pain in the thigh or leg secondary to trauma may indicate a femoral, tibial, or fibula fracture. Pain local to the calcaneus may indicate a calcaneal fracture.

SUGGESTED DIAGNOSTIC IMAGING
- Plain film radiography
  - AP hip view
  - AP frog leg view
  - AP pelvis
- Bone scan
- MRI

13

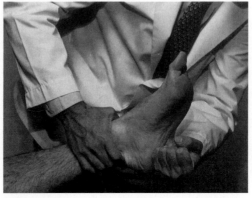

Figure 13-29

HIP CONTRACTURE TESTS

CLINICAL DESCRIPTION

A hip joint contracture is a condition of soft tissue stiffness that restricts joint motion. This may be caused by immobilization due to spasticity, paralysis, ossification, or bone or joint trauma. A frequently moved joint is unlikely to develop a contracture deformity. Contractures occur from loss of elasticity, leading to fixed shortening of soft tissue. The involved tissues may include the joint capsule, ligaments, or muscle tendon units. Hip contractures are difficult to treat; therefore, prevention by daily movement of the affected joint is paramount to treatment of a contracted joint.

CLINICAL SIGNS AND SYMPTOMS
- Stiff hip joint
- Limited hip range of motion
- Inability to position joint in the neutral position
- Hip joint pain on range of motion

Thomas Test (6)

Sensitivity/Reliability Scale

0   1   2   3   4

PROCEDURE

Instruct the supine patient to approximate each knee to the chest one at a time. Palpate the quadriceps muscles on the unflexed leg (Fig. 13-30).

RATIONALE

If the patient significantly flexes the opposite knee and tightness is palpated on the side of the involuntary flexed knee, a hip flexion contracture is indicated (Fig. 13-31). If no tightness in the rectus femoris muscle exists, the probable cause of restriction is at the hip joint structure or joint capsule.

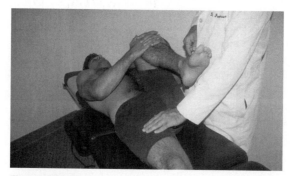

Figure 13-30

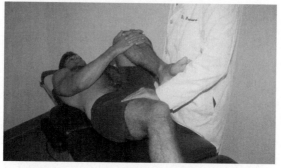

Figure 13-31

Rectus Femoris Contracture Test (5)

PROCEDURE

Instruct the patient to lie supine on the examination table with the leg off the table and flexed to 90°. Instruct the patient to flex the opposite knee to his chest and hold it. Palpate the quadriceps muscles of the leg that is flexed off the table for tightness (Fig. 13-32).

RATIONALE

If the patient involuntarily extends the knee of the leg that is flexed off the table and tightness is palpated in that thigh (Fig. 13-33), a hip flexion contracture is indicated. If there is no tightness in the rectus femoris muscle, the probable cause of restriction is at the hip joint structure or joint capsule.

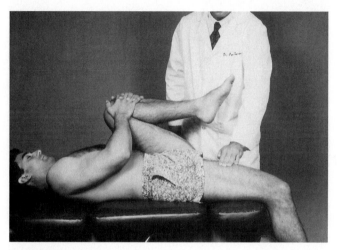

Figure 13-32

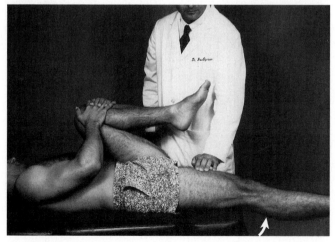

Figure 13-33

13

Ely's Test (7)

Sensitivity/Reliability Scale

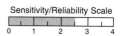

Procedure

Instruct the patient to lie prone on the examination table. Then grasp the patient's ankle and passively flex the knee to the buttock (Fig. 13-34).

Rationale

If the patient has a tight rectus femoris muscle or hip flexion contracture, the hip on the same side will flex (Fig. 13-35), raising the buttock off the table. This spontaneous flexion of the hip reduces the traction pressure on the rectus femoris muscle induced by the passive knee flexion.

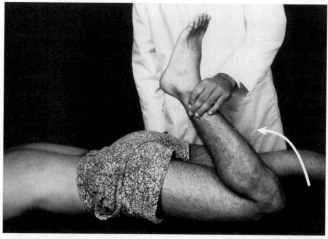

Figure 13-34

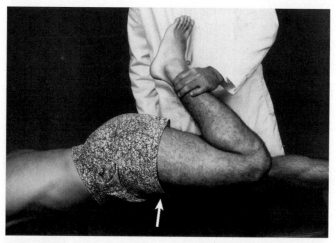

Figure 13-35

Ober's Test (8)

Sensitivity/Reliability Scale

0   1   2   3   4

PROCEDURE

With the patient side-lying, abduct the patient's leg (Fig. 13-36) and then release it (Fig. 13-37). Perform this test bilaterally.

RATIONALE

The tensor fasciae latae and iliotibial band abduct the hip. If the leg fails to descend smoothly, suspect contracture of the tensor fasciae latae muscle or iliotibial band.

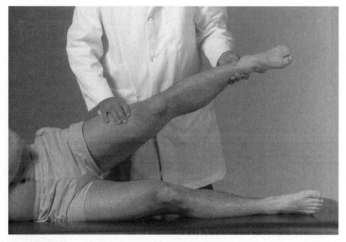

Figure 13-36

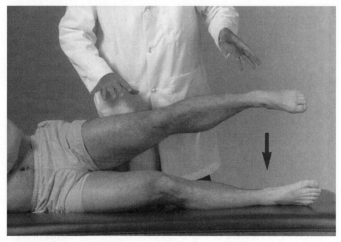

Figure 13-37

13

Piriformis Test (9)

Sensitivity/Reliability Scale

0   1   2   3   4

PROCEDURE

Instruct the patient to lie on the side opposite the leg being tested. Instruct the patient to flex the hip to 60° with the knee fully flexed (Fig. 13-38). With one hand, stabilize the hip; with the other hand, press down on the knee (Fig. 13-39).

RATIONALE

If the piriformis muscle is tight, pain will be elicited when the knee is pressed because this action further tightens the piriformis muscle. If sciatic pain sets in, the piriformis muscle may be pinching the sciatic nerve. In 15% of the population the sciatic nerve passes through the piriformis muscle.

SUGGESTED DIAGNOSTIC IMAGING

- Plain film radiography
  - AP hip view
  - AP frog leg view
  - AP pelvis

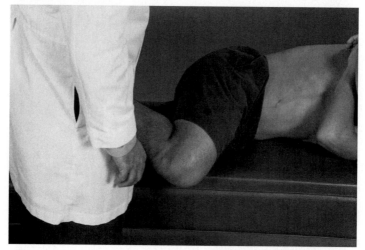

Figure 13-38

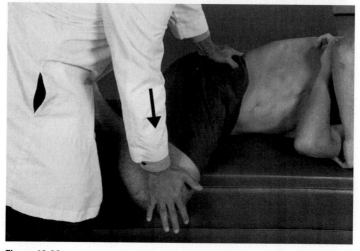

Figure 13-39

GENERAL HIP JOINT LESIONS

CLINICAL DESCRIPTION

The hip is a ball and socket joint in which the stability of the joint is enhanced by the capsule and the strong ligaments that surround the joint. The joint is weight bearing and subject to various insults and disease processes. Some of the most common problems associated with the hip joint are osteoarthritis, sprains, fractures, dislocations, bursitis, tendinitis, synovitis, and avascular necrosis of the femoral head. The following tests help to determine whether a general lesion of the hip is present. Further diagnostic testing based on the outcome of these tests can help to determine the exact pathology.

> ### CLINICAL SIGNS AND SYMPTOMS
> - Hip pain
> - Shortened extremity
> - Externally rotated extremity
> - Referred pain to medial thigh

Patrick Test (Faber) (10)

Sensitivity/Reliability Scale

0   1   2   3   4

PROCEDURE

With the patient supine, flex the leg and place the foot flat on the table. Grasp the femur and press it into the acetabular cavity (Fig. 13-40). Next, cross the patient's leg to the opposite knee. Stabilize the opposite anterior superior iliac spine and press down on the knee of the hip that is being tested (Fig. 13-41).

RATIONALE

This test forces the femoral head into the acetabular cavity, giving maximal congruence to the articular surfaces. Pain in the hip indicates an inflammatory process in the hip joint. Pain secondary to trauma may indicate a fracture in the acetabular cavity, rim of the acetabular cavity, or femoral neck. Pain may also indicate avascular necrosis of the femoral head. Faber stands for flexion, abduction, and external rotation. This is the position of the hip when the test begins.

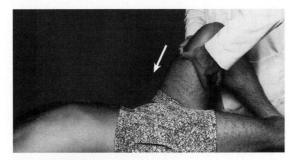

Figure 13-40

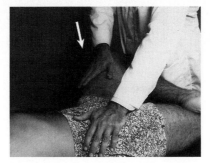

Figure 13-41

Trendelenburg Test (11)

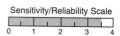

PROCEDURE

With the patient standing, grasp the patient's waist and place your thumbs on the posterior superior iliac spine of each ilium. Next, instruct the patient to flex one leg at a time (Fig. 13-42).

RATIONALE

When the patient is standing with one leg flexed, the patient is supported by an intact hip joint with its associated ligaments and muscles on that side. If the patient cannot stand on one leg because of pain and/or because the opposite pelvis falls or fails to raise, this is considered a positive test. This result may indicate a weak gluteus medius muscle opposite the side of hip flexion, and it tests the integrity of the hip joint and associated musculature and ligaments on the opposite side of hip flexion. A positive outcome of this test often indicates hip joint pathology.

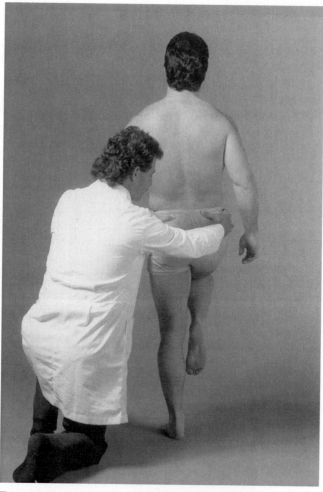

Figure 13-42

Scouring Test (12)

Sensitivity/Reliability Scale

0   1   2   3   4

PROCEDURE

With the patient supine, flex the patient's hip to 90°, fully flex the knee, and internally rotate the hip (Fig. 13-43). Assuming the patient has no injury or pathology to the knee, apply downward and lateral pressure on the knee (Fig. 13-44).

RATIONALE

This test is similar to the Patrick test, stressing the anteromedial and posterolateral aspect of the joint capsule. Pain and/or a grating sensation indicates a positive test. This result may indicate an inflammatory process in the acetabular joint, such as osteoarthritis. Pain secondary to trauma may indicate a fracture of the acetabular cavity or rim.

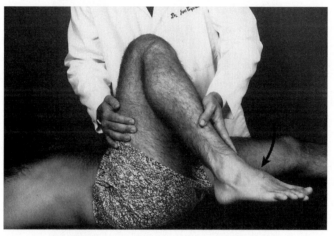

Figure 13-43

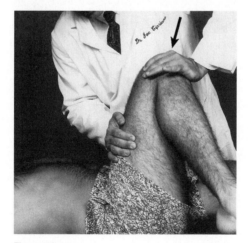

Figure 13-44

13

Laguerre's Test (13)

Sensitivity/Reliability Scale

0   1   2   3   4

PROCEDURE

With the patient supine, flex the hip and knee to 90°. Rotate the thigh outward and the knee medially. Press down on the knee with one hand, and pull up on the ankle with the other hand (Fig. 13-45).

RATIONALE

This test externally forces the head of the femur into the acetabular cavity, stressing the anterior aspect of the joint capsule. This test may indicate an inflammatory process in the acetabular joint, such as osteoarthritis. Pain secondary to trauma may indicate a fracture of the acetabular cavity or rim.

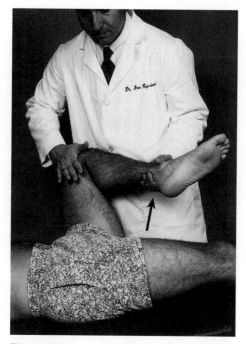

Figure 13-45

Hibb's Test

See the section on General Sacroiliac Joint Lesions in Chapter 12.

SUGGESTED DIAGNOSTIC IMAGING
- Plain film radiography
    AP hip view
    AP frog leg view
    AP pelvis
- Bone scan
- MRI

References

1. American Academy of Orthopaedic Surgeons. The Clinical Measurement of Joint Motion. Chicago: AAOS, 1994.
2. Boone DC, Azen SP. Normal range of motion of joints in male subjects. J Bone Joint Surg Am 1979;61:756–759.
3. Hensinger RN. Congenital dislocation of the hip. Summit, NJ: CIBA Clinical Symposia 1979;31(1).
4. Tachdjian MO. Pediatric Orthopedics. Philadelphia: Saunders, 1972.
5. Magee DJ. Orthopedic physical assessment. 3rd ed. Philadelphia: Saunders, 1997.
6. Hoppenfeld S. Physical Examination of the Spine and Extremities. New York: Appleton-Century-Crofts, 1976:137.
7. Gruebel-Lee DM. Disorders of the Hip. Philadelphia: JB Lippincott, 1983.
8. Ober FB. The role of the iliotibial and fascia lata as a factor in the causation of low-back disabilities and sciatica. J Bone Joint Surg 1936;18:105.
9. Saudek CE. The Hip. Orthopedic and Sports Physical Therapy. St. Louis: Mosby, 1990.
10. Kenna C, Murtagh J. Patrick or Faber test. Aust Fam Physician 1989;18:375.
11. Trendelenburg F. Dtsch Med Wschr 21, 1895;21–24 (RSM translation).
12. Maitland GD. The Peripheral Joints: Examination and Recording Guide. Adelaide, Australia: Vergo, 1973.
13. Lee D. The Pelvic Girdle. Edinburgh: Churchill Livingstone, 1989.

General References

Alderink GJ. The sacroiliac joint: review of anatomy, mechanics and function. J Orthop Sports Phys Ther 1991;13:71.

Beetham WP, Polley HF, Slocumb CH, et al. Physical Examination of the Joints. Philadelphia: Saunders, 1965.

Chung SMK. Hip Disorders in Infants and Children. Philadelphia: Lea & Febiger, 1981.

Cyriax J. Textbook of Orthopaedic Medicine. 2nd ed. Vol 1. London: Bailliéré Tindal, 1982.

Haycock CE. Sports Medicine for the Athletic Female. Oradell, NJ: Medical Economics, 1980.

Kapandji LA. The Physiology of the Joints. Vol. 2. Lower Limb. New York: Churchill Livingstone, 1970.

Maquet PGJ. Biomechanics of the Hip. New York: Springer-Verlag, 1985.

McRae R. Clinical Orthopedic Examination. New York: Churchill Livingstone, 1976.

Mercier LR. Practical Orthopedics. St. Louis: Mosby, 1991.

Moore KL, Dalley AF. Clinically oriented anatomy. 4th ed. Baltimore: Lippincott Williams & Wilkins, 1999.

Noble HB, Hajek MR, Porter M. Diagnosis and treatment of iliotibial band tightness in runners. Phys Sports Med 1984;10:67.

Phillips EK. Evaluation of the hip. Phys Ther 1975; 55:975–981.

Post M. Physical examination of the musculoskeletal system. Chicago: Year Book Medical, 1987.

Rydell N. Biomechanics of the hip joint. Clin Orthop 1973;92:6.

Singleton MC. The Hip Joint: Clinical Oriented AnatomyA Review. Common Disorders of the Hip. New York: Haworth, 1986.

Steinberg GG, Akins AM, Baran, DT. Orthopaedics in Primary Care. 3rd ed. Baltimore: Lippincott Williams & Wilkins, 1999.

Steinberg ME. The Hip and Its Disorders. Philadelphia: Saunders, 1991.

Subotnick17 SI. Sports Medicine of the Lower Extremity. 2nd ed. New York: Churchill Livingstone, 1999.

Wells PE. The examination of the pelvic joints. In: Grieve GP, ed. Modern Manual Therapy of the Vertebral Column. Edinburgh: Churchill Livingstone, 1986.

13

14

KNEE ORTHOPAEDIC TESTS

Knee Orthopaedic Examination

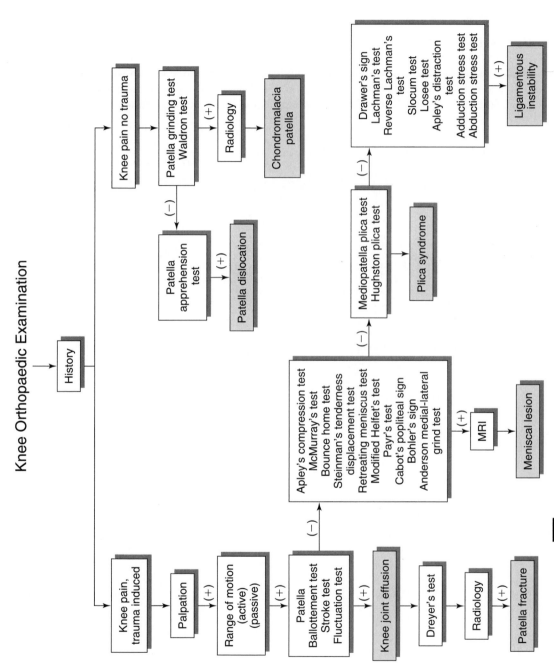

PALPATION

Anterior Aspect

Patella, Quadriceps Femoris Tendon, and Patella Ligament

DESCRIPTIVE ANATOMY

The suprapatellar tendon anchors the patella to the anterior aspect of the knee superiorly. This tendon is an extension of the quadriceps muscle and it continues inferiorly as the patellar ligament (Fig. 14-1). The patellar ligament is thick, strong, and continuous with the fibrous capsule of the knee joint, and it attaches to the tibial tuberosity. These structures, which are superficial and easily palpable, function as a lever to extend the leg when the quadriceps muscle contracts.

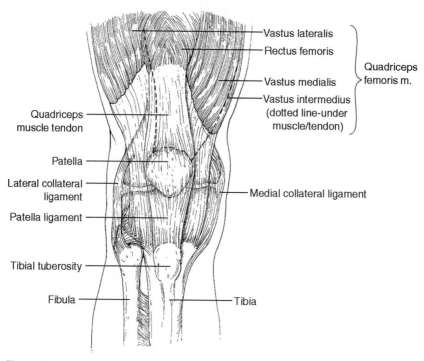

Figure 14-1

PROCEDURE

With the patient supine and the knee extended, palpate the patella and its margins (Fig. 14-2). Note any tenderness, inflammation, temperature differences, and/or roughness. Tenderness and pain from direct trauma may indicate periosteal contusion or fracture of the patella. Swelling and an increase in temperature suggest prepatellar bursitis. Roughness at the margins of the patella may indicate chondromalacia patellae, or degeneration of the undersurface of the patella.

Next, palpate the quadriceps femoris tendon (Fig. 14-3). Tenderness may indicate tendinitis caused by overuse or strain resulting from overstress. Continue palpation inferior to the patella which is the patellar ligament. Palpate from the apex of the patella, which is the inferior margin, down to the tibial tubercle, which is the attachment of the patellar ligament (Fig. 14-4). Note any pain, tenderness, swelling, or temperature differences. Any of these findings may indicate ligament sprain. If symptoms are local to the tibial tuberosity, suspect Osgood-Schlatter disease, an enlargement of the tibial tuberosity, in the adolescent; it is common in young adults.

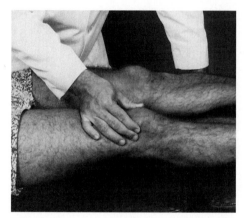

Figure 14-2

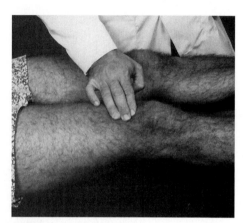

Figure 14-3

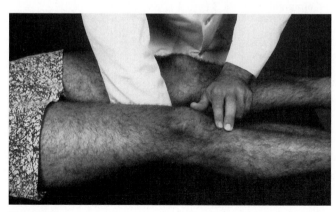

Figure 14-4

14

Anterior Knee Bursa

Descriptive Anatomy

The clinically important bursae in the anterior aspect of the knee are the suprapatellar bursa, prepatellar bursa, superficial infrapatellar bursa, and deep infrapatellar bursa (Fig. 14-5). The suprapatellar bursa, an extension of the synovial capsule, lies between the femur and the quadriceps femoris tendons. It allows for movement of the quadriceps tendon over the distal end of the femur. The prepatellar bursa is superficial to the patella between the skin and anterior surface of the patella. It allows movement of the skin over the underlying patella. The superficial infrapatellar bursa is between the tibial tuberosity and the skin. It allows for movement of the skin over the tibial tuberosity. The deep infrapatellar bursa lies between the patellar ligament and the tibia. This allows for movement of the patellar ligament over the tibia.

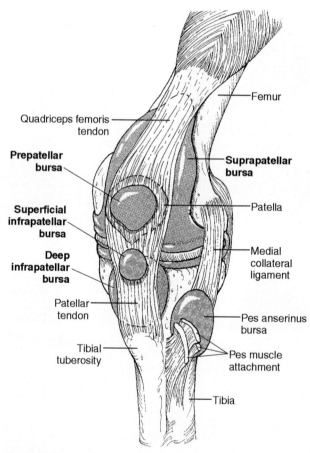

Figure 14-5

PROCEDURE

Palpate the suprapatellar bursa above the patella (Fig. 14-6). Note any thickening, tenderness, or temperature differences. These signs may indicate bursitis in the suprapatellar bursa or pathology in the quadriceps femoris tendon. Next, palpate the prepatellar bursa, which is superficial to the patella (Fig. 14-7). Note any thickening, swelling, tenderness, or temperature differences. These signs may indicate prepatellar bursitis (housemaid's knee). Palpate the superficial and deep infrapatellar bursa (Fig. 14-8). Note any thickening, swelling, tenderness, or temperature differences. Any of these may indicate infrapatellar bursitis or patellar ligament pathology.

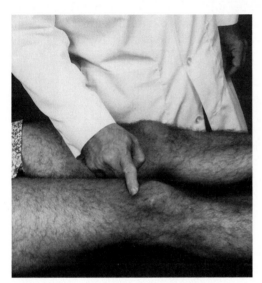

Figure 14-6

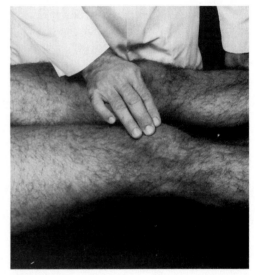

Figure 14-7

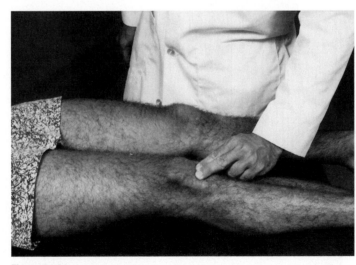

Figure 14-8

14

Quadriceps Femoris Muscle

DESCRIPTIVE ANATOMY

The quadriceps femoris consists of four muscles: rectus femoris, vastus lateralis, vastus medialis, and vastus intermedius (Fig. 14-9). The primary action of these muscles is to extend the leg at the knee. They all unite to form the quadriceps tendon, which inserts into the patella.

PROCEDURE

Palpate the entire length of the quadriceps muscle, noting any swelling, tenderness, temperature differences, or masses (Fig. 14-10). Tenderness and/or swelling may indicate muscle strain or hematoma. Point tenderness at the upper aspect of the muscle may indicate active trigger points and may refer pain to the knee. A hard mass secondary to trauma may indicate myositis ossificans, which is an ossification of muscle tissue.

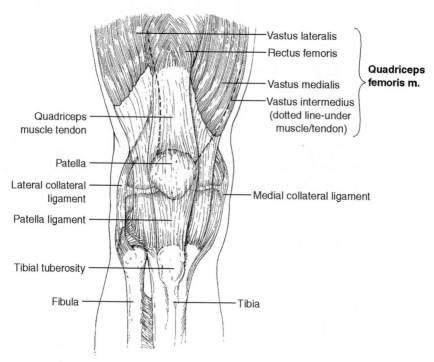

Figure 14-9

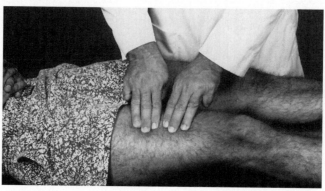

Figure 14-10

Medial Aspect

Medial Femoral Condyle, Tibial Plateau, and Joint Line

DESCRIPTIVE ANATOMY

The medial femoral condyle is a bony prominence on the medial aspect of the distal femur, which is the attachment of the medial collateral ligament. The medial tibial plateau and joint line are important palpable landmarks of the medial aspect of the knee. The medial aspect of the meniscus is in the joint line, and the coronary ligament attaches the meniscus to the tibial plateau (Fig. 14-11).

PROCEDURE

With the knee in 90° of flexion, palpate the medial femoral condyle with your index and middle fingers (Fig. 14-12). Note any tenderness or pain. These signs may indicate a sprain, avulsion, or calcification (Pellegrini-Stieda disease) of the medial collateral ligament. Next, palpate the tibial plateau and medial joint line. Note any tenderness or pain. These signs may indicate a tear of the medial meniscus or sprain of the coronary ligament.

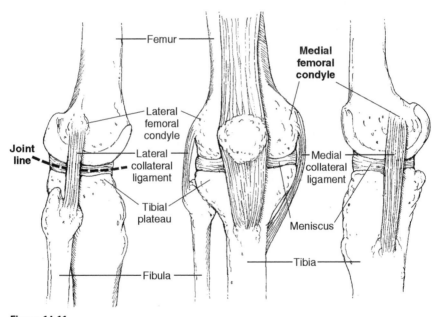

Figure 14-11

14

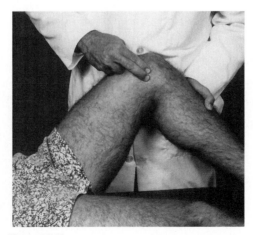

Figure 14-12

Medial Collateral Ligament

DESCRIPTIVE ANATOMY

The medial collateral, or tibial collateral, ligament is a strong, broad, flat band that extends from the medial epicondyle of the femur to the medial condyle and upper medial aspect of the tibia (Fig. 14-13). It contributes to the medial stability of the knee. Its fibers are attached to the medial meniscus and the fibrous capsule of the knee.

PROCEDURE

With the patient supine and the leg extended, palpate the medial collateral ligament from the medial epicondyle of the femur to the medial condyle of the tibia with your index and middle fingers (Fig. 14-14). Note any pain, tenderness, or defect in the ligament. Pain and tenderness may indicate a sprain of the ligament. A deficit secondary to trauma may indicate a tear of the ligament, which is usually associated with capsular and meniscal damage. A defect at either the medial femoral epicondyle or the medial tibial condyle suggests an avulsion fracture secondary to trauma.

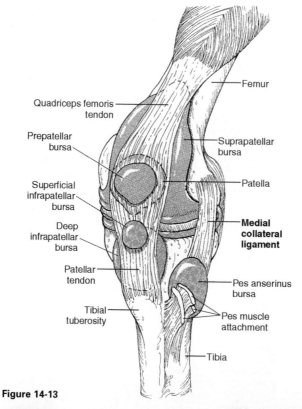

Figure 14-13

Figure 14-14

Lateral Aspect

Lateral Femoral Condyle and Joint Line

DESCRIPTIVE ANATOMY

The lateral femoral condyle is a bony prominence on the lateral aspect of the distal femur, which is the attachment of the lateral collateral ligament and iliotibial band. This structure is important for the lateral stability of the knee. The lateral joint line is an important palpable landmark of the lateral aspect of the knee. The lateral aspect of the meniscus and the coronary ligament, which attaches the meniscus to the tibia, are in the joint line (Fig. 14-15).

PROCEDURE

With the knee in 90° of flexion, palpate the lateral femoral condyle with your index and middle fingers (Fig. 14-16). Note any tenderness or pain. These signs may indicate sprain, avulsion, or calcification of the lateral collateral ligament. Next, palpate the lateral joint line. Note any tenderness or pain. These signs may indicate a tear of the lateral meniscus or strain of the coronary ligament.

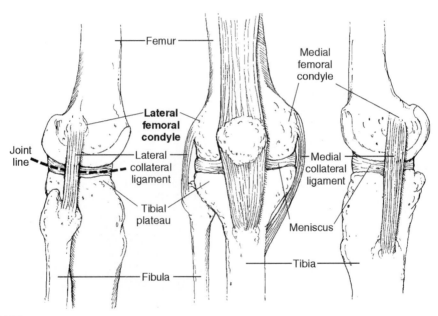

Figure 14-15

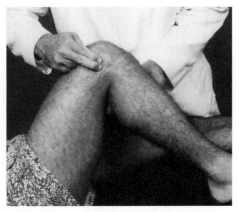

Figure 14-16

Lateral Collateral Ligament and Iliotibial Band

DESCRIPTIVE ANATOMY

The lateral collateral ligament is a round cord that extends from the lateral epicondyle of the femur to the head of the fibula (Fig. 14-15). This structure is important for the lateral stability of the knee. In contrast to the medial collateral ligament, the fibers are not attached to the meniscus. The tendon of the popliteus muscle passes deep to the ligament, separating it from the meniscus of the knee. The iliotibial band is a continuation of the tensor fasciae latae muscle, and it attaches to the lateral condyle of the tibia (Fig. 14-17). This band helps keep the knee extended during standing and is important for lateral stability of the knee.

PROCEDURE

With the patient either supine or sitting, instruct the patient to cross one leg over the other (Fig. 14-18). With your index and middle finger, palpate the lateral collateral ligament of the top leg from the lateral epicondyle of the femur to the head of the fibula. Note any pain, tenderness, or defect. Pain and tenderness may indicate a sprain or calcification of the ligament. A defect secondary to trauma may indicate a tear or avulsion of the lateral collateral ligament. Next, palpate the entire length of the iliotibial band from halfway between the hip and knee on the lateral aspect to the lateral condyle of the tibia (Fig. 14-19). Note any pain, tenderness, or defects of the iliotibial band. Pain and tenderness may indicate a strain of the band. A defect secondary to trauma may indicate a tear or avulsion of the band from the lateral condyle of the tibia.

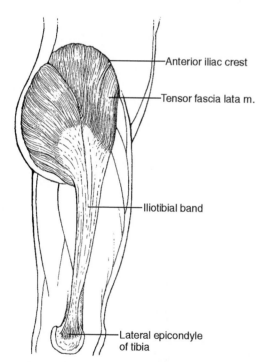

Figure 14-17

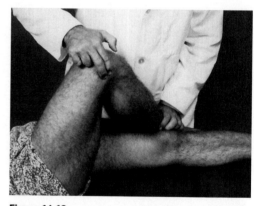

Figure 14-18

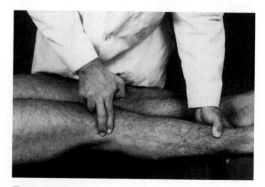

Figure 14-19

Posterior Aspect

Popliteal Fossa and Associated Structures

DESCRIPTIVE ANATOMY

The popliteal fossa is surrounded by the biceps femoris tendon on the superior lateral border and the tendons of the semimembranosus and semitendinosus on the superior medial border. The inferior borders are bounded by the two heads of the gastrocnemius muscles. The posterior tibial nerve, popliteal artery, and popliteal vein cross the popliteal fossa (Fig. 14-20).

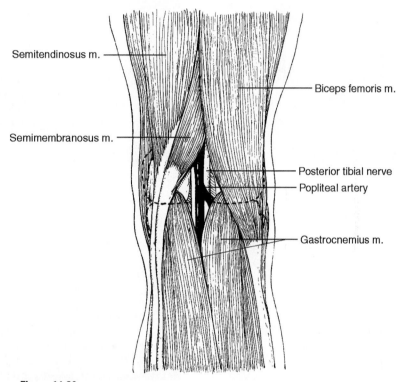

Figure 14-20

14

PROCEDURE

With the knee slightly flexed, palpate the popliteal fossa for swelling or tenderness (Fig. 14-21). These signs may indicate Baker's cyst, a pressure diverticulum of the synovial sac protruding through the joint capsule of the knee. Next, palpate the biceps femoris tendon (Fig. 14-22), semi-membranosus tendon, semitendinosus tendon (Fig. 14-23), and both heads of the gastrocnemius muscle (Fig. 14-24) for tenderness, swelling, and continuity. This tenderness and swelling may indicate a strain of the respective tendons or muscles. Loss of continuity may indicate an avulsion of the respective muscles or tendons.

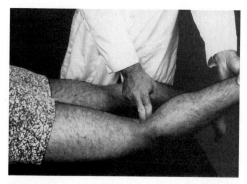

Figure 14-21

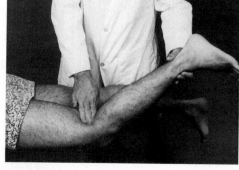

Figure 14-22

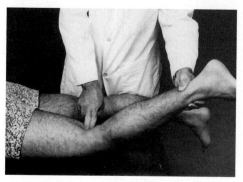

Figure 14-23

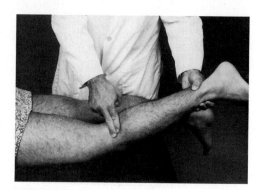

Figure 14-24

KNEE RANGE OF MOTION

Flexion (1)

With the patient prone and the leg extended, place the goniometer in the sagittal plane with the center at the knee joint (Fig. 14-25). Instruct the patient to flex the leg as far as possible while following the leg with one arm of the goniometer (Fig. 14-26).

NORMAL RANGE (2)

Normal range is 141° ± 6.5° or greater from the 0 or neutral position.

Muscles	*Nerve Supply*
Biceps femoris	Sciatic
Semimembranosus	Sciatic
Semitendinosus	Sciatic
Gracilis	Obturator
Sartorius	Femoral
Popliteus	Tibial
Gastrocnemius	Tibial
Plantaris	Superior gluteal

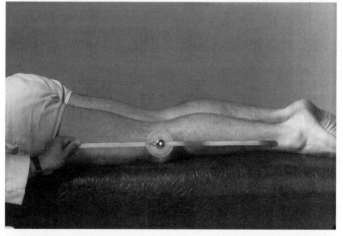

Figure 14-25

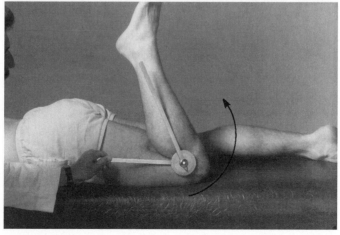

Figure 14-26

14

Extension (1)

With the patient seated, foot on the floor, place the goniometer in the sagittal plane with the center at the knee (Fig. 14-27). Instruct the patient to extend the leg as far as possible while following the leg with one arm of the goniometer (Fig. 14-28). Note that this test starts with the leg in 90° of flexion and you want the knee to extend to the 0 or neutral position.

NORMAL RANGE (2)

Normal range is 0 ± 2°.

Muscles	*Nerve Supply*
Rectus femoris	Femoral
Vastus medialis	Femoral
Vastus intermedius	Femoral
Vastus lateralis	Femoral

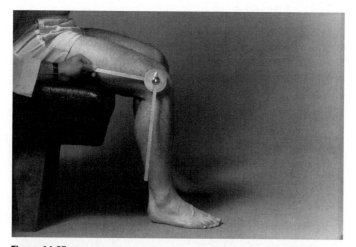

Figure 14-27

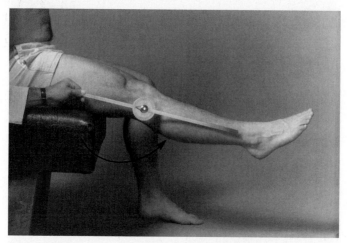

Figure 14-28

MENISCUS INSTABILITY

CLINICAL DESCRIPTION

The menisci are C-shaped disks of fibrocartilage that are interposed between the condyles of the femur and the tibia. The functions of the meniscus are many. Its primary function is load transmission or weight bearing, and the secondary function is shock absorption during gait. The menisci are also thought to contribute to joint stability and lubrication. Finally, because of the nerve endings in the anterior and posterior horns, proprioception provides a feedback mechanism for joint position.

A tear or loss of the menisci, either partial or complete, hinders their ability to function and predisposes the joint to degenerative changes. A twisting injury to the knee with the foot in a weight-bearing position is the most common injury to the meniscus. Because the outer 20% of the menisci have a vascular supply, peripheral injuries may heal. The inner 80% of the menisci are avascular, so inner meniscal injuries rarely heal.

> ### CLINICAL SIGNS AND SYMPTOMS
> - Local medial or lateral joint pain
> - Limited knee range of motion
> - Crepitus upon movement
> - Joint effusion
> - Knee buckling
> - Pain on walking up and down stairs
> - Pain on squatting

Apley's Compression Test (3)

Sensitivity/Reliability Scale

0   1   2   3   4

PROCEDURE

With the patient prone, flex the leg to 90°. Stabilize the patient's thigh with your knee. Grasp the patient's ankle and place downward pressure while you internally (Fig. 14-29) and externally (Fig. 14-30) rotate the leg.

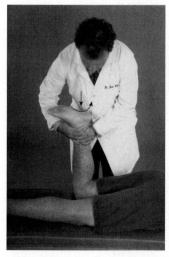

Figure 14-29

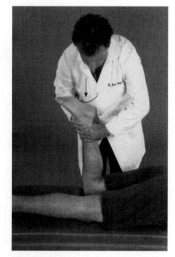

Figure 14-30

14

RATIONALE

The menisci, which are asymmetric fibrocartilaginous disks, separate the tibial condyles from the femoral condyles. When the knee is flexed, the meniscus distorts to maintain the congruence between the tibial and femoral condyles. Flexion of the knee applies downward pressure with internal and external rotation stress to the already distorted meniscus. Pain or crepitus on either side of the knee indicates a meniscus injury on that side.

McMurray's Test (4)

Sensitivity/Reliability Scale

0   1   2   3   4

PROCEDURE

With the patient supine, flex the leg (Fig. 14-31). Externally rotate the leg as you extend (Fig. 14-32); internally rotate as you extend (Fig. 14-33).

RATIONALE

Flexion and extension of the knee distort the meniscus to maintain the congruence between the tibial and femoral condyles. Flexing and extending the knee with internal and external rotation further stress the already distorted meniscus. A palpable or audible click indicates an injury of the meniscus.

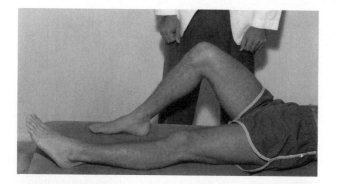

Figure 14-31

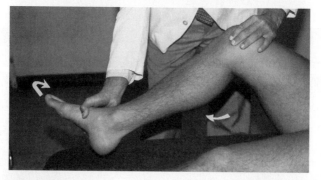

Figure 14-32

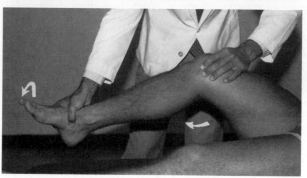

Figure 14-33

Bounce Home Test (5)

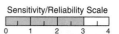

PROCEDURE

With the patient supine, instruct the patient to flex the leg. When the leg is flexed, cup your hand around the patient's heel (Fig. 14-34) and instruct him to relax his muscles and allow the knee to drop (Fig. 14-35).

RATIONALE

Extension of the knee entails medial rotation of the femur on the tibia. If the meniscus is injured, rotation of the femur on the tibia may be blocked and the patient may not be able to extend the knee fully. A rubbery end feel on full extension is also a positive sign.

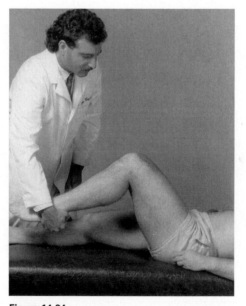

Figure 14-34

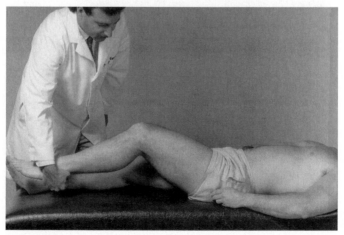

Figure 14-35

14

Steinman's Tenderness Displacement Test (6)

Sensitivity/Reliability Scale

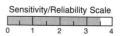

0   1   2   3   4

PROCEDURE

With the patient supine, flex the patient's hip and knee to 90°. Place your thumb and index finger on the medial and lateral knee joint lines, respectively (Fig. 14-36). With your opposite hand, grasp the patient's ankle and alternately flex and extend the knee while palpating the entire joint line (Fig. 14-37).

RATIONALE

When the knee is extended, the meniscus moves anteriorly, and when the knee is flexed, the meniscus moves posteriorly. If the pain seems to move anteriorly when the knee is extended or posteriorly when the knee is flexed, suspect a tear or injury of the meniscus.

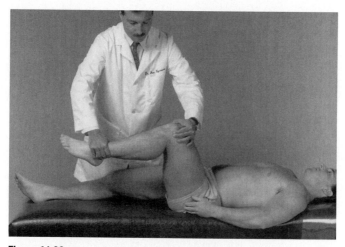

Figure 14-36

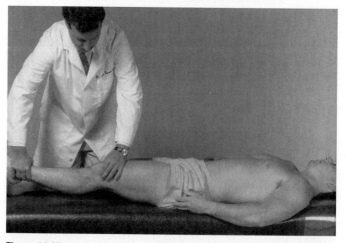

Figure 14-37

Retreating Meniscus Test (7)

PROCEDURE

With the patient supine and the patient's hip and leg flexed to 90°, palpate the meniscus on the medial joint line anterior to the medial collateral ligament. With your opposite hand, rotate the leg medially and laterally while noting whether the meniscus that you are palpating is still present or has disappeared (Figs. 14-38 and 14-39).

RATIONALE

When the knee is flexed to 90°, the femur should rotate medially on the tibia. If the meniscus does not disappear while you are rotating the leg, suspect a torn meniscus, because rotation of the tibia is blocked.

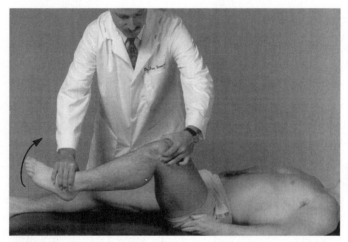

Figure 14-38

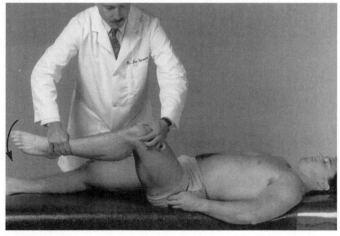

Figure 14-39

14

Modified Helfet's Test (7)

Sensitivity/Reliability Scale

0   1   2   3   4

PROCEDURE

With the patient seated, foot on the floor, note the location of the tibial tuberosity in relation to the midline (Fig. 14-40). Passively extend the patient's leg and again note the location of the tibial tuberosity in relation to the patella (Fig. 14-41).

RATIONALE

In the normal knee, the tibial tuberosity is at the midline when the knee is in 90° of flexion. When the knee is extended, the tibial tuberosity moves in line with the lateral border on the patella. If this does not occur, suspect a tear of the meniscus because rotation of the tibia is blocked.

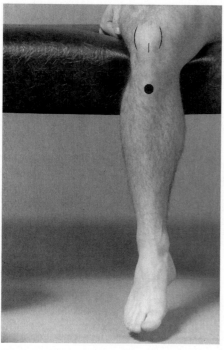

Figure 14-40

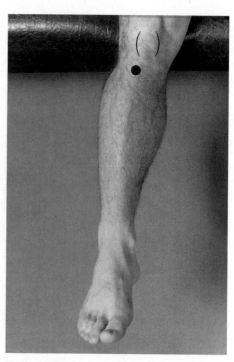

Figure 14-41

Cabot's Popliteal Sign (8)

Sensitivity/Reliability Scale

0   1   2   3   4

PROCEDURE

With the patient supine, instruct the patient to abduct the thigh and cross the leg of the affected knee (Fig. 14-42). Grasp the ankle with one hand, and with the other hand palpate the joint line with your thumb and index finger (Fig. 14-43). Ask the patient to straighten the knee isometrically against your resistance.

RATIONALE

Resisting extension of the knee in the figure-4 position stresses the meniscus. Pain on the joint line indicates a tear or pathology of the meniscus.

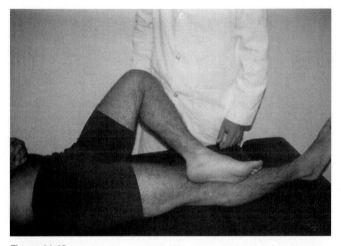

Figure 14-42

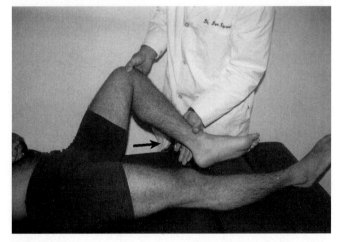

Figure 14-43

14

Bohler's Sign (8)

Sensitivity/Reliability Scale
0   1   2   3   4

PROCEDURE

With the patient supine, stabilize the medial thigh with one hand and place a valgus force on the lateral aspect of the leg with your opposite hand (Fig. 14-44). Next, stabilize the lateral knee and place a varus force on the medial aspect of the leg (Fig. 14-45).

RATIONALE

Placing a lateral or medial pressure on the knee distracts the joint capsule and meniscus on the opposite side of the pressure. Pain on the side opposite joint pressure may indicate a lesion of the joint capsule or meniscus.

NOTE

This test is similar to the adduction and abduction stress test for collateral ligament defect. If this test is positive, evaluate for collateral ligament defect opposite the side of pressure.

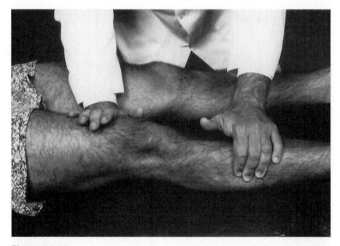

Figure 14-44

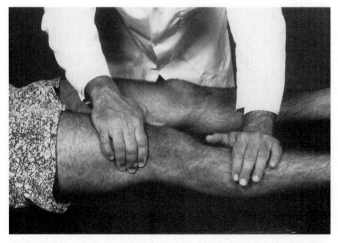

Figure 14-45

Anderson Medial–Lateral Grind Test (9)

PROCEDURE

With the patient supine, grasp the leg of the affected knee and place it between your trunk and arm. With your opposite thumb and index finger, palpate the anterolateral and medial joint lines. Place a valgus stress on the knee as it is flexed passively (Fig. 14-46) and a varus stress on the knee as it is extended passively (Fig. 14-47). Use a circular movement and increase valgus and varus stresses after each complete circle.

RATIONALE

This movement stresses the meniscus on the medial side with valgus stress and on the lateral side with varum stress. Pain and/or grinding on movement may indicate a meniscus tear or pathology.

> **SUGGESTED DIAGNOSTIC IMAGING**
> - Plain film radiography
>   Anteroposterior (AP) knee view
>   Lateral knee view
> - Magnetic resonance imaging (MRI)

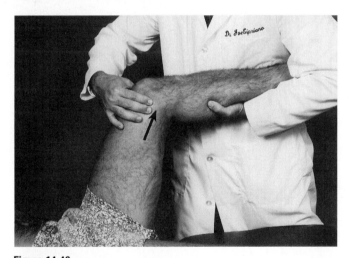

Figure 14-46

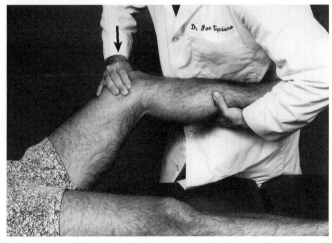

Figure 14-47

14

PLICA TESTS

Clinical Description

The synovial plica is a redundant fold in the synovial lining of the knee, extending from the fat pad medially under the quadriceps tendon superiorly to the lateral retinaculum (Fig. 14-48). This plica may become inflamed, thickened, and/or fibrotic from trauma or overuse, resulting in clinical symptoms. If the plica is inflamed, a more complex patellofemoral problem may be present.

Clinical Signs and Symptoms

- Anterior knee pain
- Anterior pain on prolonged knee flexion
- Knee pain diminishing with increased activity
- Popping or snapping upon knee flexion or extension

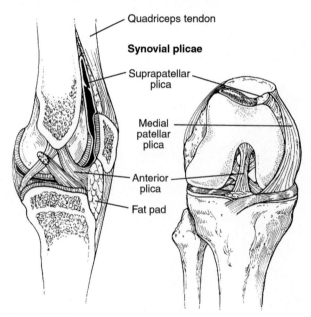

Quadriceps tendon

Synovial plicae

Suprapatellar plica

Medial patellar plica

Anterior plica

Fat pad

Figure 14-48

Mediopatella Plica Test (10)

Sensitivity/Reliability Scale

0   1   2   3   4

PROCEDURE

With the patient supine, flex the affected leg to 30°. With the other hand, move the patella medially (Fig. 14-49).

RATIONALE

Moving the patella medially with the leg in 30° of flexion pinches the plica between the medial femoral condyle and the patella. Pain may indicate that the plica is adhered to the patella and is inflamed. The plica is the remnant of an embryonic septum that makes up the knee joint capsule.

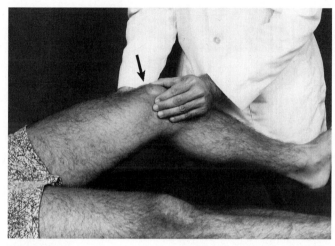

Figure 14-49

14

Hughston Plica Test (11)

Sensitivity/Reliability Scale
0   1   2   3   4

PROCEDURE

With the patient supine, grasp the patient's leg. Flex and medially rotate the leg. With your opposite hand, move the patella medially with the heel of your hand and palpate the medial femoral condyle with the fingers of the same hand (Fig. 14-50). Flex and extend the knee while feeling for popping of the plical band under your fingers (Fig. 14-51).

RATIONALE

Popping under your fingers may indicate that the plica is attached to the patella, and it may be inflamed. The incidence of patella plica varies from 18% to 60% of the population, according to different authors.

SUGGESTED DIAGNOSTIC IMAGING
- Knee MRI

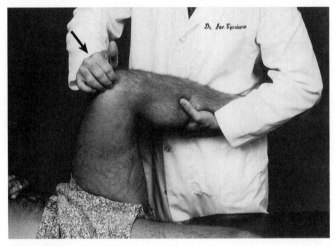

Figure 14-50

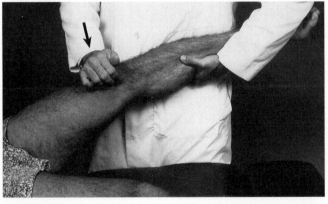

Figure 14-51

LIGAMENTOUS INSTABILITY

CLINICAL DESCRIPTION

Ligaments are vital to the stability of the knee. The major ligaments of the knee are the anterior and posterior cruciate and the medial and lateral collateral ligaments (Fig. 14-52). Ligament injuries are among the most serious knee disorders. A delay in diagnosis and treatment may lead to a chronically unstable knee, which predisposes the knee to early degeneration. Ligament instability is usually due to a traumatic stress to the knee while the knee was bearing weight. A valgus stress may sprain or tear the medial collateral ligament. A varus stress may sprain or tear the lateral collateral ligament. Both of these stresses with a rotational force may also sprain or tear the anterior and/or posterior cruciate ligaments.

CLINICAL SIGNS AND SYMPTOMS

- Knee pain
- Limited range of motion
- Difficulty in weight bearing in acute stage
- Joint effusion
- Knee giving out; chronic unstable knee

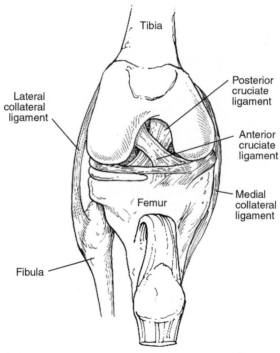

Figure 14-52

14

Drawer Sign (12–14)

Sensitivity/Reliability Scale

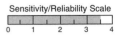

0   1   2   3   4

PROCEDURE

With the patient supine, flex the leg and place the foot on the table (Fig. 14-53). Grasp behind the flexed knee and pull (Fig. 14-54) and push (Fig. 14-55) on the leg. The hamstring tendons must be relaxed for this test to be accurate.

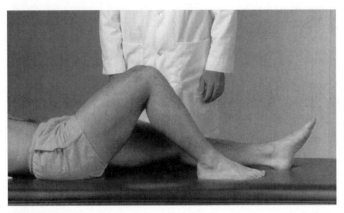

Figure 14-53

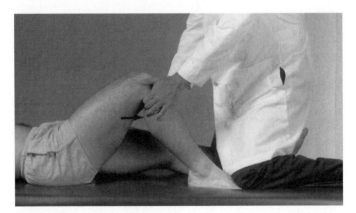

Figure 14-54

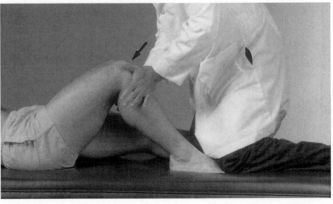

Figure 14-55

RATIONALE

If there is more than 5 mm of tibial movement on the femur when the leg is pulled, an injury or tear of some degree to one or more of the following structures is indicated:

- Anterior cruciate ligament (Fig. 14-56)
- Posterolateral capsule
- Posteromedial capsule
- Medial collateral ligament (if more than 1 cm of movement)
- Iliotibial band
- Posterior oblique ligament
- Arcuate-popliteus complex

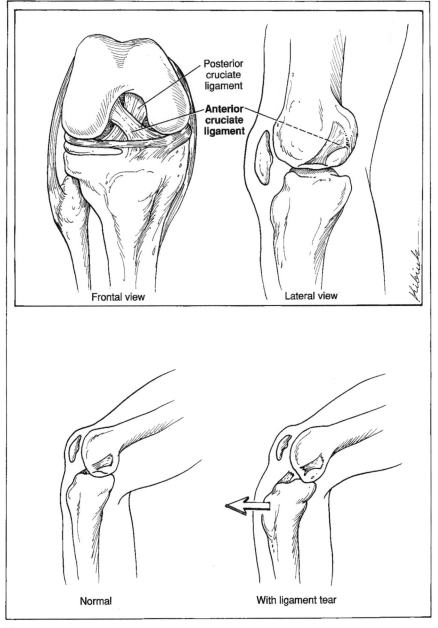

Figure 14-56

If excessive movement occurs when the leg is pushed, an injury to one of the following structures is indicated:

- Posterior cruciate ligament (Fig. 14-57)
- Arcuate–popliteus complex
- Posterior oblique ligament
- Anterior cruciate ligament

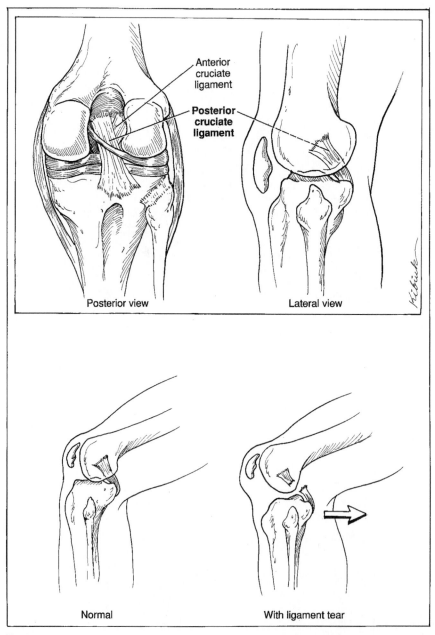

Figure 14-57

Lachman's Test (14)

Sensitivity/Reliability Scale

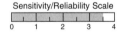

0   1   2   3   4

PROCEDURE

With the patient supine and the knee in 30° of flexion, grasp the patient's thigh with one hand to stabilize it. With the opposite hand, grasp the tibia and pull it forward (Fig. 14-58).

RATIONALE

If a softened feel and anterior translation of the tibia is present when the tibia is moved forward, then a tear of any of the following ligaments is suspect:

- Anterior cruciate ligament
- Posterior oblique ligament

This is the most reliable test for anterior cruciate ligament rupture because the knee does not need to flex to 90°, as with the anterior drawer sign; there is less meniscal impingement; and the hamstrings are less likely to spasm.

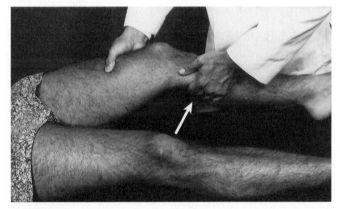

Figure 14-58

Reverse Lachman's Test (8)

Sensitivity/Reliability Scale

0   1   2   3   4

PROCEDURE

With the patient prone, flex the leg to 30°. With one hand, stabilize the posterior thigh, making sure that the hamstring muscles are relaxed. With your opposite hand, grasp the tibia and push it posteriorly (Fig. 14-59).

RATIONALE

Posterior pressure on the tibia stresses the posterior cruciate ligament. A soft end feel and a posterior translation of the tibia indicate an injury or tear to the posterior cruciate ligament.

14

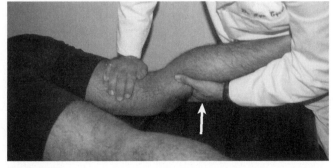

Figure 14-59

Slocum Test (15)

Sensitivity/Reliability Scale

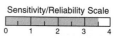

0   1   2   3   4

Procedure

With the patient supine, place the patient's foot on the examination table in 30° of internal rotation. Stabilize the patient's foot with your knee, grasp the tibia with your hand, and pull the tibia toward you (Fig. 14-60).

Rationale

This test is similar to the anterior drawer sign except that in this test, the foot is in 30° of internal rotation. If tibial translation and a soft end feel occur when the tibia is drawn forward, suspect instability or a tear of any of the following ligaments:

- Anterior cruciate
- Posterolateral capsule
- Fibular collateral ligament
- Iliotibial band

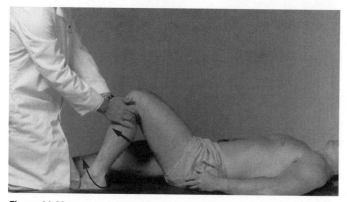

Figure 14-60

Losee Test (16)

Sensitivity/Reliability Scale
0   1   2   3   4

PROCEDURE

With the patient supine, grasp the patient's leg with one hand, externally rotate it, and brace it against your abdomen. Flex the leg 30° to relax the hamstring muscles (Fig. 14-61). With your opposite hand, grasp the knee with your thumb behind the fibular head and your fingers over the patella. Place valgus force against the lateral aspect of the knee and forward pressure behind the fibular head while extending the knee (Fig. 14-62).

RATIONALE

Externally rotating the leg in 30° of flexion and applying a valgus force compress the structure in the lateral compartment of the knee. This compression may accentuate anterior subluxation of the tibia. While extending the knee and applying a valgus force, look for a palpable clunk. This clunk may indicate anterior subluxation of the tibia, which is a reproduction of the patient's previous instability experience. It indicates injury or tear to one or more of the following structures:

- Anterior cruciate ligament
- Posterolateral joint capsule
- Arcuate–popliteus complex
- Lateral collateral ligament
- Iliotibial band

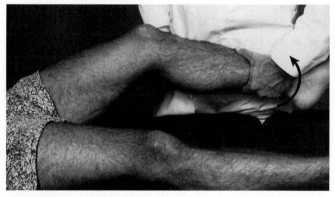

Figure 14-61

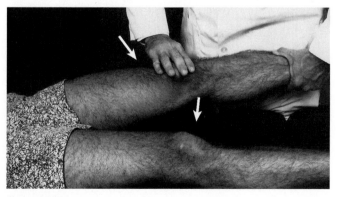

Figure 14-62

14

Apley's Distraction Test (17)

Sensitivity/Reliability Scale

0   1   2   3   4

PROCEDURE

With the patient prone, flex the leg to 90°. Stabilize the patient's thigh with your knee. Pull on the patient's ankle while internally (Fig. 14-63) and externally (Fig. 14-64) rotating the leg.

RATIONALE

Distraction of the knee takes pressure off the meniscus and puts strain on the medial and lateral collateral ligaments. Pain on distraction indicates nonspecific ligament injury or instability.

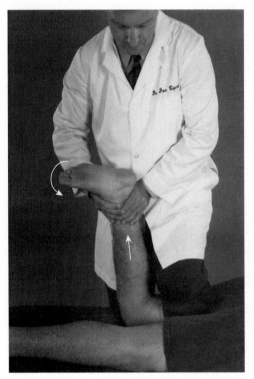

Figure 14-63

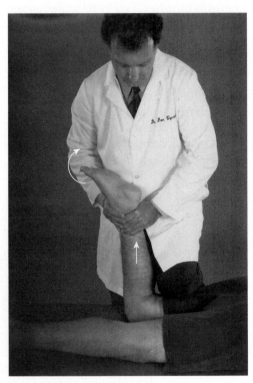

Figure 14-64

Adduction Stress Test (5)

Sensitivity/Reliability Scale

0   1   2   3   4

PROCEDURE

With the patient supine, stabilize the medial thigh. Grasp the lower leg and push it medially (Fig. 14-65). Also perform this test with the knee in 20° to 30° of flexion (Fig. 14-66).

RATIONALE

If the tibia moves an excessive medial amount away from the femur (Box 14-1) when the knee is in full extension, there may be a tear of any of the following ligaments:

- Tibial collateral ligament
- Posterior meniscofemoral ligament
- Posterior medial capsule
- Anterior cruciate ligament
- Posterior cruciate ligament

If the foregoing is positive when the knee is flexed 20° to 30°, any of the following ligaments may be unstable:

- Tibial collateral ligament
- Posterior meniscofemoral ligament
- Posterior cruciate ligament

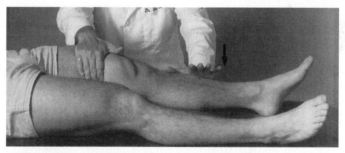

Figure 14-65

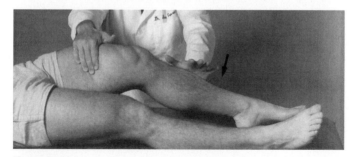

Figure 14-66

14

Box 14-1	Medial Stability Rating Scale
Grade 0	No joint opening
Grade 1+	Less than 0.5 cm joint opening
Grade 2+	0.5 to 1.0cm joint opening
Grade 3+	More than 1 cm joint opening

Abduction Stress Test (5)

Sensitivity/Reliability Scale

0   1   2   3   4

PROCEDURE

With the patient supine, stabilize the lateral thigh. Grasp the lower leg and pull it laterally (Fig. 14-67). Then perform this test in 20° to 30° of flexion (Fig. 14-68).

RATIONALE

If the tibia moves an excessive amount away from the femur (Box 14-2) when the knee is in full extension, there may be a tear of any of the following ligaments:

- Fibular collateral ligament
- Posterolateral capsule
- Posterior cruciate ligament
- Anterior cruciate ligament

If the foregoing is positive when the knee is flexed 20° to 30°, then the following ligaments may be unstable:

- Fibular collateral ligament
- Posterolateral capsule
- Iliotibial band

SUGGESTED DIAGNOSTIC IMAGING
- Plain film radiography
  AP knee view
  Lateral knee view
- Knee MRI

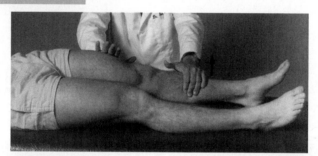

Figure 14-67

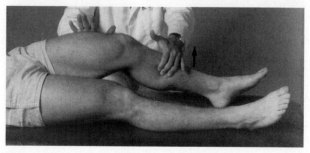

Figure 14-68

Box 14-2	Lateral Stability Rating Scale
Grade 0	No joint opening
Grade 1+	Less than 0.5 cm joint opening
Grade 2+	0.5 to 1.0 cm joint opening
Grade 3+	More than 1cm joint opening

PATELLOFEMORAL DYSFUNCTION

The patella protects the anterior aspect of the knee joint. It also functions as a fulcrum that increases the mechanical advantage of the quadriceps muscle. The patella lies in the trochlear groove. With normal flexion and extension the patella tracks smoothly within the groove. Many causes of anterior knee pain and dysfunction may be caused by an abnormality of the patella tracking in the trochlear groove or direct trauma to the patella. Patellofemoral abnormalities include fractures, dislocations, malalignment syndrome, chondromalacia patellae, and patellofemoral arthritis.

> **CLINICAL SIGNS AND SYMPTOMS**
> - Anterior knee joint pain
> - Knee joint effusion
> - Popping sensation
> - Joint crepitus
> - Discomfort with stair climbing
> - Knee buckling

Patella Grinding Test

Sensitivity/Reliability Scale

0 1 2 3 4

PROCEDURE

With the patient supine, move the patella medially and laterally while pressing down (Fig. 14-69).

RATIONALE

Pain under the patella indicates chondromalacia patellae, retropatellar arthritis, or a chondral fracture. Osteochondritis of the patella also elicits pain on the patella. Pain over the patella may indicate prepatellar bursitis.

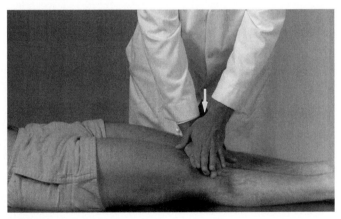

Figure 14-69

14

Patella Apprehension Test (17)

Sensitivity/Reliability Scale

0   1   2   3   4

PROCEDURE

With the patient supine, manually displace the patella laterally (Fig. 14-70).

RATIONALE

A look of apprehension on the patient's face and a contraction of the quadriceps muscle indicates a chronic tendency to lateral patella dislocation. Pain is also present with this test.

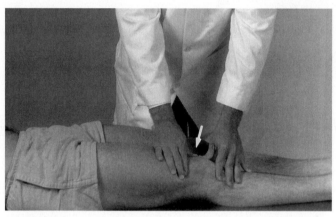

Figure 14-70

Dreyer's Test

Sensitivity/Reliability Scale

0   1   2   3   4

PROCEDURE

With the patient supine, instruct him or her to raise the leg actively (Fig. 14-71). If the patient cannot raise the leg, stabilize the quadriceps tendon just above the knee. At this point, instruct the patient to raise the leg again (Fig. 14-72).

RATIONALE

If the patient can raise the leg the second time, suspect a traumatic fracture of the patella. The rectus femoris muscle, which is a primary hip flexor, is attached to the patella by the quadriceps tendon. If the patella is fractured, the quadriceps tendon is not stabilized. Stabilizing the quadriceps tendon manually allows hip flexion to occur.

> **SUGGESTED DIAGNOSTIC IMAGING**
> - Plain film radiography
>   AP knee view
>   Lateral patella view
>   Axial patella view
> - Computed tomography (CT)
> - Magnetic Resonance Imaging (MRI)

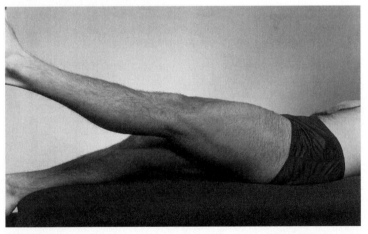

Figure 14-71

14

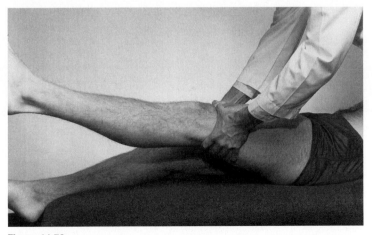

Figure 14-72

KNEE JOINT EFFUSION

CLINICAL DESCRIPTION

Effusion in and around the knee may be caused by trauma, infection, degenerative joint disease, rheumatoid arthritis, gout, or pseudogout. The fluid may contain blood, fat, lymphocytes, and crystals such as urate, pyrophosphate, and oxalate. Analysis of the effusion is beyond the scope of this book. The following physical tests attempt to determine whether fluid is present around the knee joint. If fluid is present, you must determine, based on the patient's history and clinical findings, whether aspiration is indicated.

> ### CLINICAL SIGNS AND SYMPTOMS
> - Knee pain on walking
> - Anterior knee inflammation
> - Knee joint warm to the touch

Patella Ballottement Test

Sensitivity/Reliability Scale

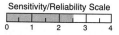

0   1   2   3   4

PROCEDURE

With one hand, encircle and press down on the superior aspect of the patella. With the other hand, push the patella against the femur with your finger (Fig. 14-73).

RATIONALE

If fluid is present in the knee, the patella will elevate when pressure is applied. When the patella is pushed down, it will strike the femur with a palpable tap.

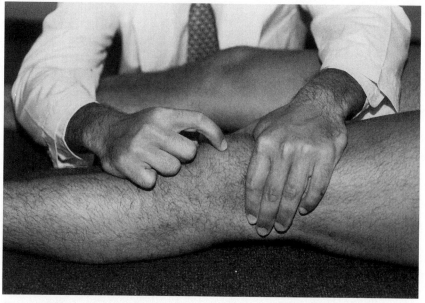

Figure 14-73

Stroke Test (5)

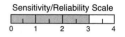

PROCEDURE

With the patient supine, stroke the medial side of the patella up toward the suprapatellar pouch two or three times with your fingers and simultaneously stroke the lateral aspect of the patella inferior with your opposite hand (Fig. 14-74).

RATIONALE

If a wave of synovial fluid is present, it will concentrate to the inferior medial border of the patella; subsequently, the area will bulge.

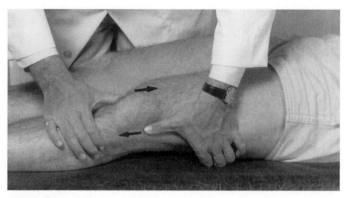

Figure 14-74

Fluctuation Test (5)

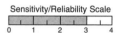

PROCEDURE

With the patient supine, grasp the thigh at the suprapatellar pouch with one hand and grasp the leg just below the patella with your opposite hand (Fig. 14-75). Press down with each hand alternately.

RATIONALE

If synovial fluid is present, you will feel it fluctuate alternately under your hand. This fluctuation indicates significant joint effusion.

> **SUGGESTED DIAGNOSTIC IMAGING**
> • None

14

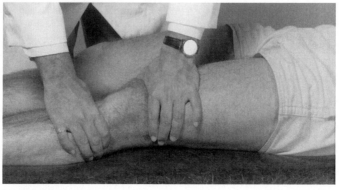

Figure 14-75

References

1. American Academy of Orthopaedic Surgeons. The Clinical Measurement of Joint Motion. Chicago: AAOS, 1994.
2. Boone DC, Azen SP. Normal range of motion of the joints in male subjects. J Bone Joint Surg Am 1979;61:756–759.
3. Apley AG. The diagnosis of meniscus injuries: some new clinical methods. J Bone Joint Surg 1947;29:78.
4. McMurray TP. The semilunar cartilages. Br J Surg 1942;29:407.
5. McGee DJ. Orthopedic Physical Assessment. 2nd ed. Philadelphia: Saunders, 1992.
6. Ricklin P, Ruttiman A, Del Buono MS. Meniscal Lesions: Diagnosis, Differential Diagnosis, and Therapy. 2nd ed. Mieller NH, trans. New York: Theme Stratton, 1983.
7. Helfet A. Disorders of the Knee. Philadelphia: JB Lippincott, 1974.
8. Strobel M, Stedtfeld HW. Diagnostic Evaluation of the Knee. Berlin: Springer-Verlag, 1990.
9. Anderson AF, Lipscomb AB. Clinical diagnosis of meniscal tears—description of a new manipulative test. Am J Sports Med 1988;14:291.
10. Mital MA, Hayden J. Pain in the knee in children: the medial plica shelf syndrome. Orthop Clin North Am 1979;10:714.
11. Houghston JC, Walsh WM, Puddu G. Patella subluxation and dislocation. Philadelphia: Saunders, 1984.
12. Butler DL, Noyes FR, Grood ES. Ligamentous restraints to anterior-posterior drawer in the human knee. J Bone Joint Surg Am 1980;62: 259.
13. Fukybayashi T, Torzilli PA, Sherman MF, et al. An in vitro biomechanical evaluation of anterior posterior motion of the knee. J Bone Joint Surg Br 1972;54:763.
14. Jonsson TB, Althoff L, Peterson J, et al. Clinical diagnosis of ruptures of the anterior cruciate ligament: a comparative study of the Lachman test and the anterior drawer sign. Am J Sports Med 1982;10:100.
15. Slocum DB, James SL, Larson RL, et al. A clinical test for anterolateral rotary instability of the knee. Clin Orthop 1976;118;63.
16. Loose RE, Jenning TR, Southwich WO. Anterior subluxation of the lateral tibial plateau: a diagnostic test and operative review. J Bone Joint Surg Am 1978;60:1015.
17. Hoppenfeld S. Physical examination of the spine and extremities. New York: Appleton-Century-Crofts, 1976:127.

General References

Bloom MH. Differentiating between meniscal and patellar pain. Phys Sports Med 1989;17(8):95–108.

Butler DL, Noyes FR, Grood ES. Ligamentous restraints to anterior-posterior drawer in the human knee. J Bone Joint Surg Am 1980;62:259.

Cailliet R. Knee Pain and Disability. Philadelphia: FA Davis, 1973.

Cipriano J. Post traumatic knee injuries. Today's Chiropractic 1985;14(5):49–51.

Clancy WG. Evaluation of acute knee injuries. American Association of Orthopedic Surgeons symposium on sports medicine: the Knee. St. Louis: Mosby, 1985.

Clancy WG, Keene JS, Goletz TH. The symptomatic dislocation of the anterior horn of the medial meniscus. Am J Sports Med 1984;12:57–64.

Cyriax J. Textbook of Orthopaedic Medicine. Vol. 1. Diagnosis of Soft Tissue Lesions. London: Bailliéré Tindall, 1982.

Frankel VH, Burstein AH, Brooks DB. Biomechanics of internal derangement of the knee. J Bone Joint Surg Am 1971;53:945.

Hardaker WT, Whipple TL, Bassett FH. Diagnosis and treatment of the plica syndrome of the knee. J Bone Joint Surg Am 1980;62:221–255.

Johnson T, Althoff B, Peterson L, et al. Clinical diagnosis of ruptures of the anterior cruciate ligament: a comparative study of the Lachman test and the anterior drawer sign. Am J Sports Med 1982;10:100.

Kapandji LA. The Physiology of the Joints. Vol. 2. Lower Limb. New York: Churchill Livingstone, 1970.

Katz KW, Fingeroth RF. The diagnostic accuracy of ruptures of the anterior cruciate ligament comparing the Lachman test, the anterior drawer sign and the pivot shift test in acute and chronic knee injuries. Am J Sports Med 1986;14:88.

Nottage WM, Sprague NF, Auerbach BJ, et al. The medial patellar plica syndrome. Am J Sports Med 1983;11:211214.

Outerbridge RE, Dunlop J. The problem of chondromalacia patellae. Clin Orthop 1975;110:177196.

Pickett JC, Radin EL. Chondromalacia of the Patella. Baltimore: Williams & Wilkins, 1983.

Slocum DB, Larson RL. Rotary instability of the knee. J Bone Joint Surg Am 1968;50:211.

Stickland A. Examination of the knee joint. Physiotherapy 1984;70:144.

Scuderi, GR: The Patella. New York: Springer-Verlag, 1995.

Torg JS, Conrad W, Nalen V. Clinical diagnosis of anterior cruciate ligament instability in the athlete. Am J Sports Med 1976;4:84.

Tria AJ. Ligaments of the Knee. New York: Churchill Livingstone, 1995.

ANKLE ORTHOPAEDIC TESTS

Ankle Orthopaedic Examination

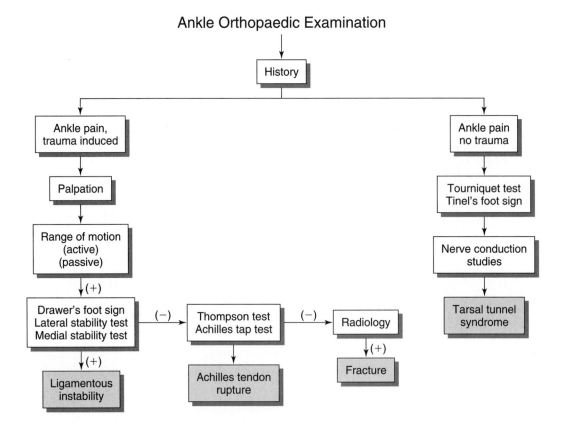

PALPATION

Medial Aspect

Medial Malleolus and Deltoid Ligament

DESCRIPTIVE ANATOMY

The medial malleolus is the most distal prominence of the tibia. It embraces the medial aspect of the talus and gives the ankle joint bony stability. Attached to the malleolus is the strong deltoid ligament, which connects with three tarsal bones: the talus, navicular, and calcaneus. The deltoid is a four-part ligament that is named according to its attachments: tibionavicular, anterior and posterior tibiotalar, and tibiocalcaneal (Fig. 15-1). The deltoid ligament strengthens and provides medial stability to the ankle joint and holds the calcaneus and navicular bones against the talus. A common injury is a forceful eversion of the foot that causes an avulsion fracture of the deltoid ligament on the medial malleolus.

PROCEDURE

With the patient's weight off that foot, palpate the medial malleolus and deltoid ligament for tenderness and/or swelling (Fig. 15-2). Tenderness and/or swelling secondary to trauma may indicate periosteal contusion, sprain, or avulsion of the deltoid ligament.

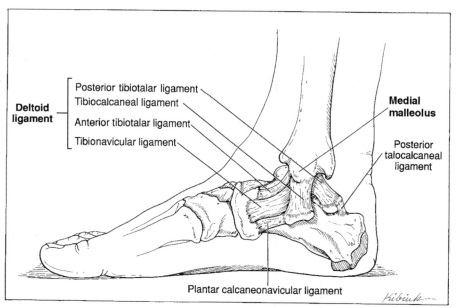

Figure 15-1

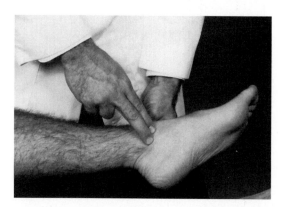

Figure 15-2

15

Tibialis Posterior, Flexor Digitorum Longus, and Flexor Hallucis Longus Tendons

DESCRIPTIVE ANATOMY

The posterior tibial tendon passes posterior to the medial malleolus and inserts into the tuberosity of the navicular bone (Fig. 15-3). The action of the muscle is to plantar-flex the ankle and invert the foot. The flexor digitorum longus tendon is posterior to the posterior tibial tendon; it closely follows the tibia and passes behind the medial malleolus (Fig. 15-3). It inserts into the distal phalanges of the lateral four digits. The action of the muscle is to plantar-flex the ankle and flex all of the joints of the last four toes. The flexor hallucis longus tendon is posterior to the flexor digitorum longus tendon, and it passes behind the ankle joint, not posterior to the medial malleolus. It inserts into the base of the distal phalanx of the great toe (Fig. 15-3). Its action is to flex the great toe.

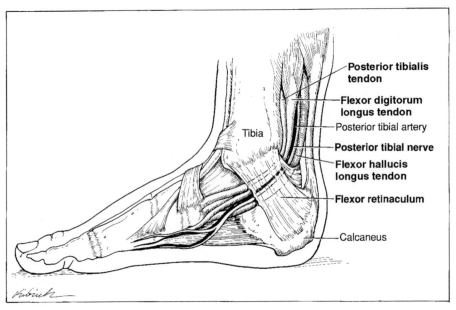

Figure 15-3

PROCEDURE

To palpate the tibialis posterior tendon, invert and plantar-flex the patient's foot. Palpate medial to the tibia posterior to the medial malleolus (Fig. 15-4). Note the continuity of the tendon and any tenderness or swelling. Tenderness and/or swelling may indicate a strain secondary to trauma or tendinitis. Loss of continuity and a valgus foot secondary to trauma may indicate a ruptured tendon.

Palpate the flexor digitorum longus tendon, which is posterior to the tibialis posterior tendon. With one hand, resist flexion of the patient's toes, and with the other hand palpate the tendon (Fig. 15-5). Note any tenderness, swelling, or crepitus. These signs may indicate a strain or tendinitis of the tendon. The flexor hallucis longus tendon is not palpable and not described in this book.

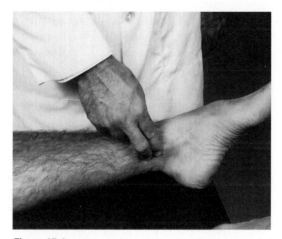

Figure 15-4

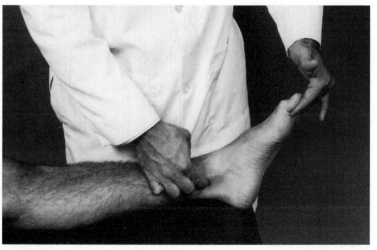

Figure 15-5

15

Posterior Tibial Artery and Tibial Nerve

DESCRIPTIVE ANATOMY

The posterior tibial artery runs between the tendons of the flexor digitorum longus and flexor hallucis longus muscles. This artery is the major blood supply to the foot. The tibial nerve is a branch of the sciatic nerve. It runs with the posterior tibial artery under the flexor retinaculum of the ankle and posterior to the medial malleolus (Fig. 15-6). The flexor retinaculum may become constricted and cause a neurovascular deficit to the foot similar to carpal tunnel in the wrist.

PROCEDURE

Using light pressure with your middle and index finger, palpate the posterior tibial artery (Fig. 15-7). Note the amplitude and compare bilaterally. A decrease in the pulse amplitude may indicate a compression of the posterior tibial artery. The tibial nerve is difficult at best to palpate and is not discussed in this book. It is an important nerve supply to the sole of the foot.

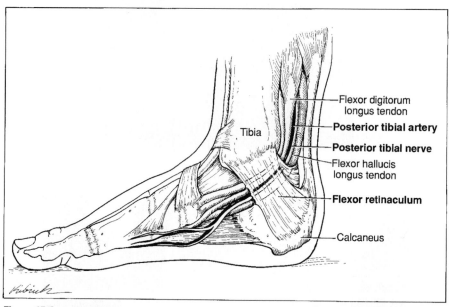

Figure 15-6

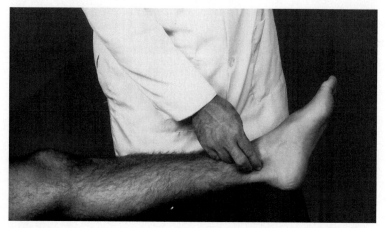

Figure 15-7

Lateral Aspect

Lateral Malleolus and Attached Ligaments

DESCRIPTIVE ANATOMY

The lateral malleolus is the protuberance at the distal end of the fibula. Attached to the malleolus are three clinically important ligaments:

- Anterior talofibular ligament
- Calcaneofibular ligament
- Posterior talofibular ligament

These ligaments provide lateral support to the ankle, but they are not as strong as the deltoid ligament on the medial aspect (Fig. 15-8). These ligaments are prone to tears in inversion injuries.

PROCEDURE

Palpate the lateral malleolus with your index and middle fingers (Fig. 15-9). Note any tenderness and/or swelling. These signs may indicate periosteal contusion, fracture, avulsion fracture, or inversion sprain of any of the previously mentioned ligaments secondary to trauma.

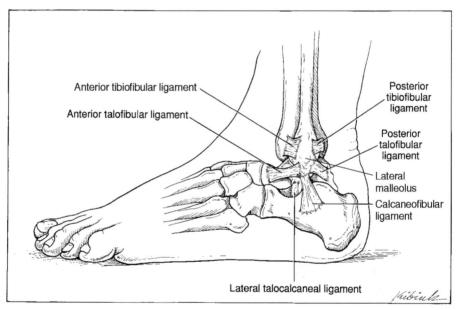

Figure 15-8

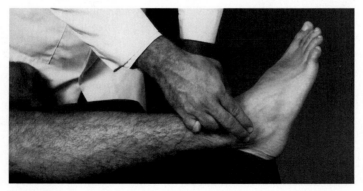

Figure 15-9

Peroneus Longus and Peroneus Brevis Tendons

DESCRIPTIVE ANATOMY

The peroneus tendons travel together behind the lateral malleolus and are held in place by the peroneal retinaculum (Fig. 15-10). The action of the muscles are to plantar flex and evert the foot.

PROCEDURE

With the patient not bearing weight, palpate behind the lateral malleolus with one hand, and passively invert (Fig. 15-11) and evert (Fig. 15-12) the foot with the other hand. Note any tenderness, swelling, or snapping. Tenderness and/or swelling may indicate tenosynovitis of either or both tendons. Tenderness with snapping may indicate a defect of the peroneal retinaculum that causes the peroneal tendons to subluxate or dislocate.

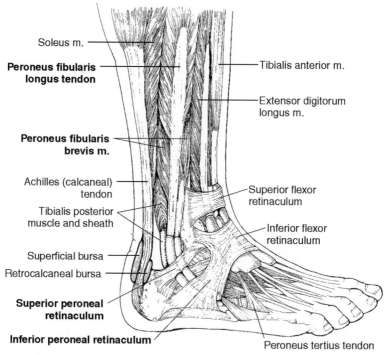

Figure 15-10

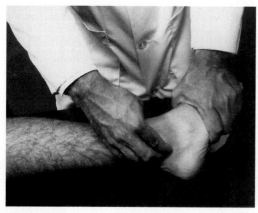

Figure 15-11

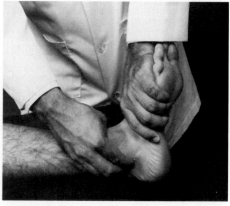

Figure 15-12

Anterior Aspect

Tibialis Anterior, Extensor Hallucis Longus, and Extensor Digitorum Longus Tendons

Descriptive Anatomy

The tibialis anterior tendon lies against the anterior surface of the tibia under the extensor retinaculum. It attaches to the medial cuneiform bone and first metatarsal (Fig. 15-13). Its action is to dorsiflex the ankle and invert the foot. The extensor hallucis longus tendon passes under the superior and inferior extensor retinacula. It inserts into the dorsal aspect of the great toe (Fig. 15-13). The action of the muscle is to dorsiflex the ankle and extend the great toe. The extensor digitorum longus tendon lies lateral to the tibialis anterior. It inserts into the middle and distal phalanges of the lateral four toes. It passes under the superior and inferior flexor retinacula (Fig. 15-13). Its action is to dorsiflex the ankle, evert the foot, and extend the lateral four toes.

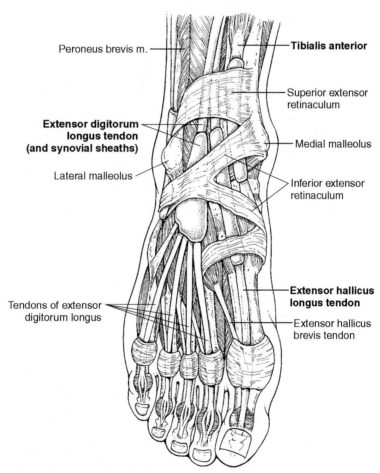

Figure 15-13

PROCEDURE

To palpate the tibialis anterior, instruct the patient to dorsiflex and invert the foot. The tendon should become prominent. Palpate the tendon for point tenderness (Fig. 15-14). Tenderness may be caused by overpronation, especially in runners. Tendinitis or a strain of the tendon also may be present. This muscle and tendon support the longitudinal arch of the foot.

To palpate the extensor hallucis longus tendon, instruct the patient to extend the great toe (Fig. 15-15). The tendon should be prominent. Palpate the tendon for point tenderness. This may indicate tendinitis or strain of the tendon.

To palpate the extensor digitorum longus tendon, instruct the patient to extend the toes. Palpate the tendon first where it crosses the ankle (Fig. 15-16), then when it divides into the four parts (Fig. 15-17) that insert into the middle phalanx. Tenderness may indicate tendonitis or tenosynovitis from overuse, especially in the runner.

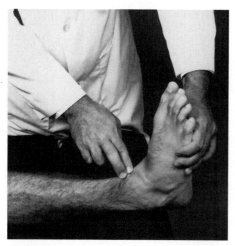

Figure 15-14

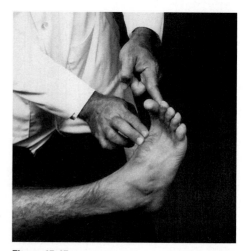

Figure 15-15

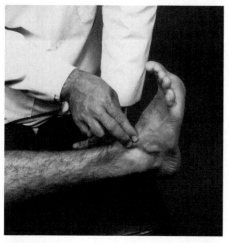

Figure 15-16

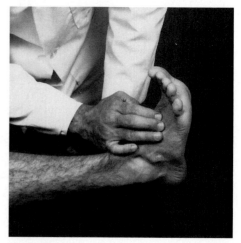

Figure 15-17

Posterior Aspect

Achilles Tendon, Calcaneal Bursa, and Retrocalcaneal Bursa

DESCRIPTIVE ANATOMY

The Achilles tendon attaches the gastrocnemius and soleus muscles to the calcaneus. It is the strongest tendon in the body but the one most frequently ruptured. Two bursae surround this tendon: the calcaneal bursa, which is superficial to the Achilles tendon and below the skin; and the retrocalcaneal bursa, which is deep to the Achilles tendon (Fig. 15-18). These bursae are normally not palpable unless they are inflamed.

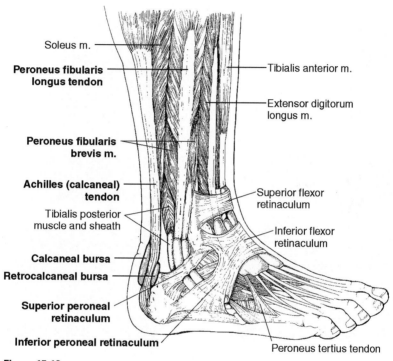

Figure 15-18

PROCEDURE

With the ankle in the neutral position, palpate the Achilles tendon with your thumb and index finger (Fig. 15-19). Next, place posterior to anterior pressure on the Achilles tendon with your thumb (Fig. 15-20). Note any pain, tenderness, increase in temperature, swelling, crepitus, and/or continuity of the tendon. Pain, tenderness, and an increase in temperature may indicate tendinitis, a strain, or a partial tear of the tendon. Loss of continuity of the tendon may indicate a complete rupture of the tendon. This is rare but may affect especially patients with a history of chronic Achilles tendinitis. Pain, tenderness, and inflammation deep to the Achilles tendon may indicate retrocalcaneal bursitis. Pain, tenderness, and swelling over the Achilles tendon and below the skin indicate calcaneal bursitis.

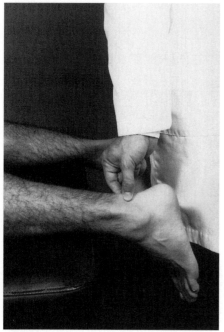

Figure 15-19

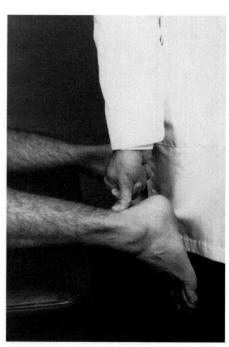

Figure 15-20

ANKLE RANGE OF MOTION

Dorsiflexion (1)

With the patient supine, place the goniometer in the sagittal plane with the center at the lateral malleolus (Fig. 15-21). Instruct the patient to flex the foot backward while following the foot with one arm of the goniometer (Fig. 15-22).

NORMAL RANGE (2)

Normal range is 13° ± 4.4° or greater from the 0 or neutral position.

Muscles	Nerve Supply
Tibialis anterior	Deep peroneal
Extensor digitorum longus	Deep peroneal
Extensor hallucis longus	Deep peroneal
Peroneus tertius	Deep peroneal

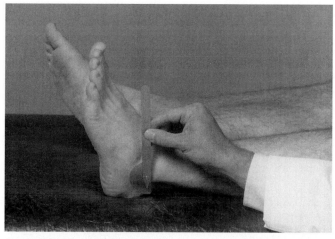

Figure 15-21

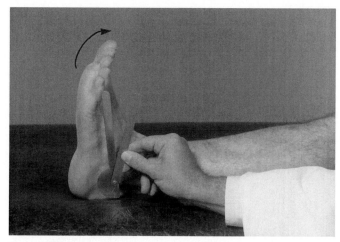

Figure 15-22

15

Plantar Flexion (1)

With the patient supine, place the goniometer in the sagittal plane with the center at the lateral malleolus (Fig. 15-23). Instruct the patient to flex the foot forward while following the foot with one arm of the goniometer (Fig. 15-24).

NORMAL RANGE (2)

Normal range is 56° ± 6.1° or greater from the 0 or neutral position.

Muscles	*Nerve Supply*
Gastrocnemius	Tibial
Soleus	Tibial
Plantaris	Tibial
Flexor digitorum longus	Tibial
Peroneus longus	Superficial peroneal
Peroneus brevis	Superficial peroneal
Flexor hallucis longus	Tibial
Tibialis posterior	Tibial

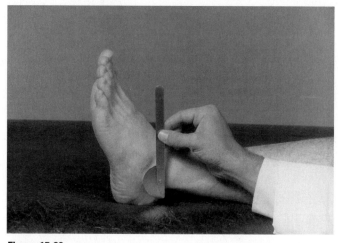

Figure 15-23

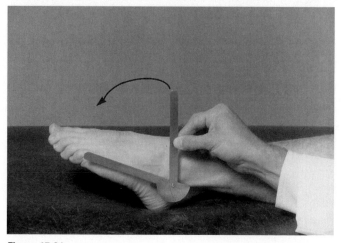

Figure 15-24

Inversion (1)

With the patient prone and the knee flexed, place the inclinometer at the base of the heel and zero out the inclinometer (Fig. 15-25). Instruct the patient to invert the foot, and record the measurement (Fig. 15-26).

NORMAL RANGE (2)

Normal range is 37° ± 4.5° or greater from the 0 or neutral position.

Muscles	*Nerve Supply*
Tibialis posterior	Tibial
Flexor digitorum longus	Tibial
Flexor hallucis longus	Tibial
Tibialis anterior	Deep peroneal
Extensor hallucis longus	Deep peroneal

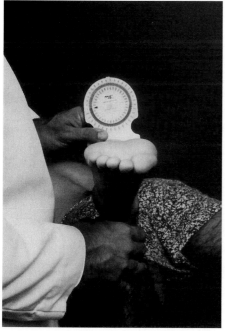

Figure 15-25

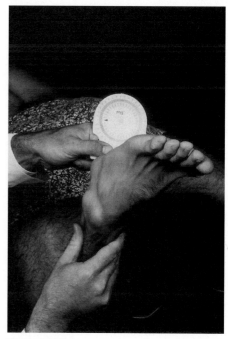

Figure 15-26

15

Eversion (1,2)

With the patient prone and the knee flexed, place the inclinometer at the base of the heel and zero out the inclinometer (Fig. 15-27). Instruct the patient to evert the foot and record the measurement (Fig. 15-28).

NORMAL RANGE

Normal range is 21° ± 5° or greater from the 0 or neutral position.

Muscles	Nerve Supply
Peroneus longus	Superficial peroneal
Peroneus brevis	Superficial peroneal
Peroneus tertius	Deep peroneal
Extensor hallucis longus	Deep peroneal

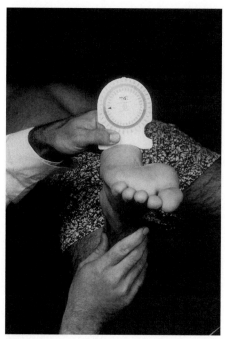

Figure 15-27

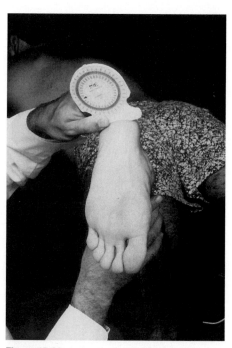

Figure 15-28

LIGAMENTOUS INSTABILITY

CLINICAL DESCRIPTION

The ankle joint is formed by the tibia, fibula, and talus, which are bound together by ligaments that provide for stability and joint movement. These are the anterior and posterior talofibular, anterior tibiofibular, calcaneofibular, and deltoid ligaments (Fig. 15-29). If any of these ligaments are torn, the tibia can separate from the fibula and the talus may become unstable. The degree to which these ligaments are torn determines the degree of talar instability. Most of theses injuries are sports related, and the most common mechanism of injury is a supination or inversion force. This occurs when the foot turns under the ankle after walking or running on uneven surfaces or when landing on an inverted foot after a jump. The most common injured ligament is the anterior talofibular ligament. Ligament laxity or instability may lead to chronic ankle sprains.

CLINICAL SIGNS AND SYMPTOMS
- Ankle swelling
- Static ankle pain
- Pain on passive motion
- Tenderness over affected ligament

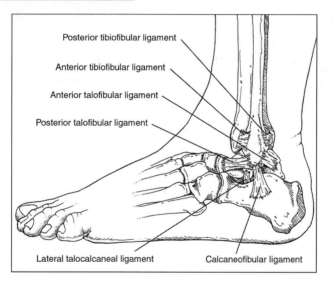

Figure 15-29

Posterior tibiofibular ligament

Anterior tibiofibular ligament

Anterior talofibular ligament

Posterior talofibular ligament

Lateral talocalcaneal ligament

Calcaneofibular ligament

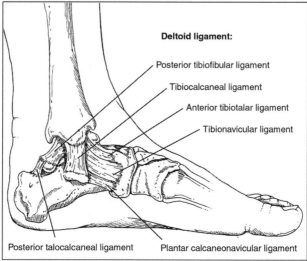

Deltoid ligament:

Posterior tibiofibular ligament

Tibiocalcaneal ligament

Anterior tibiotalar ligament

Tibionavicular ligament

Posterior talocalcaneal ligament

Plantar calcaneonavicular ligament

15

Drawer's Foot Sign (3)

Sensitivity/Reliability Scale
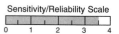
0   1   2   3   4

Procedure

With the patient supine, stabilize the ankle with one hand. With your opposite hand, grasp and press posterior on the tibia (Fig. 15-30). Next, grasp the anterior aspect of the foot with one hand and the posterior aspect of the tibia with the other, and pull anterior (Fig. 15-31).

Rationale

Gapping secondary to trauma when the tibia is pushed indicates a tear of the anterior talofibular ligament. Gapping when the tibia is pulled indicates a posterior talofibular ligament tear (Fig. 15-32).

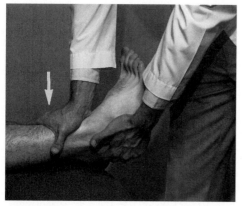

Figure 15-30

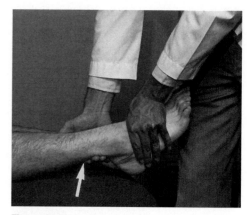

Figure 15-31

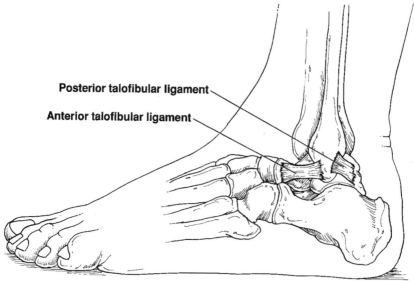

Posterior talofibular ligament

Anterior talofibular ligament

Figure 15-32

Lateral Stability Test (3)

Sensitivity/Reliability Scale

0   1   2   3   4

Procedure

With the patient supine, grasp the patient's foot and passively invert it (Fig. 15-33).

Rationale

If gapping secondary to trauma is present, suspect a tear of the anterior talofibular and/or calcaneofibular ligament (Fig. 15-34).

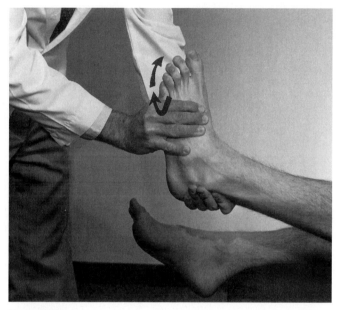

Figure 15-33

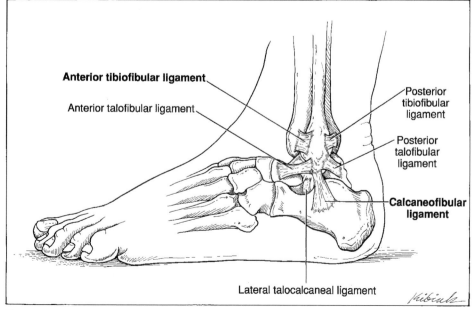

Anterior tibiofibular ligament

Anterior talofibular ligament

Posterior tibiofibular ligament

Posterior talofibular ligament

Calcaneofibular ligament

Lateral talocalcaneal ligament

Figure 15-34

15

Medial Stability Test (3)

Sensitivity/Reliability Scale

0   1   2   3   4

PROCEDURE

With the patient supine, grasp the foot and passively evert it (Fig. 15-35).

RATIONALE

If gapping secondary to trauma is present, suspect a tear of the deltoid ligament (Fig. 15-36).

> **SUGGESTED DIAGNOSTIC IMAGING**
>
> - Plain film radiography
>   Anteroposterior (AP) ankle view
>   Mortise view
>   Lateral view
>   Stress views
> - Magnetic resonance imaging (MRI)

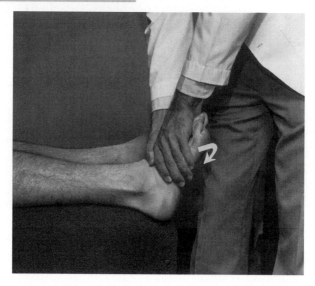

Figure 15-35

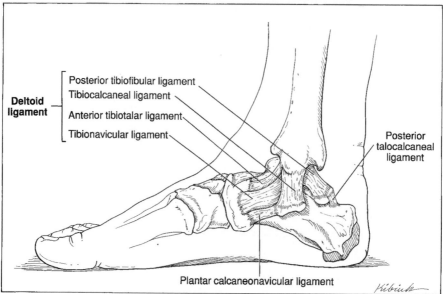

Posterior tibiofibular ligament
Tibiocalcaneal ligament
Deltoid ligament
Anterior tibiotalar ligament
Tibionavicular ligament

Posterior talocalcaneal ligament

Plantar calcaneonavicular ligament

Figure 15-36

TARSAL TUNNEL SYNDROME

CLINICAL DESCRIPTION

Tarsal tunnel syndrome occurs when the posterior tibial nerve becomes entrapped in its tunnel as it passes behind the medial malleolus to enter the foot. The tunnel may be compressed either intrinsically or extrinsically. Space-occupying lesions account for 50% of cases. Direct trauma and repetitive dorsiflexion account for a significant portion of the other 50%. A severe flat foot can unduly stretch the posterior tibial nerve, causing tarsal tunnel syndrome. Other causes, such as fracture callus, ganglion of the tendon sheath, lipoma, exostosis, engorged venus plexus, and excessive pronation of the hind foot, should be investigated.

> ### CLINICAL SIGNS AND SYMPTOMS
> - Intermittent paresthesia of plantar aspect of the foot
> - Pain on foot inversion and/or eversion of the foot
> - Pain radiating to medial aspect of the leg
> - Pain made worse by activity and improved by rest

Tourniquet Test (4)

PROCEDURE

Sensitivity/Reliability Scale

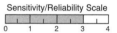

Wrap a sphygmomanometer cuff around the affected ankle and inflate it to just above the patient's systolic blood pressure. Hold for 1 to 2 minutes (Fig. 15-37).

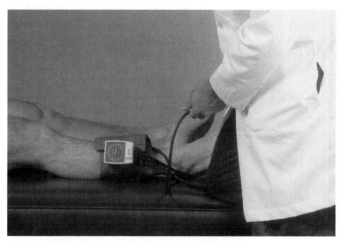

Figure 15-37

15

RATIONALE

Tarsal tunnel syndrome is compression of the posterior tibial nerve beneath the flexor retinaculum at the ankle (Fig. 15-38). Compression of the area by the cuff accentuates the narrowing of the tunnel, increasing the patient's pain. If pain is elicited or existing pain is exacerbated, suspect a compromise of the tarsal tunnel.

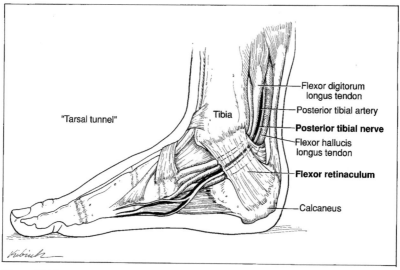

"Tarsal tunnel"

Tibia

Flexor digitorum longus tendon
Posterior tibial artery
Posterior tibial nerve
Flexor hallucis longus tendon
Flexor retinaculum
Calcaneus

Figure 15-38

Tinel's Foot Sign

Sensitivity/Reliability Scale

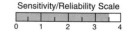

0   1   2   3   4

PROCEDURE

Tap the area over the posterior tibial nerve with a neurological reflex hammer (Fig. 15-39).

RATIONALE

Paresthesias radiating to the foot indicate an irritation to the posterior tibial nerve that may be caused by a constriction at the tarsal tunnel.

> **SUGGESTED DIAGNOSTIC TEST**
> • Nerve conduction velocity of the posterior tibial nerve

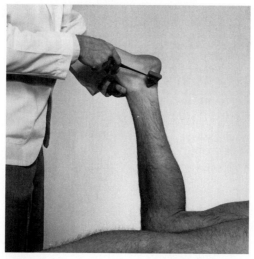

Figure 15-39

ACHILLES TENDON RUPTURE

CLINICAL DESCRIPTION

Achilles tendon rupture generally occurs in adults aged 30 to 50. It is usually spontaneous in athletes, who account for most of these injuries. Some authors suggest that this is due to decreased vascularity of the Achilles tendon as the patient ages. The mechanism that causes rupture is forced dorsiflexion of the foot as the soleus and gastrocnemius contract. Rupture occurs usually 2 to 6 cm from the insertion of the Achilles tendon into the calcaneus. As the proximal aspect of the tendon retracts, there is usually a palpable defect of the tendon.

CLINICAL SIGNS AND SYMPTOMS
- Severe posterior ankle pain
- Inability to stand on toes
- Posterior leg and heel swelling
- Posterior leg and heel ecchymosis

Thompson's Test (5)

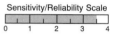
Sensitivity/Reliability Scale
0   1   2   3   4

PROCEDURE

Instruct the prone patient to flex the knee. Squeeze the calf muscles against the tibia and fibula (Fig. 15-40).

RATIONALE

When the calf muscles are squeezed, the gastrocnemius and soleus muscles mechanically contract. These muscles are attached to the Achilles tendon, which in turn plantar-flexes the foot. If the Achilles tendon is ruptured, contraction of the gastrocnemius and soleus muscles will not plantar-flex the foot.

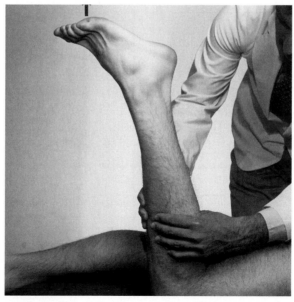

Figure 15-40

15

Achilles Tap Test

PROCEDURE

Tap the Achilles tendon with a neurological reflex hammer (Fig. 15-41).

RATIONALE

Exacerbation of pain and a loss of plantarflexion indicate an Achilles tendon rupture.

NOTE

The patient must be neurologically sound for this test to be valid.

SUGGESTED DIAGNOSTIC IMAGING
- Plain film radiography
   AP ankle view
   Lateral view
- Ankle MRI

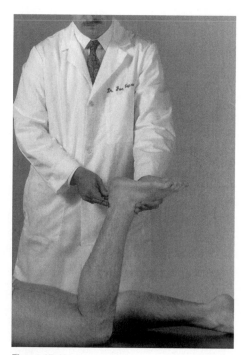

Figure 15-41

References

1. American Academy of Orthopaedic Surgeons. The clinical measurement of joint motion. Chicago: AAOS, 1994.
2. Boone DC, Azen SP. Normal range of motion of joint in male subjects. J Bone Joint Surg Am 1979;61:756–759.
3. Hoppenfeld S. Physical Examination of the Spine and Extremities. New York: Appleton-Century-Crofts, 1976:127.
4. McRae R. Clinical Orthopedic Examination. New York: Churchill Livingstone, 1976.
5. Thompson T, Doherty J. Spontaneous rupture of the tendon of Achilles: a new clinical diagnostic test. Anat Res 1967;158:126.

General References

Anderson BC. Office Orthopedics For Primary Care. 2nd ed. Philadelphia: Saunders, 1999.

Colter JM. Lateral ligamentous injuries of the ankle. In: Hamilton WC, ed. Traumatic disorders of the ankle. New York: Springer Verlag, 1984.

Cox JS, Brand RL. Evaluation and treatment of lateral ankle sprains. Sports Med 1977;5:51.

Dvorkin ML. Oddice Orthopaedics. Norwalk, CT: Appleton & Lang, 1993.

Gates SJ, Mooar PA. Musculoskeletal Primary Care. Baltimore: Lippincott Williams & Wilkins, 1999.

Kapandji LA. The Physiology of the Joints. Vol. 2. Lower Limb. New York: Churchill Livingstone, 1970.

Kelikian H. Disorders of the Ankle. Philadelphia: Saunders, 1985.

Lam SJ. Tarsal tunnel syndrome. Lancet 1962; 2:1354.

Mennell JM. Foot Pain. Boston: Little, Brown, 1969.

Post M. Physical examination of the musculoskeletal system. Chicago: Year Book Medical, 1987.

Soma CA, Mandelbaum BR. Achilles tendon disorders. Clin Sports Med 1994;13(4):118.

15

16

MISCELLANEOUS ORTHOPAEDIC TESTS

PERIPHERAL ARTERIAL INSUFFICIENCY

Peripheral arterial insufficiency may involve both the upper and lower extremities. It may be due to obstruction, traumatic occlusion, arthrosclerosis, diabetes, Buerger's disease, or Raynaud's phenomenon. The patients who develop arterial insufficiency generally demonstrate one of three clinical patterns: (*a*) cold, cyanosed, livid and/or painful digits (Raynaud's phenomenon); (*b*) digital ischemia; or (*c*) crampy pain on exercise (claudication). There is usually prolonged venous filling time following elevation of the extremity. The impaired flow or arterial insufficiency may be adequate to serve the metabolic activities of the muscles at rest but does not maintain the circulation necessary to the increased metabolic rates of exercise. Therefore, exercise testing, such as flexing and extending the arms and legs or walking, may reproduce the patient's symptoms. Diagnosis is based on the combination of physical examination and vascular diagnostic testing, such as angiography, plethysmography, thermography, and vascular ultrasound.

CLINICAL SIGNS AND SYMPTOMS
- Extremity pain
- Cold extremities
- Decreased pulse amplitude
- Pallor or rubor
- Hair loss
- Shiny skin
- Claudication
- Gangrene

Buerger's Test

Sensitivity/Reliability Scale

0   1   2   3   4

PROCEDURE

With the patient supine, instruct him or her to elevate one leg at a time. The patient must consecutively dorsiflex and plantar-flex the raised foot for a minimum of 2 minutes (Figs. 16-1 and 16-2). The leg is then lowered and hung off the side of the table with the patient seated (Fig. 16-3).

RATIONALE

Elevating and flexing the foot diminishes the blood flow in the lower extremity. When the leg is lowered and hung off the table, the lower leg and foot should fill with blood. This turns the foot a pinkish color, and the veins distend. This process takes less than 1 minute. If it takes longer, the test is positive for arterial compromise to the lower extremity.

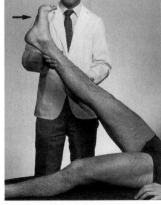

Figure 16-1

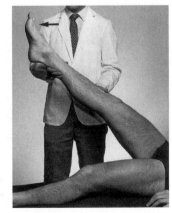

Figure 16-2

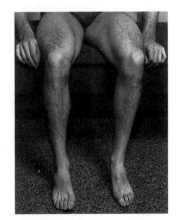

Figure 16-3

16

Allen's Test (1,2)

Sensitivity/Reliability Scale
0 1 2 3 4

PROCEDURE

With the patient seated, occlude the radial and ulnar arteries with both thumbs (Fig. 16-4). Then instruct the patient to open and close the fist to express blood from the tissue (Fig.16-5). At that point, instruct the patient to open the hand as you release the pressure to the radial artery (Fig. 16-6). Repeat the test with the pressure released to the ulnar artery (Fig. 16-7).

RATIONALE

Consecutively opening and closing the fist diminishes the blood flow in the hand, causing blanching. When pressure on one of the arteries is released, the hand should fill with blood, which turns it a pinkish color, and the veins distend. A delay of more than 10 seconds in returning a pinkish color to the hand indicates either ulnar artery insufficiency or radial artery insufficiency. The artery being tested is the one not being manually occluded.

SUGGESTED DIAGNOSTIC IMAGING

- Peripheral vascular ultrasound
- Thermography
- Plethysmography
- Angiography

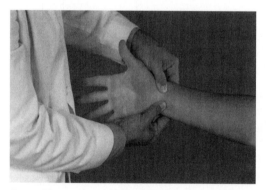

Figure 16-4

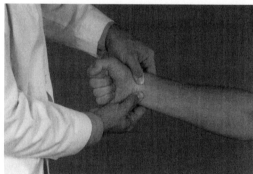

Figure 16-5

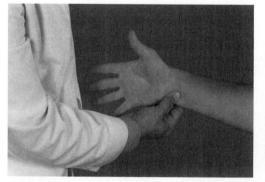

Figure 16-6

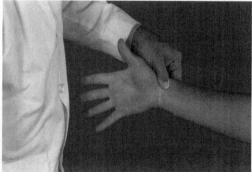

Figure 16-7

DEEP VEIN THROMBOSIS

Deep vein thrombosis (DVT) is a cordlike clot formation that usually arises in the deep veins of the calf muscles. This venous occlusion results in edema and dependent cyanosis. The cause may be iatrogenic or result from a mechanical trauma that injured the endothelium of the veins, hypercoagulability associated with malignant tumor or oral contraceptives, or stasis that occurs with prolonged bed rest. If left untreated, approximately 20% of thrombi may extend into the proximal venous system and pose a serious and even life-threatening risk of a pulmonary embolism: 90% of pulmonary emboli originate in the deep venous system of the legs.

CLINICAL SIGNS AND SYMPTOMS
- Leg pain
- Leg swelling
- Leg tenderness
- Local temperature elevation
- Discoloration
- Venous distension
- Palpable cord (thrombosed vessel)

Homan's Sign

Sensitivity/Reliability Scale
0   1   2   3   4

PROCEDURE

With the patient supine, dorsiflex the foot and squeeze the calf (Fig. 16-8) (3).

RATIONALE

Deep-seated pain at the posterior leg or calf may indicate thrombophlebitis. Dorsiflexing the foot places a dynamic stretch on the gastrocnemius muscle and tension of the deep veins. The addition of squeezing the calf compresses the surrounding tissue against the thrombus, stimulating a nociceptive response.

SUGGESTED DIAGNOSTIC IMAGING
- Peripheral vascular ultrasound
- Plethysmography
- Venography

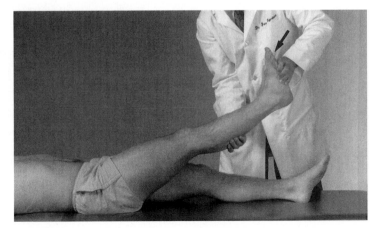

Figure 16-8

16

SYMPTOM MAGNIFICATION ASSESSMENT

Symptom magnification is usually misrepresentation of the patient's symptoms, feigned for secondary gain. This is a very difficult assessment. Although this condition is most common in the setting of workers compensation and personal injury cases, the secondary gain may not be financial alone. It may occur if individuals desire a less strenuous job at work. They may gain control over fellow workers or family members. The injured party may allow others to do work that the patient would normally do.

The possibility of symptom magnification should be raised when major discrepancies or inconsistencies appear in the patient's condition. These inconsistencies are most noted in history and physical examination. Some examples of these inconsistencies: (*a*) dramatized complaints that are vague or global, (*b*) overemphasized gait or postural abnormalities, (*c*) resistance to evaluation or rehabilitation, and (*d*) lack of motivation to develop new skills or lack of treatment compliance.

Once the information has been collected, a determination of symptom magnification may be made. This is difficult because very few symptom magnification cases are totally without pain or fear of being placed in a job perceived as potentially harmful. Second opinions are quite useful if you suspect symptom magnification. Concurrence by more that one physician is prudent in these cases.

> **CLNICAL SIGNS AND SYMPTOMS**
>
> - Discrepancy between patient's presentation and degree of reported pain
> - Negative workup for organic problems by multiple physicians
> - Dramatized complaints that are vague or global
> - Overemphasized gait or posture
> - Resistance to evaluation
> - Resistance to rehabilitation

Hoover's Sign (3,4)

Sensitivity/Reliability Scale

0　1　2　3　4

PROCEDURE

With the patient supine, instruct him or her to lift the affected leg while you place one hand under the heel on the unaffected side (Fig. 16-9).

RATIONALE

The patient who is magnifying the symptoms will not raise the affected leg, and no posterior pressure will be put on the unaffected heel. If the patient is genuinely trying to raise the leg but cannot do so, you should feel pressure from the unaffected heel.

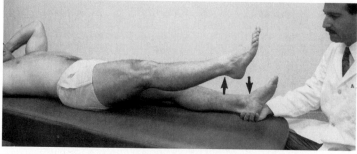

Figure 16-9

Burn's Bench Test

Sensitivity/Reliability Scale

0   1   2   3   4

PROCEDURE

Instruct the patient to kneel on the examination table. Have the patient bend at the waist to touch the floor while you stabilize the legs (Fig. 16-10).

RATIONALE

Patients with low back pain will be able to perform this test because no strenuous activity of the back is involved. The stress is placed on the posterior leg muscles. If the patient with low back pain cannot perform the test, suspect magnification of the symptoms.

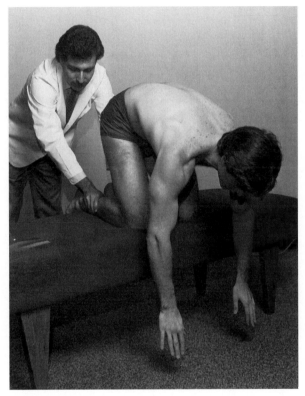

Figure 16-10

16

Magnuson's Test

Sensitivity/Reliability Scale

0   1   2   3   4

PROCEDURE

Instruct the seated patient to point at the site of the pain (Fig. 16-11). Next, distract the patient by performing some irrelevant test. Then instruct the patient to point at the site of the pain again (Fig. 16-12).

RATIONALE

The patient with real pain will point to the specific site of pain both times. The patient who is magnifying the symptoms usually does not indicate the exact same site twice.

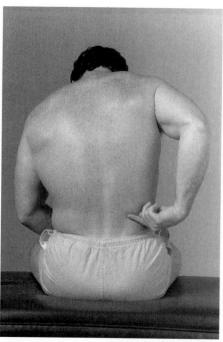

Figure 16-11

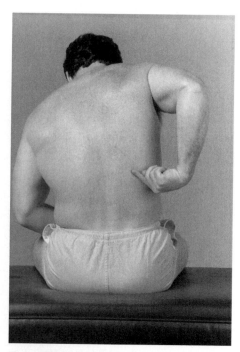

Figure 16-12

Mannkopf's Maneuver

PROCEDURE

With the patient seated, obtain the resting pulse rate (Fig. 16-13). Then irritate the patient's complaint by poking at it with your finger (Fig. 16-14). Next, retake the pulse rate.

RATIONALE

The sympathetic system controls vasoconstriction and heart rate. When the area of pain is provoked, the patient with true pain will undergo a fight or flight phenomenon, increasing the heart rate and blood pressure. In the patient who has true pain, the pulse rate will increase by 10% or more. This reaction is carried out below the conscious level and is not under the patient's control. If the heart rate does not increase, the patient may be magnifying the symptoms.

> SUGGESTED DIAGNOSTIC IMAGING
> • Based on area of complaint

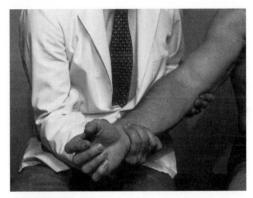

Figure 16-13

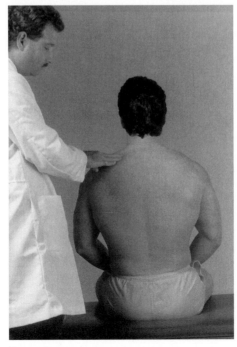

Figure 16-14

MENINGEAL IRRITATION AND INFLAMMATION

CLINICAL DESCRIPTION

Irritation of the meninges is a local condition usually caused by mechanical pressure to a specific section of the meninges, such as a herniated intervertebral disc, spinal stenosis, or tumor. Inflammation of the meninges or meningitis is usually caused by infection, either bacterial or viral. It usually develops from hematogenous spread through the bloodstream from a distant infected location or by contiguous spread from a local structure, such as the nasopharynx. The infection causes an exudation of cells and proteins into the subarachnoid space. The meningeal reaction spreads through the central nervous system (CNS), involving the meninges covering the spinal cord as well as the brain.

CLINICAL SIGNS AND SYMPTOMS

- Meningeal Irritation
  - Local neck or back pain
  - Radicular pain to an extremity
  - Decreased or lost extremity sensation
  - Decreased or lost extremity motor function
  - Loss of bladder or bowel functions
- Meningitis
  - Violent headache
  - Stiff, painful neck
  - Elevated temperature
  - Mental status change

Kernig's Test (5–7)

Sensitivity/Reliability Scale

0   1   2   3   4

PROCEDURE

With the patient supine, instruct him or her to flex the hip and knee to 90° with the lower leg parallel to the table (Fig. 16-15). Then instruct the patient to extend the knee on the side that is being tested (Fig. 16-16).

RATIONALE

With the hip and knee flexed, the sciatic nerve and the dural sac are relaxed. Extension of the knee puts traction on the sciatic nerve, hence ultimately the dural sac or meninges. Inability to straighten the leg or pain while straightening the leg indicates meningeal irritation or nerve root involvement.

NOTE

If bacterial meningitis is present, the patient may have head pain that increases with sudden neck movements, neck stiffness, nuchal rigidity, and an elevated temperature. This test will also elicit radicular pain in the patient with sciatic radiculopathy.

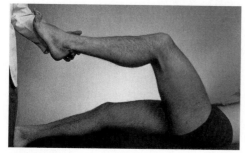

Figure 16-15

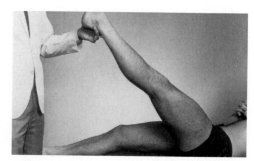

Figure 16-16

Brudzinski's Sign (8)

PROCEDURE

With the patient supine, flex the patient's neck to the chest (Fig. 16-17).

RATIONALE

Flexing the neck places traction on the dural sac and spinal cord. Irritation of the dural sac causes pain at the level of irritation. Flexing the knees reduces the traction on the spinal cord and meninges. If the patient flexes the knees, the test is positive and indicates meningeal irritation or nerve root involvement (Fig. 16-18).

NOTE

Suspect bacterial meningitis if the patient has head pain that is increased with sudden neck movements, neck stiffness, nuchal rigidity, and an elevated temperature. This test will also elicit radicular pain in the patient with sciatic radiculopathy.

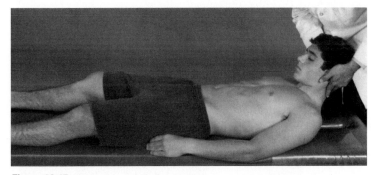

Figure 16-17

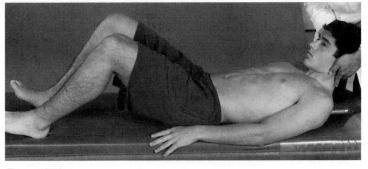

Figure 16-18

16

Lhermitte's Sign

Sensitivity/Reliability Scale

0   1   2   3   4

PROCEDURE

With the patient seated, instruct the patient to passively flex his head to his chest (Fig. 16-19).

RATIONALE

Flexing the neck stretches the spinal cord and meninges. Sharp pain radiating down the spine or into the upper or lower extremities may indicate nerve root, dural, or meningeal irritation. It also may indicate cervical myelopathy or multiple sclerosis.

> **SUGGESTED DIAGNOSTIC IMAGING AND TESTING**
>
> - Meningeal Irritation
>   Plain film radiography
>   Computed tomography (CT)
>   Magnetic resonance imaging (MRI)
> - Meningitis
>   Cerebrospinal fluid examination

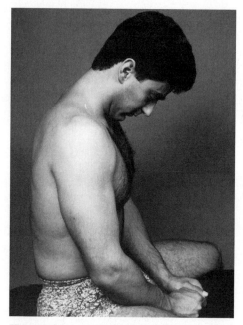

Figure 16-19

LEG MEASUREMENTS

CLINICAL DESCRIPTION

Measurement of the lower extremities is performed to evaluate a true anatomical leg length discrepancy versus an apparent or false leg length discrepancy. A true shortened lower limb may be due to congenital defect of development, impaired epiphyseal growth, or fracture. An apparent or false shortened leg may be due to a functional pelvic tilt, scoliosis, or an adduction or abduction deformity of the hip. Each may cause a distinct biomechanical defect leading to lower back pain or local lower extremity joint pain. Evaluation and correction may relieve lower back or local lower extremity joint pain, especially when findings of examination of the lower back and lower extremity joints are unremarkable.

> **CLINICAL SIGNS AND SYMPTOMS**
> - Shortened lower extremity
> - Lower back pain
> - Hip, knee, or ankle pain

Actual Leg Length

Sensitivity/Reliability Scale

0   1   2   3   4

PROCEDURE

With the patient standing, take a tape measure and measure bilaterally from the anterior superior iliac spine to the floor (Fig. 16-20).

RATIONALE

This is a true measurement of the patient's lower extremity. Compare the measurements. Any difference indicates an anatomic short leg.

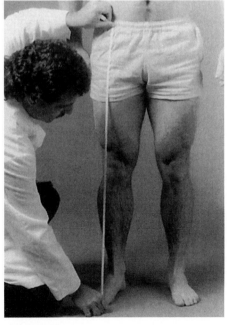

Figure 16-20

16

Apparent Leg Length

Sensitivity/Reliability Scale

0   1   2   3   4

PROCEDURE

With the patient supine, measure bilaterally the distance between the umbilicus and the medial malleolus (Fig. 16-21).

RATIONALE

Any difference in the two measurements indicates a functional leg deficiency that may be caused by muscular or ligamentous contracture deformities.

> **SUGGESTED DIAGNOSTIC IMAGING**
> * Radiographic scanogram

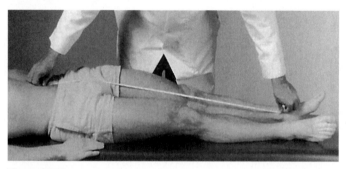

Figure 16-21

References

1. Allen EV, Barker NW, Hines EA Jr. Peripheral Vascular Disease. 4th ed. Philadelphia: Saunders, 1972:37–38.
2. Allen EV. Thromboangiitis obliterans: methods of diagnosis of chronic occlusive arterial lesions distal to the wrist. Am J Med Sci 1929;178: 238–239.
3. Arieff AJ, Tigay EI, Kurtz JF, et al. The Hoover sign: an objective sign of pain and/or weakness in the back or lower extremities. Arch Neurol 1961;5:673.
4. Hoover CF. A new sign for the detection of malingering and functional paralysis of the lower extremities. JAMA 1928;51:746–749.
5. Kernig W. Concerning a little noted sign of meningitis. Arch Neurol 1969;21:216.
6. Wartenberg R. The signs of Brudzinski and of Kernig. J Pediatr 1950;37:679.
7. Brody IA, Williams KH. The sign of Kernig and Brudzinski. Arch Neurol 1969;21:216.
8. Brudzinski J. A new sign of the lower extremities in meningitis of children (neck sign). Arch Neurol 1969;21:216.

General References

American Society for Surgery of the Hand. The Hand: Examination and Diagnosis. Aurora, CO: ASSH, 1978.

Borenstein D, Wiesel SW, Boden SD. Neck Pain: Medical Diagnosis and Comprehensive Management. Philadelphia: Saunders, 1996.

Edgar VA, Barker NW, Hines EA Jr. Peripheral Vascular Disease. Philadelphia: Saunders, 1946:57–58.

Hoppenfeld S. Physical Examination of the Spine and Extremities. New York: Appleton-Century-Crofts, 1976:127.

Woerman AL, Binder-Macleod SA. Leg-length discrepancy assessment: accuracy and precision in five clinical methods of evaluation. J Orthop Sports Phys Ther 1984;5:230.

CRANIAL NERVES

Twelve pairs of cranial nerves exit from the brain and brainstem. These nerves innervate the face, head, and neck, controlling all motor and sensory functions in these areas, including vision, hearing, smell, and taste. The cranial nerves may be affected by cranial trauma, infections, aneurysm, stroke, degenerative diseases (multiple sclerosis), upper motor neuron lesions, lower motor neuron lesions, increased intracranial pressure, and abnormal masses or tumors.

An important anatomic feature of cranial nerves is bilateral and unilateral innervation. In bilateral innervation, relatively equal distributions of right and left brain hemisphere innervation govern the function of a specific facial part. Movements that are performed in bilateral synchrony, such as swallowing and moving the forehead, are innervated bilaterally. In unilateral innervation, the contralateral hemisphere innervates the specific body part. Fine movements of the face are examples of unilateral cranial nerve innervation.

The many types of cranial nerve lesions produce a number of syndromes. Unilaterally affected cranial nerves V, VII, and VIII may indicate a cerebellopontine angle lesion. Unilaterally affected cranial nerves III, IV, V, and VI may indicate a cavernous sinuous lesion. Unilaterally affected cranial nerves IX, X, and XI may indicate a jugular foramen syndrome. Bilaterally affected cranial nerves X, XI, and XII may indicate bulbar or pseudobulbar palsy. Multiple cranial nerve abnormalities are shown in Figure 17-1.

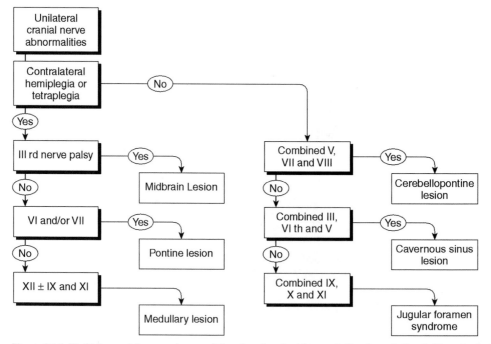

Figure 17-1. Multiple cranial nerve abnormalities. Reprinted with permission from Fuller G. Neurological Examination Made Easy. London: Churchill Livingstone, 1993.

OLFACTORY NERVE (I)

PROCEDURE

The olfactory nerve is responsible for the sense of smell. To test this nerve, obtain some aromatic substances, such as coffee, tobacco, or peppermint oil. Instruct the patient to close one nostril. Place the substance under the open nostril and ask what the patient smells, if anything (Fig. 17-2). Repeat the procedure for the opposite nostril.

RATIONALE

If the patient cannot smell or identify the smell unilaterally, suspect a lesion of the olfactory nerve. If the patient cannot smell or identify the smell bilaterally, consider a nonorganic problem or a bilateral cranial nerve I lesion.

NOTE

A diminished or almost absent sense of smell is common in the elderly. It will be apparent if loss of smell is bilateral and the cranium has undergone no trauma. Other nonneurogenic lesions, such as sinus infection, deviated septum, and lesions caused by smoking, may also cause a loss of smell, either unilaterally or bilaterally.

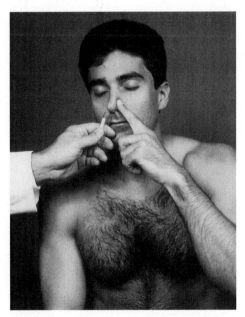

Figure 17-2

17

OPTIC NERVE (II)

PROCEDURE

The optic nerve is responsible for visual acuity and peripheral vision. To test for visual acuity, ask the patient to cover one eye and read the smallest print possible on a Snellen chart (Fig. 17-3). Repeat the test with the opposite eye. Note the results. This is not a test for visual acuity for refractive error; it tests the acuity for optic nerve involvement. This test may be performed with the patient wearing glasses or contact lenses.

To test for peripheral vision, ask the patient to cover one eye with the hand and keep a fixed gaze on your nose with the uncovered eye. Directly motion a large cross with your finger from superior to inferior and from right to left (Fig. 17-4). Instruct the patient to tell you when he or she begins to see your finger. Repeat with the opposite eye and record the results.

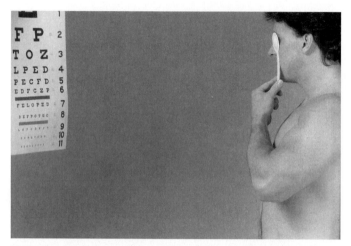

Figure 17-3

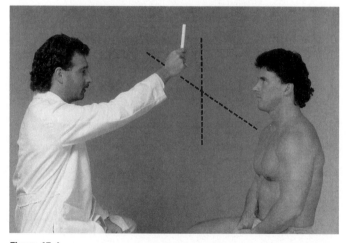

Figure 17-4

RATIONALE

Any loss of vision, from complete unilateral or bilateral loss of vision to loss of half fields of vision (hemianopsia) or a partial defect in the field of vision (scotoma), indicates an optic nerve lesion. Temporal lobe lesions can produce superior contralateral quadrantanopsia. Occipital lobe lesions can produce a contralateral homonymous hemianopsia with macular sparing. Figure 17-5 shows a schematic of the neural pathway from the brain to the retina and demonstrates the location of the lesion and its effect on vision. Also associated with the schematic is a flow chart of field defects (Fig. 17-6).

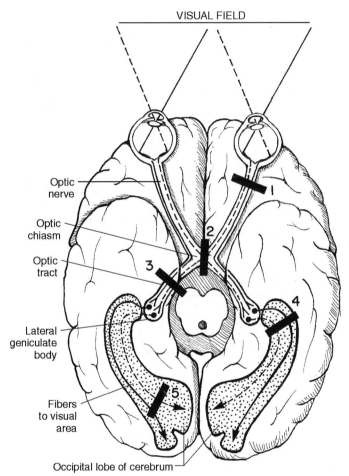

VISUAL FIELD

Optic nerve

Optic chiasm

Optic tract

Lateral geniculate body

Fibers to visual area

Occipital lobe of cerebrum

Figure 17-5

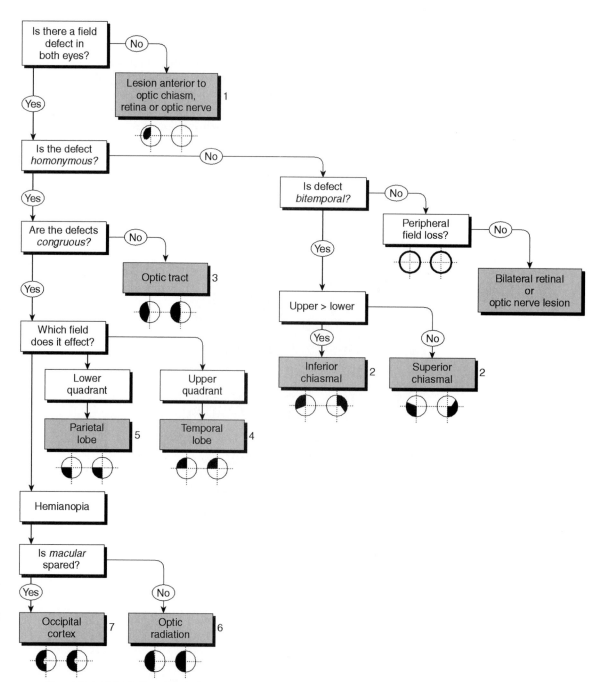

Figure 17-6. Field defects. Reprinted with permission from Fuller G, ed. *Neurological Examination Made Easy.* London: Churchill Livingstone, 1993.

OPHTHALMOSCOPIC EXAMINATION

PROCEDURE

With an ophthalmoscope, look into the patient's eye. Bring the scope 1 to 2 cm from the eye and encourage the patient to fix the gaze at a distant point (Fig. 17-7). Use the focus ring to correct for your vision and the patient's vision. If you or the patient is myopic and is not using glasses or contact lenses, turn the focus ring dial counterclockwise to focus on the eye. If you or the patient is presbyopic, turn the focus dial clockwise to focus on the eye. Look at the optic disc, blood vessels, and retinal background.

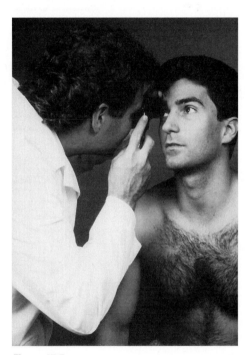

Figure 17-7

17

RATIONALE

Visualize the optic nerve, the optic disc, and the optic cup for swelling and atrophy (Fig. 17-8).

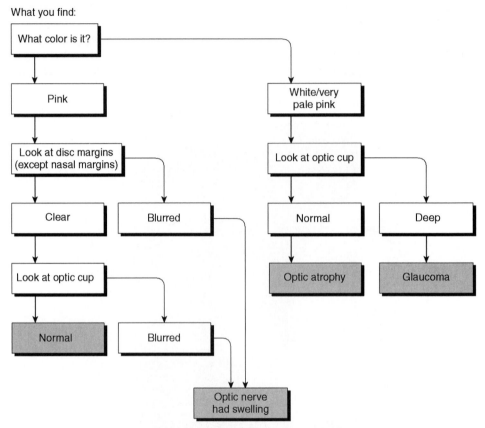

Figure 17-8. Optic disc abnormalities. Reprinted with permission from Fuller G. Neurological Examination Made Easy. London: Churchill Livingstone, 1993.

OCULOMOTOR, TROCHLEAR, AND ABDUCENS NERVES (III, IV, VI)

PROCEDURE

Cranial nerves III, IV, and VI are all associated with ocular and pupillary motility and are tested together for simplicity. Cranial nerve III also innervates the levator palpebrae muscles, which are responsible for movement of the eyelids. First, look at the patient's eyelids and note any ptosis. After inspection of the eyelids, inspect the eye globes for alignment. Dysfunction of cranial nerve III, IV, or VI may be responsible for deviations of eye alignment. Next, inspect the pupils and determine their size and shape. Then test the pupillary reflex by flashing a light into one of the patient's eyes (Fig. 17-9). Look at the pupils one at a time for contraction or dilation.

To test ocular movements, have the patient follow either your finger or a moving object through the entire field of vision in all axes. Observe for nystagmus and/or inability to move the eye in a particular axis (Fig. 17-10). Also, test for convergence by having the patient look at a distant object and continue to focus on it as you move that object closer to the patient. The pupil should constrict and converge as the object approaches. Look at both pupils in both instances.

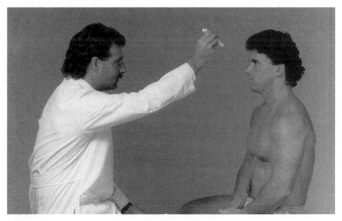

Figure 17-9

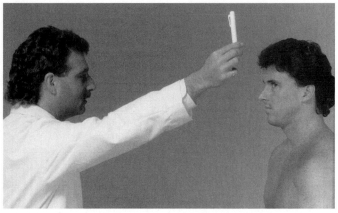

Figure 17-10

17

RATIONALE

An oculomotor nerve lesion causes ptosis of the eyelid with inability to open the lid. Eye alignment may be down and lateral. Also, the patient will be unable to move the eyeball upward, inward, or downward because of weakness of the medial, superior, and inferior rectus muscles and the inferior oblique muscle. The pupil is usually dilated, and the pupillary reflex is absent. The most frequent cause of a cranial nerve III paralysis is an aneurysm in the circle of Willis. Other conditions may also cause the pupil to dilate and the pupillary reflex to become absent (Fig. 17-11).

A trochlear nerve lesion causes superior and lateral deviation of the eye with inability to move the eyeball downward and inward because of weakness of the superior oblique muscle.

An abducens nerve lesion causes inability to move the eyeball outward because of weakness of the lateral rectus muscle. Figure 17-12 shows lateral rectus muscle defects of alignment.

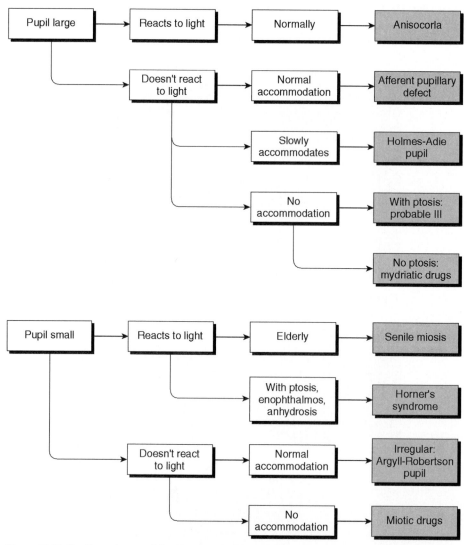

Figure 17-11. Pupillary abnormalities. Reprinted with permission from Fuller G. Neurological Examination Made Easy. London: Churchill Livingstone, 1993.

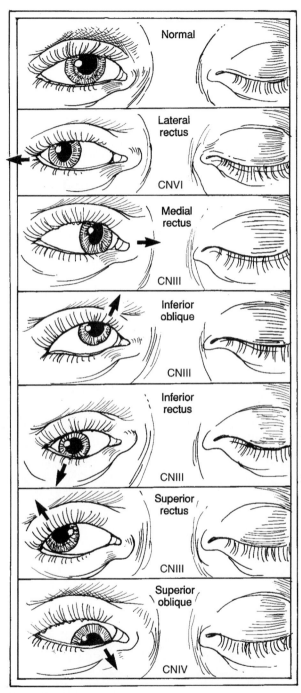

Figure 17-12

TRIGEMINAL NERVE (V)

The trigeminal nerve is composed of motor and sensory portions. The motor portion innervates the muscles of mastication. These muscles are the masseter, pterygoid, and temporal muscles. The sensory portion is divided into three branches: the ophthalmic (V1), maxillary (V2), and mandibular branches (V3).

Motor

PROCEDURE FOR THE MASSETER, PTERYGOID, AND TEMPORALIS MUSCLES

To test the motor portion that innervates the masseter muscle, instruct the patient to simulate a bite while you palpate the masseter muscle and attempt to open the patient's jaw with your thumbs (Fig. 17-13). To test the pterygoid muscle, instruct the patient to deviate the jaw against your resistance (Fig. 17-14). To test the temporalis muscle, instruct the patient to clench the jaw while you palpate the temporalis muscles with your fingers (Fig. 17-15). Note whether muscle contraction is symmetrical.

RATIONALE

A weak masseter or pterygoid muscle may indicate a trigeminal nerve lesion. A difference in muscle tension of the temporalis muscle is also an indication of a trigeminal motor lesion. In bilateral paralysis, the jaw may not close tightly. In unilateral lesions, the jaw deviates toward the side of the lesion when the patient opens the mouth.

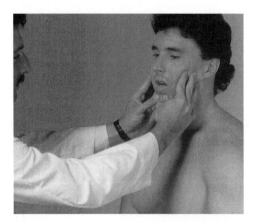

Figure 17-13

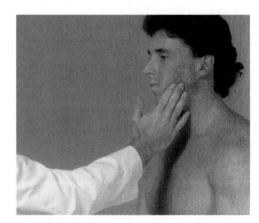

Figure 17-14

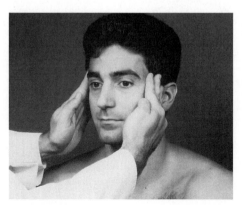

Figure 17-15

Reflex

Corneal Reflex

PROCEDURE

Instruct the patient to gaze upward and inward while you touch the cornea with a strand of cotton, approaching from the lateral side (Fig. 17-16). Be careful not to touch the eyelash or conjunctiva. The patient should blink when the cornea is touched. The corneal reflex has sensory fibers from the trigeminal nerve and motor fibers from the facial nerve.

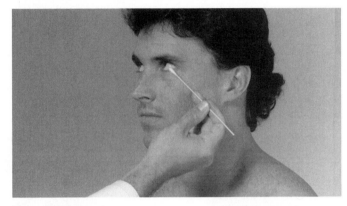

Figure 17-16

Jaw Reflex

PROCEDURE

Instruct the patient to open the mouth slightly. Place your thumb or index finger just lateral to the midline of the patient's chin, and press down. With a neurological reflex hammer, tap down on your finger to open the jaw (Fig. 17-17). The normal response is to close the jaw rapidly.

RATIONALE

The corneal and jaw jerk reflexes have a sensory component from the trigeminal nerve. The jaw jerk reflex has a motor component to the trigeminal nerve. The corneal reflex has a motor component from the facial nerve. If the corneal reflexes are absent, suspect a lesion of either the sensory portion of the trigeminal nerve or the motor component of the facial nerve. If the jaw jerk reflex is absent, suspect a lesion of the trigeminal nerve.

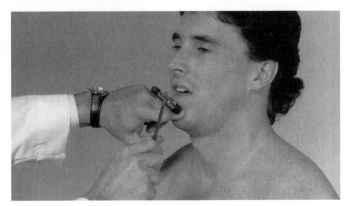

Figure 17-17

17

Sensory

PROCEDURE

To test for sensory deficit, instruct the patient to close the eyes. Touch the forehead, cheek, and chin with a pin for pain sensation; a piece of cotton for the sensation of light touch; and small test tubes of hot and cold water for thermal sensation (Figs. 17-18 to 17-20). Perform these procedures to both sides of the face and ask the patient to compare the sensations bilaterally. Next, instruct the patient to open the mouth and touch the tongue, the inside of both cheeks, and the hard palate with a wooden tongue depressor (Fig. 17-21). Instruct the patient to give a signal, such as raising the hand, on feeling the sensation.

RATIONALE

A decrease in the sensation of light touch, pain, and/or temperature from one side to the other indicates a lesion of the sensory portion of the affected branch of the trigeminal nerve. Lesions of the ophthalmic, maxillary, or mandibular branch of the trigeminal nerve produces decreased sensation of the forehead, cheek, or chin, respectively.

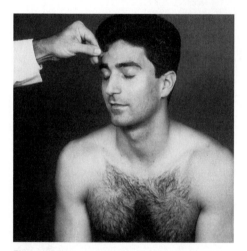

Figure 17-18

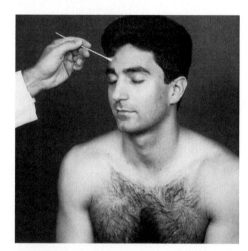

Figure 17-19

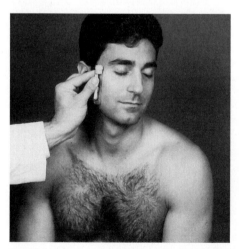

Figure 17-20

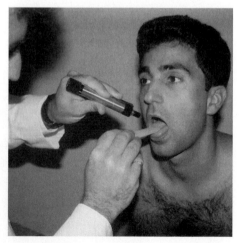

Figure 17-21

Motor

PROCEDURE

The facial nerve has both motor and sensory fibers. The motor fibers innervate the muscles of the face and platysma. Observe the patient's face for abnormal movements, such as tics or tremors. Note the degree of change of expression or lack of change.

To test for motor function, observe the face in repose. Then instruct the patient to frown, raise the eyebrows, close the eyes, show the teeth, smile, and whistle or puff the cheeks (Figs.17-22 to 17-25).

FACIAL NERVE (VII)

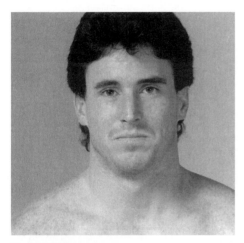

Figure 17-22

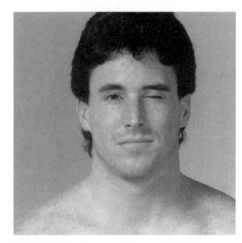

Figure 17-23

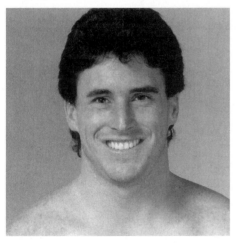

Figure 17-24

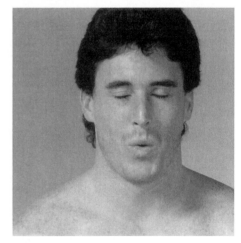

Figure 17-25

17

RATIONALE

Facial nerve lesions may stem from upper motor neurons or lower motor neurons. These neurons may be distinguished by the various facial expressions. An upper motor neuron lesion generally has no effect on the forehead and eyelids. In a lower motor neuron lesion, when the eyebrows are raised and lowered, the forehead does not wrinkle. Showing the teeth and whistling are absent in both upper and lower motor neuron lesions. Smiling may not elevate the mouth in a lower motor neuron lesion, but a symmetrical smile may occur in an upper motor neuron lesion. Inability of the patient to perform these movements indicates a lesion of the motor portion of the facial nerve (Fig. 17-26).

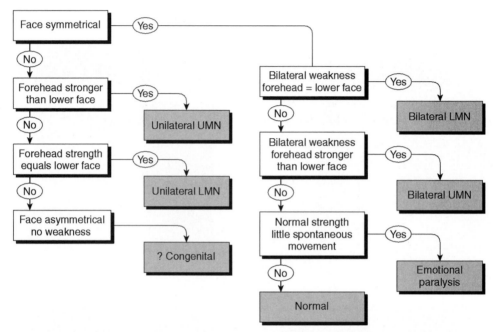

Figure 17-26. Facial nerve abnormalities. Reprinted with permission from Fuller G. Neurological Examination Made Easy. London: Churchill Livingstone, 1993.

Sensory

PROCEDURE

Instruct the patient to close the eyes and protrude the tongue. Apply solutions of sugar, salt, and/or vinegar to one side and on the anterior two-thirds of the tongue (Fig. 17-27). Instruct the patient to identify each substance without retracting the tongue. This can be done by having the patient point to a list of various substances on a card or on a sheet of paper. Instruct the patient to rinse the mouth; then apply another substance on the opposite side.

RATIONALE

Inability to taste and/or identify the substances may indicate a lesion of the sensory portion of the facial nerve.

NOTE

Complete loss of taste in facial nerve lesions is rare. It is most common for the patient to have a spontaneous or perverted taste as opposed to complete loss of taste. If complete loss of taste is noted, consider nonneurogenic causes, such as viral infection, aging, smoking, and toxic or metabolic disease.

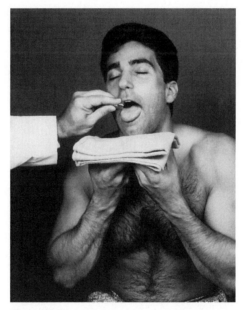

Figure 17-27

17

AUDITORY NERVE (VIII)

The auditory nerve is composed of a cochlear portion and a vestibular portion. The cochlear portion is responsible for hearing, and the vestibular portion is responsible for balance. The cochlear portion is tested by evaluating the patient's hearing. The most accurate way to test hearing is with an audiometer. If one is not available, place a ticking watch close to the patient's ear and see whether he or she can hear it. Weber's and Rinne's tests indicate cochlear lesions. Vestibular lesions are also determined by veering and past pointing tests and by observing the patient for nystagmus.

Weber's Test: Cochlear Nerve

PROCEDURE

Place a vibrating 256-Hz tuning fork on top of the patient's head (Fig. 17-28). Ask the patient whether he or she hears the sound equally in both ears.

RATIONALE

The test is normal if the patient hears the sound equally in both ears. If the sound is louder in one ear than in the other, suspect a conduction problem, such as a blockage of the ear canal or middle ear disease on the side of the louder sound. If a nerve lesion is present, the sound will be heard only in the normal ear. This hearing problem could be caused by otosclerosis, Ménière's disease, meningitis, cerebellopontine tumors, trauma, or a demyelinating lesion.

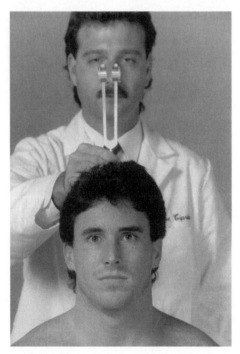

Figure 17-28

Rinne's Test: Cochlear Nerve

PROCEDURE

Place a vibrating tuning fork on the mastoid process (Fig. 17-29). Ask the patient to say when the sound disappears. After the sound disappears, place the tuning fork next to but not touching the ear (Fig. 17-30). Ask the patient again to say when the sound fades out.

RATIONALE

Normally, air conduction is twice as loud as bone conduction—a Rinne positive. In conduction lesions and nonneurogenic lesions, bone conduction is greater than air conduction—a Rinne negative. In auditory nerve lesions, air conduction is greater than bone conduction.

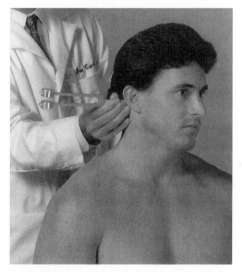

Figure 17-29

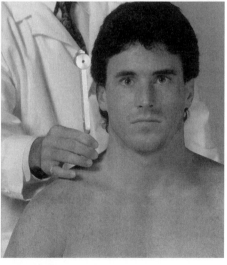

Figure 17-30

17

Veering Test: Vestibular Nerve

PROCEDURE

Instruct the patient to walk with the eyes closed (Fig. 17-31).

RATIONALE

Veering in walking or a positive Romberg's test indicates a unilateral vestibular lesion. See Chapter 19 for Romberg's test.

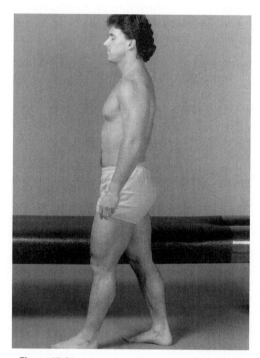

Figure 17-31

Past Pointing Test: Vestibular Nerve

PROCEDURE

With the patient's eyes open, instruct the patient to elevate the extended arm over the head with index finger extended (Fig. 17-32). Next, instruct the patient to touch your extended index finger, which you hold near the patient at hip level (Fig. 17-33). Repeat the test with the patient's eyes closed.

RATIONALE

If the patient has a vestibular lesion, the patient's arm will drift, and he or she will have difficulty placing the finger on yours with eyes closed.

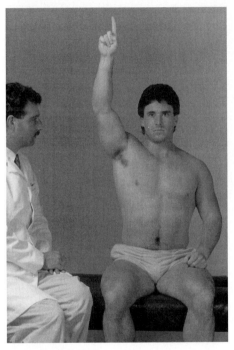

Figure 17-32

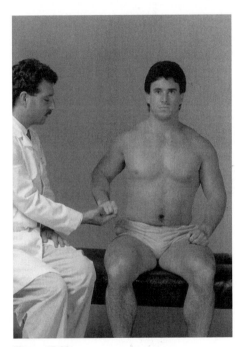

Figure 17-33

17

Labyrinthine Test for Positional Nystagmus

PROCEDURE

With the patient seated, inspect the eyes and note any nystagmus (Fig. 17-34). Nystagmus is a slow drift of the eye in one direction with a fast correction in the opposite direction. It is described in the direction of the fast phase. Next, have the patient lie supine and inspect for nystagmus for 30 seconds (Fig. 17-35). Assist the patient to turn to one side and stabilize the head. Note any nystagmus for 30 seconds (Fig. 17-36). Repeat with the patient turned to the opposite side. Have the patient extend the head over the examination table, and inspect for nystagmus for 30 seconds (Fig. 17-37). Allow sufficient time between tests for the patient with nystagmus to recover.

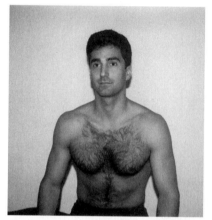

Figure 17-34

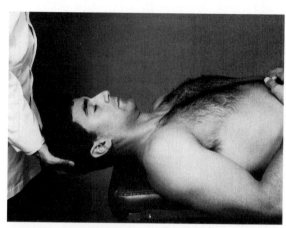

Figure 17-35

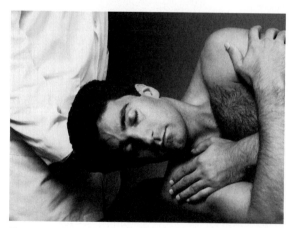

Figure 17-36

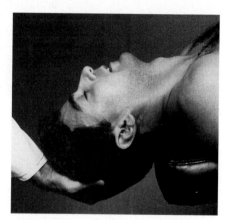

Figure 17-37

RATIONALE

A patient with persistent nystagmus that changes direction with changes in the head position and that appears on repeated maneuvers suggests brainstem or posterior fossa pathology. A delayed, mild, rapidly disappearing response that produces nystagmus in only one direction and cannot be repeated suggests benign postural vertigo (Fig. 17-38).

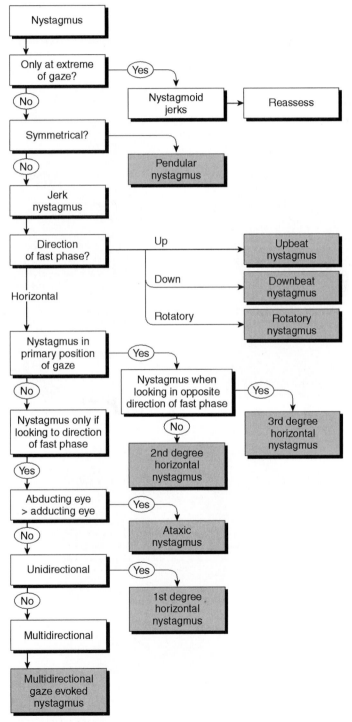

Figure 17-38. Nystagmus. Reprinted with permission from Fuller G. Neurological Examination Made Easy. London: Churchill Livingstone, 1993.

GLOSSOPHARYNGEAL AND VAGUS NERVES (IX, X)

The glossopharyngeal and vagus nerves are clinically inseparable because of their overlap and are therefore tested together. The glossopharyngeal nerve conveys taste from the posterior tongue and has sensory innervation to the tonsillar pillars, soft palate, and pharyngeal wall. The vagus nerve overlaps the functions of the glossopharyngeal nerve and innervates the larynx. Note any hoarseness or change in voice tone. The vagus nerve controls activity in the cardiac, respiratory, and gastrointestinal systems; however, these functions are difficult to assay because of the variable suprasegmental and hormonal influences.

Motor function is assessed by having the patient say "ah" and observing the palate for deviation. Place a tongue depressor on the patient's tongue and observe palatal deviation (Fig. 17-39). If deviation exists, it will be toward the normal side. Next, ask the patient to swallow rapidly while you palpate the trachea (Fig. 17-40). Fatigue on continued swallowing may be seen in a patient who has myasthenia gravis. You may also ask the patient to puff the cheeks with air (Fig. 17-41). Leakage through the nose indicates weakness in the muscle of the soft palate. This weakness is also a sign of a lesion in cranial nerve IX or X. The leakage can be stopped by pinching the nose.

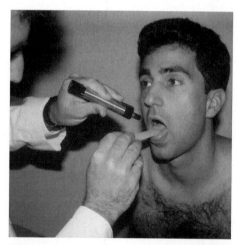

Figure 17-39

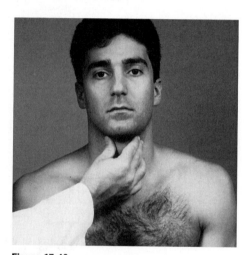

Figure 17-40

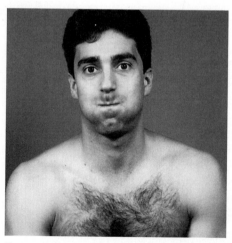

Figure 17-41

Sensory

PROCEDURE

Instruct the patient to close the eyes and protrude the tongue. Apply a bitter-tasting solution on one side of the posterior third of the tongue (Fig. 17-42). Instruct the patient to identify each substance without retracting the tongue. This can be done by having the patient point out one of a list of substances on a card or sheet of paper.

RATIONALE

Inability to taste and/or identify the substances indicates a lesion of the sensory portion of the glossopharyngeal and/or vagus nerve.

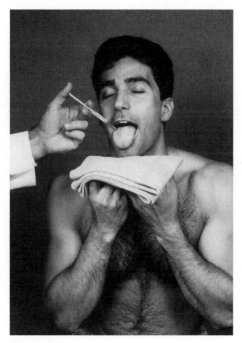

Figure 17-42

Reflex

Gag Reflex

PROCEDURE

With a throat stick, touch the posterior pharyngeal wall, first on one side and then on the other (Fig. 17-43). Observe the movement of the palate and the patient when he or she gags. Also, ask the patient whether the stimulus feels the same on both sides or is stronger on one side than on the other.

RATIONALE

Deviation of the palate to one side and/or an asymmetrical feeling of the stimulus indicates a lesion of the glossopharyngeal and/or vagus nerves. If the patient has had a tonsillectomy, a slight asymmetry of palatal movement may be normal.

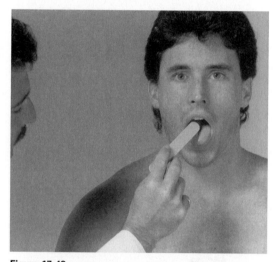

Figure 17-43

SPINAL ACCESSORY NERVE (XI)

The spinal accessory nerve innervates the trapezius and the sternocleidomastoideus muscles. To assess the spinal accessory nerve, test the trapezius and sternocleidomastoideus muscles.

Trapezius Muscle Test

PROCEDURE

With the patient seated, apply pressure to the patient's shoulders bilaterally and ask him or her to shrug against your resistance (Fig. 17-44). Grade each side according to the muscle grading chart in Chapter 4.

RATIONALE

A grade 0 to 4 indicates a spinal accessory nerve lesion. Suspect a strained or weak trapezius muscle if the sternocleidomastoideus muscle has reasonably normal strength.

Sternocleidomastoideus Muscle Test

PROCEDURE

With the patient seated, place your hand on the lateral aspect of the patient's jaw and instruct him or her to turn the head toward your hand against resistance (Fig. 17-45). Grade each side according to the muscle grading chart in Chapter 4.

RATIONALE

A grade 0 to 4 indicates a spinal accessory nerve lesion. A strained or weak sternocleidomastoideus muscle is suspect if the trapezius muscle is of reasonably normal strength.

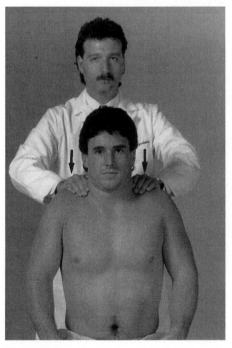

Figure 17-44

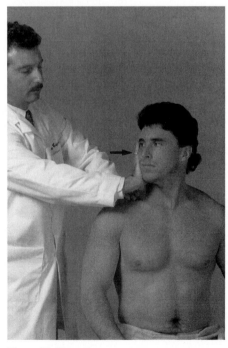

Figure 17-45

17

HYPOGLOSSAL NERVE (XII)

The hypoglossal nerve is purely motor and is responsible for the movement of the tongue.

PROCEDURE

Place your hand on the patient's cheek and instruct the patient to press the tip of the tongue against the cheek under your hand (Fig. 17-46). Have the patient do this bilaterally. Instruct the patient to protrude the tongue (Fig. 17-47).

RATIONALE

If the pressure under your hand by the patient's tongue is unequal, suspect a unilateral hypoglossal nerve lesion, which will exhibit a deviation of the tongue toward the side of the lesion.

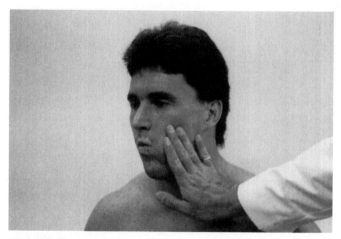

Figure 17-46

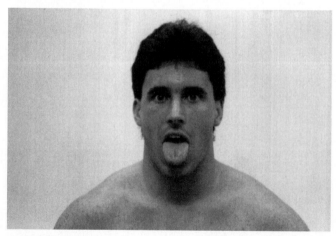

Figure 17-47

General References

Barrows HS. Guide to Neurological Assessment. Philadelphia: JB Lippincott, 1980.

Bickerstaff ER. Neurological Examination in Clinical Practice. 4th ed. Boston: Blackwell Scientific, 1980.

Chusid JG. Correlative neuroanatomy and functional neurology. 17th ed. Los Altos: Lange Medical, 1976.

Colling RD. Illustrated Manual of Neurologic Diagnosis. 2nd ed. Philadelphia: JB Lippincott, 1982.

DeJong RN. The Neurologic Examination. 4th ed. Hagerstown, MD: Harper & Row, 1979.

DeMyer W. Technique of the Neurologic Examination: A Programmed Text. 3rd ed. New York: McGraw-Hill, 1980.

Devinsky O, Feldmann E. Examination of the Cranial and Peripheral Nerves. New York: Churchill Livingstone, 1988.

Fuller G. Neurological Examination Made Easy. London: Churchill Livingstone, 1993.

Mancall E. Essentials of the Neurologic Examination. 2nd ed. Philadelphia: FA Davis, 1981.

Merritt HH. A Textbook of Neurology. 4th ed. Philadelphia: Lea & Febiger, 1967.

VanAllen MW, Rodnitzky RL. Pictorial Manual of Neurologic Tests. 2nd ed. Chicago: Year Book Medical, 1981.

17

18

REFLEXES

PATHOLOGICAL UPPER EXTREMITY REFLEXES

This chapter discusses various pathological reflexes that usually are present in corticospinal disease and higher cortical dysfunction, such as stroke, tumor, demyelinating diseases, and vasculitis. If no corticospinal pathology or other higher cortical dysfunction is present, these reflexes should be absent. These reflexes are not graded on the Wexler scale but are referred to as being either present or absent. Babinski's and Rossolimo's foot signs are considered normal in infants.

Hoffman's Sign

PROCEDURE

With the patient's forearm pronated, grasp the patient's hand and middle finger. With your opposite hand, flick the distal end of the patient's middle finger, stretching the flexor and eliciting a stretch reflex (Fig. 18-1).

RATIONALE

A positive sign is elicited if the patient flexes the thumb and forefinger (Fig. 18-2). A positive sign indicates a hyperactive reflex only. If this sign is present, it may be one indicator of pyramidal tract disease.

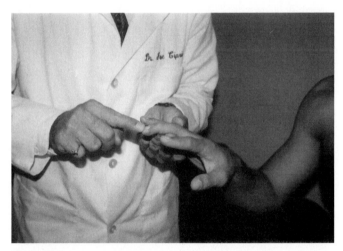

Figure 18-1

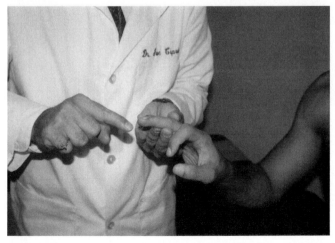

Figure 18-2

18

Tromner's Sign

PROCEDURE

Grasp the patient's wrist and tap the plantar surface of the tip of the index and middle digits (Fig. 18-3).

RATIONALE

A positive sign is elicited if the patient flexes all of the fingers (Fig. 18-4). A positive sign indicates a hyperactive reflex only. If this sign is present, it may be one indicator of corticospinal tract disease.

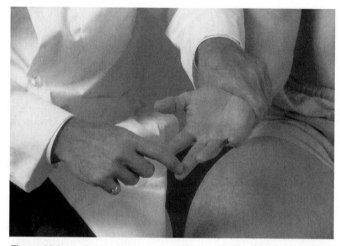

Figure 18-3

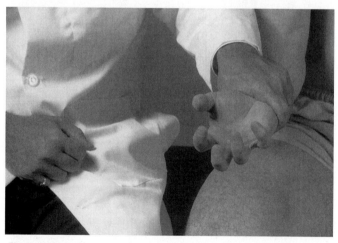

Figure 18-4

Rossolimo's Hand Sign

PROCEDURE

With a neurological reflex hammer, tap the palmar surface of the metacarpophalangeal joint (Fig. 18-5).

RATIONALE

A positive sign is elicited if the patient flexes all of the fingers (Fig. 18-6). This sign is present in pyramidal tract disease.

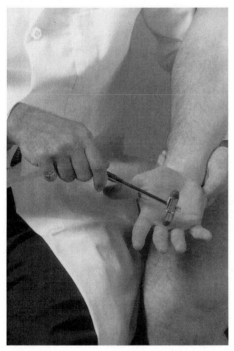

Figure 18-5

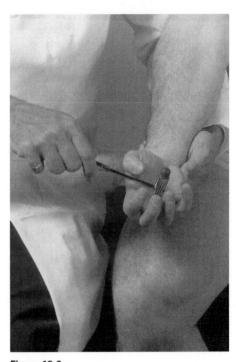

Figure 18-6

18

Chaddock's Wrist Sign

Procedure

Grasp the patient's wrist, putting pressure on the palmaris longus tendon (Fig. 18-7).

Rationale

A positive sign is elicited if the patient flexes the wrist and extends the fingers (Fig. 18-8). This sign is present in pyramidal tract disease.

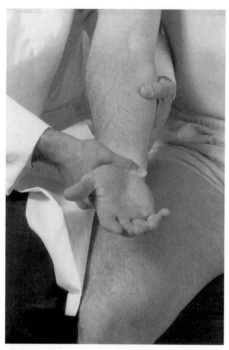

Figure 18-7

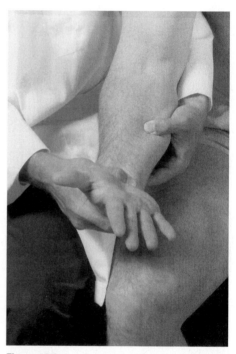

Figure 18-8

PATHOLOGICAL LOWER EXTREMITY REFLEXES

Babinski's Sign

PROCEDURE

With the patient supine, stroke the sole of the foot with a blunt object like the handle of a neurological reflex hammer. Begin with the lateral aspect of the heel and move superiorly and medially to the big toe (Fig. 18-9).

RATIONALE

This sign is very important in the neurological examination. A positive sign is evident if the patient dorsiflexes the great toe and fans the rest of the digits (Fig. 18-10). This sign is a classic indication of a corticospinal motor system lesion. It may be present in normal infants aged 12 to 16 months.

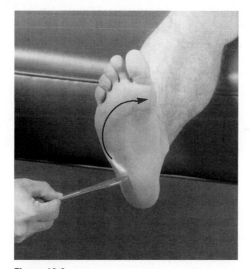

Figure 18-9

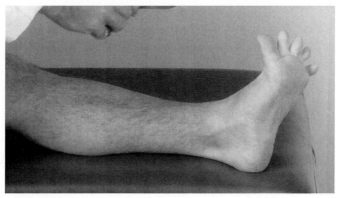

Figure 18-10

18

Oppenheim's Sign

PROCEDURE

With the patient supine, stroke the medial side of the tibia with a blunt object (Fig. 18-11).

RATIONALE

Extension of the great toe is a positive sign (Fig. 18-12). If this reflex is present, suspect a corticospinal motor system lesion.

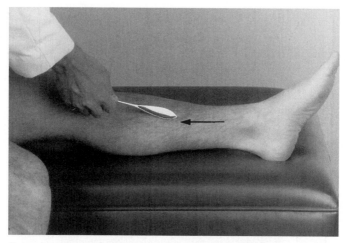

Figure 18-11

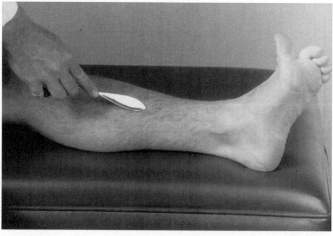

Figure 18-12

Chaddock's Foot Sign

PROCEDURE

With the patient supine, stroke the lateral malleolus with a blunt object (Fig. 18-13).

RATIONALE

Extension of the great toe indicates a positive sign (Fig. 18-14). If this reflex is present, suspect a corticospinal motor system lesion.

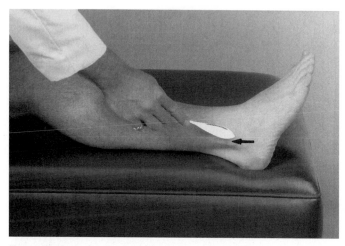

Figure 18-13

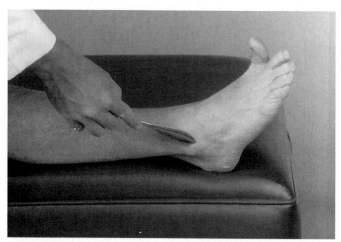

Figure 18-14

18

Rossolimo's Foot Sign

Procedure

With the patient supine, tap the metatarsal heads of the patient's feet with a neurological reflex hammer (Fig. 18-15).

Rationale

Plantar flexion of the toes indicates a positive sign (Fig. 18-16). This sign is considered normal in children aged 2 months to 3 years. In other age groups, if this sign and a Babinski sign are present, suspect pyramidal tract disease.

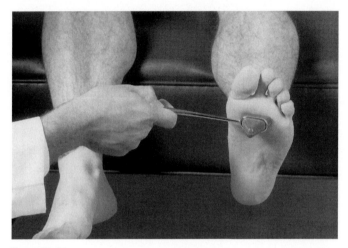

Figure 18-15

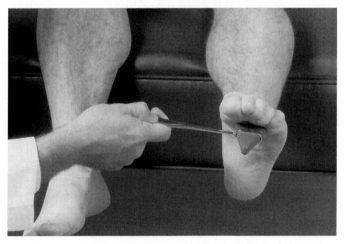

Figure 18-16

Schaeffer's Sign

PROCEDURE

With the patient supine and the feet overhanging the examination table, squeeze the Achilles tendon (Fig. 18-17).

RATIONALE

Extension of the great toe is a positive sign (Fig. 18-18). If this sign is present, suspect a lesion of the pyramidal tract.

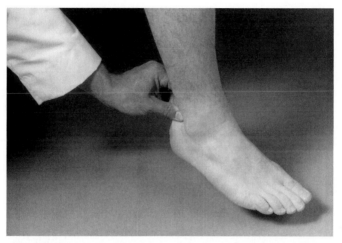

Figure 18-17

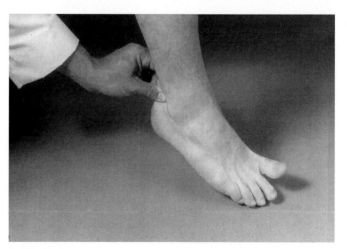

Figure 18-18

SUPERFICIAL CUTANEOUS REFLEXES

Superficial cutaneous reflexes are polysynaptic. They are mediated through a reflex arc but are controlled inherently by the corticospinal system. These reflexes are also not graded by the Wexler scale but are either present or absent. Unlike the pathological reflexes, these reflexes are normally present if there is no lesion of the corticospinal tract. The superficial corneal, pharyngeal, and palatal reflexes belong in this group but are discussed in Chapter 17.

Upper Abdominal Reflex

PROCEDURE

With the patient supine, scrape the skin from medial to lateral above the umbilicus with the blunt end of a neurological reflex hammer (Fig. 18-19) and evaluate bilaterally.

RATIONALE

A deviation of the umbilicus to the stroked side is a normal response. If the umbilicus does not move unilaterally or if the response is delayed, the response is absent. The reflex may be absent in obese patients and pregnant women. This absent reflex is normal, but only if it is absent bilaterally. An absent unilateral response indicates a T7 to T9 nerve root lesion or disease of the corticospinal system. If you suspect the latter, perform other corticospinal system tests to verify your findings.

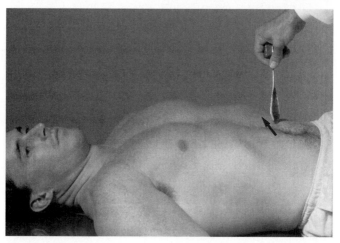

Figure 18-19

Lower Abdominal Reflex

PROCEDURE

With the patient supine, scrape the skin from medial to lateral below the umbilicus with the blunt end of a neurological reflex hammer (Fig. 18-20) and evaluate bilaterally.

RATIONALE

A deviation of the umbilicus to the stroked side is a normal response. If the umbilicus does not move unilaterally or if the response is delayed, the response is absent. The reflex may be absent in obese patients and pregnant women. This absence is normal, but only if the reflex is absent bilaterally. An absent unilateral response indicates a T10 to T12 nerve root lesion or disease of the corticospinal system. If you suspect the latter, perform other corticospinal system tests to verify your findings.

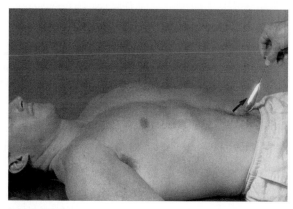

Figure 18-20

Superficial Gluteal Reflex

PROCEDURE

With the patient prone, scrape the buttock with the blunt end of a neurological reflex hammer (Fig. 18-21). Perform this test bilaterally.

RATIONALE

A contraction of the gluteal muscle on the side of the scraping is a normal response. If the reflex is absent unilaterally, suspect an L4 or L5 nerve root lesion or a corticospinal system lesion. If you suspect the latter, perform other corticospinal system tests to verify your evaluation.

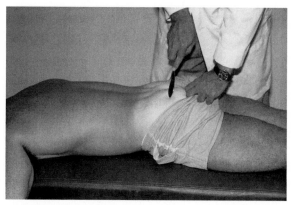

Figure 18-21

18

Corneal Reflex
See Chapter 17.

Pharyngeal Reflex
See Chapter 17.

Palatal Reflex
See Chapter 17.

General References

Adams C. Neurology in Primary Care. Philadelphia: FA Davis, 2000.

Aminoff MJ, Greenberg DA, Simon RP. Clinical Neurology. 3rd ed. Stamford, CT: Appleton & Lange, 1996.

Barrows HS. Guide to Neurological Assessment. Philadelphia: JB Lippincott, 1980.

Bickerstaff ER. Neurological Examination in Clinical Practice. 4th ed. Boston: Blackwell Scientific, 1980.

Bronisch FW. The Clinically Important Reflexes. New York: Grune & Stratton, 1952.

Chusid JG. Correlative Neuroanatomy and Functional Neurology. 16th ed. Los Altos, CA: Lange Medical, 1976.

Colling RD. Illustrated Manual of Neurologic Diagnosis. 2nd ed. Philadelphia: JB Lippincott, 1982.

DeJong RN. The Neurologic Examination. 4th ed. Hagerstown, MD: Harper & Row, 1979.

DeMyer W. Technique of the Neurologic Examination: A Programmed Text. 3rd ed. New York: McGraw-Hill, 1980.

Devinsky O, Feldmann E. Examination of the Cranial and Peripheral Nerves. New York: Churchill Livingstone, 1988.

Heilman NM, Watson RT, Green M. Handbook for Differential Diagnosis of Neurologic Signs and Symptoms. New York: Appleton-Century-Crofts, 1977.

Lapides J, Babbitt JM. Diagnostic value of bulbocavernosus reflex. JAMA 1956;162:971.

Mancall E. Essentials of the Neurologic Examination. 2nd ed. Philadelphia: FA Davis, 1981.

Merritt HH. A Textbook of Neurology. 4th ed. Philadelphia: Lea & Febiger, 1967.

Swanson P. Signs and Symptoms in Neurology. Philadelphia: JB Lippincott, 1989.

VanAllen MW, Rodnitzky RL. Pictorial Manual of Neurologic Tests. 2nd ed. Chicago: Year Book Medical, 1981.

CEREBELLAR FUNCTION TESTS

Cerebellar dysfunction is an interruption of the integration of afferent sensory feedback and efferent motor output. Loss of joint position sense can produce some uncoordination, which can be substantially worse when the eyes are closed. The following tests attempt to evaluate the patient's coordination and joint position sense.

If any of the tests are positive, suspect an ipsilateral cerebellar syndrome. This syndrome may be caused by demyelination, vascular disease, trauma, tumor, or abscess. If any of the tests are positive bilaterally, suspect a bilateral cerebellar syndrome. This syndrome may be caused by alcohol consumption, demyelination, or vascular disease.

UPPER EXTREMITY

Finger–Nose Test

PROCEDURE

With the patient standing or sitting with eyes closed, ask him or her to touch both index fingers to the nose simultaneously (Fig. 19-1).

RATIONALE

The patient should be able to perform this procedure smoothly and easily. If the patient cannot perform this procedure, cerebellar function is impaired.

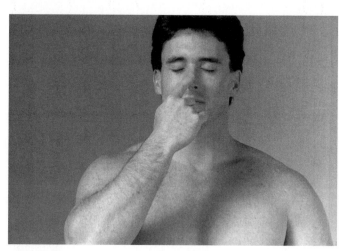

Figure 19-1

Finger–Finger Test

PROCEDURE

Ask the patient to place his or her finger on your finger. Repeat this several times with the patient's eyes open and closed (Figs. 19-2 and 19-3).

RATIONALE

The patient should be able to perform this procedure smoothly and easily. If the patient cannot perform this procedure, cerebellar function is impaired.

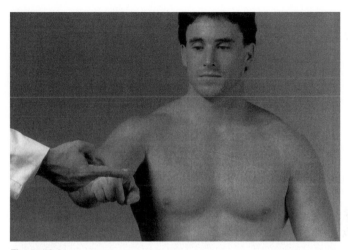

Figure 19-2

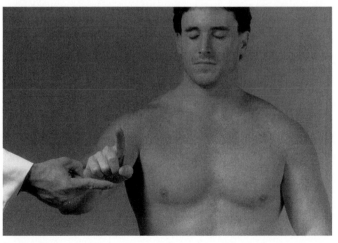

Figure 19-3

Pronation–Supination Test

PROCEDURE

Ask the standing patient to extend the arms forward. Next, ask the patient to pronate and supinate the arms rapidly (Figs. 19-4 and 19-5).

RATIONALE

The patient should be able to perform these movements smoothly and with an even rhythm. If the patient cannot perform the movements or performs them in a spastic or uncoordinated manner, suspect cerebellar dysfunction.

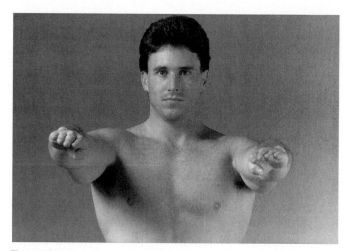

Figure 19-4

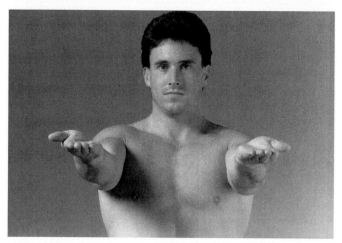

Figure 19-5

Patting Test

PROCEDURE

Instruct the seated patient to pat the hand rapidly and repeatedly on the thigh (Fig. 19-6).

RATIONALE

The patient should be able to perform this movement briskly and with equal amplitude. If the patient cannot perform this movement or performs it in a slow, spastic, or uncoordinated manner, suspect cerebellar dysfunction.

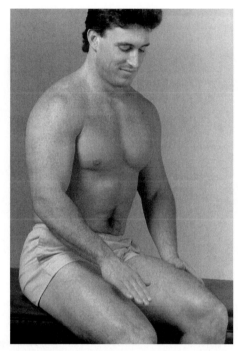

Figure 19-6

Dexterity Test

PROCEDURE

Ask the patient to touch each fingertip with the thumb of the same hand sequentially (Figs. 19-7 and 19-8).

RATIONALE

These movements are usually done in a smooth and coordinated manner. If the patient cannot perform these movements or performs them in a spastic or uncoordinated manner, suspect cerebellar dysfunction.

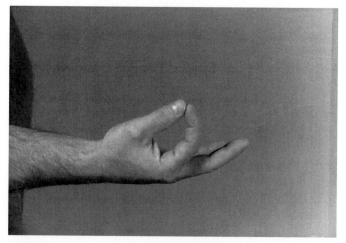

Figure 19-7

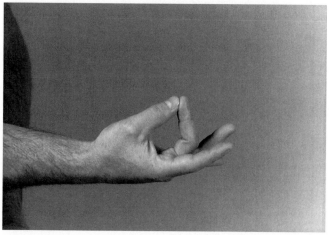

Figure 19-8

LOWER EXTREMITY

Heel–Knee Test

PROCEDURE

With the patient supine, ask the patient to place one foot on the opposite knee (Fig. 19-9). Then ask the patient to slide the foot down the shin (Fig. 19-10).

RATIONALE

These movements are usually done in a smooth and coordinated manner. If the patient cannot perform these movements or performs them in a spastic or uncoordinated manner, suspect cerebellar dysfunction.

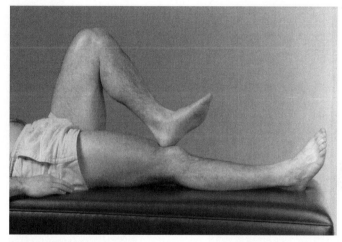

Figure 19-9

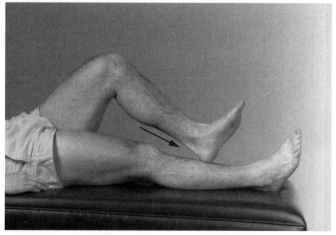

Figure 19-10

19

Patting Test

PROCEDURE

Ask the patient to tap the foot rapidly and repeatedly on the floor (Figs. 19-11 and 19-12).

RATIONALE

The patient should be able to perform this movement briskly and with equal amplitude. If the patient cannot perform this movement or performs it in a slow, spastic, or uncoordinated manner, suspect cerebellar dysfunction.

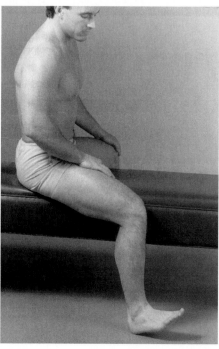

Figure 19-11

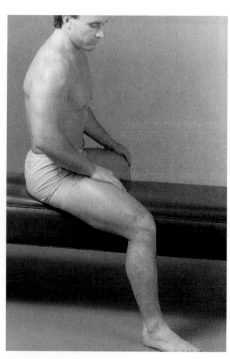

Figure 19-12

Figure-Eight Test

PROCEDURE

With the patient supine, ask the patient to draw a figure-eight in the air with the great toe (Fig. 19-13).

RATIONALE

These movements are usually done in a smooth and coordinated manner. If the patient cannot perform these movements or performs them in a spastic or uncoordinated manner, suspect cerebellar dysfunction.

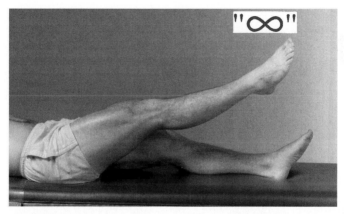

Figure 19-13

Romberg's Test

PROCEDURE

Instruct the patient to stand. Observe the patient for any swaying. While the patient is still standing, instruct him or her to close the eyes (Fig. 19-14).

RATIONALE

This is not a cerebellar test per se, but swaying with eyes closed suggests a posterior column disorder. A patient with cerebellar dysfunction will sway with eyes open, but the swaying will be exaggerated with eyes closed.

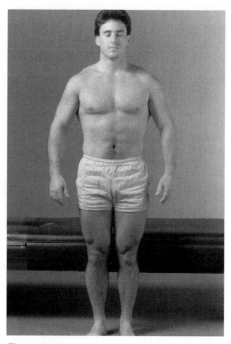

Figure 19-14

General References

Barrows HS. Guide to Neurological Assessment. Philadelphia: JB Lippincott, 1980.

Bickerstaff ER. Neurological Examination in Clinical Practice. 4th ed. Boston: Blackwell Scientific, 1980.

Chusid JG. Correlative Neuroanatomy and Functional Neurology. 16th ed. Los Altos, CA: Lange Medical, 1976.

Colling RD. Illustrated Manual of Neurologic Diagnosis. 2nd ed. Philadelphia: JB Lippincott, 1982.

DeJong RN. The Neurologic Examination. 4th ed. Hagerstown, MD: Harper & Row, 1979.

Greenberg DA, Aminoff MJ, Simon RP. Clinical Neurology. 2nd ed. Norwalk: Appleton & Lange, 1993.

Heilman NM, Watson RT, Green M. Handbook for Differential Diagnosis of Neurologic Signs and Symptoms. New York: Appleton-Century-Crofts, 1977.

Klein R, Mayer-Gross W. The Clinical Examination of Patients With Organic Cerebral Disease. Springfield, IL: Charles C. Thomas, 1957.

Mancall E. Essentials of the neurologic examination. 2nd ed. Philadelphia: FA Davis, 1981.

Merritt HH. A Textbook of Neurology. 4th ed. Philadelphia: Lea & Febiger, 1967.

Scheinberg P. An Introduction to Diagnosis and Management of Common Neurologic Disorders. 3rd ed. New York: Raven, 1986.

Steegmann AT. Examination of the Nervous System: A Student's Guide. Chicago: Year Book Medical, 1970.

Swanson P. Signs and Symptoms in Neurology. Philadelphia: JB Lippincott, 1989.

VanAllen MW, Rodnitzky RL. Pictorial Manual of Neurologic Tests. 2nd ed. Chicago: Year Book Medical, 1981.

INDEX

Page numbers in *italics* denote figures.